# CHRISTIAAN
# BARNARD
## THE SURGEON
## WHO DARED

# CHRISTIAAN BARNARD

## THE SURGEON WHO DARED

### THE MAN AND THE STORY OF HEART TRANSPLANTATION

DAVID K. C. COOPER MD, PHD, FRCS, FACS

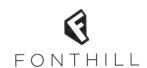

FONTHILL

Fonthill Media Language Policy

Fonthill Media publishes in the international English language market. One language edition is published worldwide. As there are minor differences in spelling and presentation, especially with regard to American English and British English, a policy is necessary to define which form of English to use. The Fonthill Policy is to use the form of English native to the author. David Cooper was born and educated in the UK; therefore, British English has been adopted in this publication.


Fonthill Media Limited
Fonthill Media LLC
www.fonthillmedia.com
office@fonthillmedia.com

First published in the United Kingdom and the United States of America 2017

British Library Cataloguing in Publication Data:
A catalogue record for this book is available from the British Library

Typeset in 10.5pt on 13pt Sabon
Printed and bound in England

*In memory of my parents and sister*

# Foreword

Sir Roy Calne FRCS, FRS
Emeritus Professor of Surgery, University of Cambridge, UK

David Cooper has produced an extremely well-researched and accurate biography on Christiaan Barnard, which I found fascinating. Particularly interesting were the obsessional ambitions that Barnard exhibited in putting together the first human heart transplant in Cape Town on 3 December 1967.

Barnard's origins were humble, poor, and very religious, his father being a small-town minister to the mixed-race community in the Dutch Reformed Mission Church. The fantastic will to win and bitter frustration and misery in failure, both developed in excessive degree, seem to be the essential ingredients of Barnard's progress. He was obviously a good and intelligent student, but what he possessed to a degree that was quite exceptional was the capacity for continuous and sustained hard work, being driven mercilessly not by external agencies, such as pressure from his family or fear of poverty, but by his own will to succeed. After preliminary excursions into general practice, a fever hospital, and internal medicine, he convinced the professor of surgery at the Groote Schuur Hospital that he was worthy of training as a surgeon.

Working in Minnesota under Professors Owen Wangensteen and C. Walton Lillehei, Barnard became interested and later proficient in the techniques of cardiac surgery, which were just then emerging, with Minneapolis being one of the major pioneering centres in this field. On his return to Cape Town, he set up a Division of Cardiac Surgery that proved very successful. His services to the community of Cape Town in providing one of the best open heart surgical teams in the world have saved many thousands of lives. He was admirably suited for this work with his industry and ability, which were grafted on to the technical knowledge he had acquired in the United States.

His research projects were intelligent and competently executed, but they have not advanced knowledge in surgery to any great extent. Transplanting the first human heart, which was covered by the media on a scale that might be expected for the outbreak of a major war, was carried out with remarkable efficiency in the technical sense, but there is no doubt that others would have succeeded at about the same time, independent of Barnard's contribution. Nevertheless, it took considerable courage to attempt this daring operation. For me, the most poignant part of Barnard's description of the operation was the loneliness of the surgeon who has removed a vital organ—therefore reaching the point of no return—and the feeling of intense relief when the organ graft takes over that vital function.

The truth is that transplantation of the heart had much in common with transplantation of other life-supporting organs and was part of a serious surgical endeavour to try to treat patients with terminal disease that continues to this day. Unlike in 1967, today, there is a high degree of success in the transplantation of all organs.

The ambition of Barnard fitted his own abilities, but could not be transferred to his teenage daughter, Deirdre, despite the most intense psychological onslaught on the young girl. She had a natural talent for water skiing and won several championships, at one point being ranked second in the world. She appeared to have the potential to become world champion but, to quote Barnard from the book, 'she did not have the killer instinct needed to become a world champion.' Barnard considered that he had 'failed to transplant into her my own hunger for victory. She was still not going to beat her fists and cry if she lost. She could laugh it off. She would never make it. She was just too damned nice.'

The crest of Barnard's surgical achievements was followed by his rapid evolution to become a celebrity on a scale never seen before nor since for a surgeon or physician. At a high-profile BBC TV programme, *Tomorrow's World*, in 1968 (in which I participated), Barnard fielded vitriolic criticism from a variety of prominent leaders, but especially those with strong religious arguments against heart transplantation and political arguments against the apartheid regime in South Africa at that time. He was articulate, logical, and eloquent in his responses. My own small contribution was to praise the science and surgical applications, but to regret the 'razzamatazz' that led surgeons all over the world to 'have a go' at heart transplantation without any background research or knowledge of immunosuppressive drug therapy. They wished to 'join the club', to grandstand that they also could perform the relatively straightforward operation.

There was envy associated with criticism of Barnard, especially in his enjoyment of the company of pretty young girls who seemed equally attracted to him. For many years, he immersed himself with relish in *la dolce vita* to such an extent that it impaired his own scientific and surgical progress. Perhaps, with some justification, he felt he had already done enough. Dubious business flurries into 'rejuvenation' therapy and a cosmetic cream were badly received by his peers, harming his reputation. After the breakup of his third marriage, the last couple of years of his life were extremely sad; he became isolated, lonely, ill, and found it very difficult to live with the ageing process, a general weakness in humanity, but one especially pertinent to the youth-loving Barnard. His only loving carer was his daughter, Deirdre, who in some ways he had treated so poorly.

Reading this book made me wonder whether a personality with an obsessive work ethic and massive ambition is an essential requirement for success on the world stage of surgery and science. If so, Christiaan Barnard certainly was a good example, but there are many instances of outstanding advances in science and surgery that have been achieved by those apparently without these characteristics.

I strongly recommend this biography as a 'warts and all' record of a meteoric surgical ascent to the pinnacle of public fame, only to be followed by a slower descent, but which was to some extent almost equally remarkable.

# Preface

It is not the critic who counts; not the man who points out how the strong man stumbled, or whether the doer of deeds could have done them better. The credit belongs to the man who is actually in the arena, whose face is marred by dust and sweat and blood; who strives valiantly, who errs and comes short again and again; who knows the great enthusiasms, the great devotions; who spends himself in a worthy cause; who, at the best, knows in the end the triumph of high achievement, and who, at the worst, if he fails, at least fails while daring greatly, so that his place shall never be with those timid souls who know neither victory nor defeat.

Theodore Roosevelt

There is nothing more difficult to take in hand, more perilous to conduct or more uncertain in its success than the introduction of a new order of things, because the innovator has for enemies all those who have done well under the old conditions and lukewarm defenders in those who may do well under the new.

Niccolo Machiavelli

## Chris Barnard: The Surgeon?

From a scroll that used to decorate the wall outside the office of Professor Christiaan Barnard in the Department of Surgery at the University of Cape Town Medical School:

The conditions necessary for the surgeon are four:
First, he should be learned.

Second, he must be expert.

Third, he must be ingenious.

Fourth, he should be able to adapt himself.

It is required for the First that the surgeon should know not only the principles of surgery but also those of medicine in theory and practice; for the Second, that he should have seen others operate; for the Third, that he should be ingenious, of good judgment and memory to recognise conditions; and for the Fourth, that he be adaptable and able to accommodate himself in circumstances.

Let the Surgeon be bold in all sure things and fearful in dangerous things; let him avoid all faulty treatment and practices.

He ought to be gracious to the sick, considerate to his associates, cautious in his prognostications.

Let him be modest, dignified, gentle, pitiful and merciful; not covetous nor an extortionist of money, but rather let his reward be according to his work, to the means of his patient, to the quality of his issue and to his own dignity.'

Guy de Chauliac (1300–1370)

## Two Poems: Chris's Philosophy of Life?

Below are two poems that Chris Barnard was fond of quoting. I first came across them more than thirty years ago when rummaging through the collection of lecture slides he kept in his office in the medical school at the University of Cape Town. Each poem was quoted on an individual slide, and had been clearly used in lectures he had given.

My guess is that Chris first heard the words of 'A Bag of Tools' in 1968 on the occasion of a symposium, published in 1969 in book form, *Experience with Human Heart Transplantation*, edited by H. A. Shapiro, when the poem was recited at a dinner one evening in a speech by the then Administrator of the Province of the Cape of Good Hope, Dr J. N. Malan.

Presumably, Chris's attachment to these poems can be interpreted as meaning that the 'philosophy' put forward in them reflected his own attitudes to life.

## 'A Bag of Tools'
R. L. Sharpe

*Isn't it strange*
*That princes and kings,*

*And clowns that caper*
*In sawdust rings,*
*And common people*
*Like you and me*
*Are builders for eternity?*
*Each is given a bag of tools,*
*A shapeless mass,*
*A book of rules;*
*And each must make –*
*Ere life is flown –*
*A stumbling block*
*Or a stepping stone.*

## 'It's All in the State of the Mind'
## Walter D. Wintle

*If you think you are beaten, you are;*
*If you think you dare not, you don't.*
*If you'd like to win, but think you can't*
*It's almost a cinch you won't.*
*If you think you'll lose, you've lost*
*For out in the world you'll find*
*Success begins with a fellow's will,*
*It's all in the state of the mind.*
*For many a race is lost*
*Ere even a race is run,*
*And many a coward fails*
*Ere ever his work's begun.*
*Think big and your deeds will grow.*
*Think small and you'll fall behind.*
*Think that you can and you will*
*It's all in the state of the mind.*
*If you think you're outclassed you are;*
*You've got to think hard to rise,*
*You've got to be sure of yourself*
*Before you can win a prize.*
*Life's battles don't always go*
*To the stronger or faster man,*
*But sooner or later the man who wins*
*Is the fellow who thinks he can.*

# Acknowledgements

I thank Sir Roy Calne, one of my former mentors, for kindly contributing the foreword to this book. I am most grateful to Dene Friedmann, a long-time colleague of Chris Barnard at Groote Schuur Hospital and a close friend of several members of his family, for reading the draft, checking facts and opinions, and adding valuable comments. I am also grateful to transplant surgeon and medical historian, David Hamilton, for kindly reading the manuscript and providing insightful comments. I thank Pat Kaley for her skilled secretarial assistance.

I thank the following surgeons, physicians, colleagues, friends, and biographers who I interviewed either in person or by telephone in the course of the preparation of this book, or who otherwise provided assistance in its preparation: Guy Alexandre, Charles Bailey, Christiaan Barnard, Leonard Bailey, Sir Brian Barratt-Boyes, Ferdinand Barends, Clyde Barker, Karin Berman, Wilfred Bigelow, Viking Bjork, Johan Brink, Ben Cosimi, Christian Cabrol, Sir Roy Calne, Aldo Castaneda, Morley Cohen, Denton Cooley, Joel Cooper, Ben Cosimi, Michael DeBakey, Frank Delmonico, Clarence Dennis, William DeVries, Richard DeWall, Arnold Diethelm, Anthony Dobell, 'Max' Dubernard, Sir Terence English, Rene Favaloro, Robert Finley, Robert Frater, O. Howard Frazier, Allan L. Friedlich, Dene Friedmann, Peter Friend, John Fung, Vincent Gott, James Hardy, Dwight Harken, Hardy Hendren, Rodney Hewitson, Charles Hufnagel, Chris Hughes, Neville Jamieson, John Kirklin, Joanna Kloppers, Henri Kreis, René Küss, Willem Kolff, F. John Lewis, C. Walton Lillehei, Richard Lower, Prescott Madlingozi, Sam Metz, Bernard Miller, G. Wayne Miller, Ben Milstein, Francis Moore, Sir Peter Morris, Randall Morris, Joseph Murray, John Najarian, Father Tom Nicholson, John Norman, Dimitri Novitzky, John Oschner, Philip Oyer, Keith Reemtsma, Bruce Reitz, Donald Ross, John Roussouw, Paul Russell, John Salaman, Ake Senning,

Ron Shapiro, Norman Shumway, Richard Simmons, Maurice Slapak, Frederick Snyders, Thomas Starzl, Terry Strom, David Sutherland, Henry Swan, Joe Tector, Paul Terasaki, Frank Thomas, Luis Toledo-Peyrera, Jan van Rood, Richard Varco, John Wallwork, Herbert Warden, Watts Webb, David White, Winston Wicomb, G. Melville Williams, and Nazih Zuhdi.

Certain figures are reproduced by permission of the New York Academy of Medicine Library, the University of Minnesota Archives, or *Time* Inc.

Many of the statements quoted in the text are from personal unpublished conversations with the people cited, particularly with Chris Barnard. When not specifically attributed in the text, the majority of the other quotations from Chris Barnard are taken from his two autobiographies, *One Life* and *The Second Life,* with the permission of the trustees of his estate. Others are from Bob Molloy's edited collections of Chris's newspaper columns, *The Best Medicine* and *The Best of Barnard.* Quotes from Deirdre Barnard, Louwtjie Barnard, Marius Barnard, and Philip Blaiberg are taken from their respective memoirs (see Selected Bibliography). If not specifically attributed in the text, the majority of the statements quoted by others are taken from my own books, *Chris Barnard: By Those Who Know Him,* and *Open Heart: The Radical Surgeons Who Revolutionized Medicine.*

# CONTENTS

1

# The Most Unforgettable Character

Christiaan Barnard, who led the surgical team that stunned the world by performing the first human-to-human heart transplant on the night of 2–3 December 1967, literally became famous overnight. The daring operation captured the public's imagination as no other before or since, and Barnard became one of the best-known people in the world. This was in part because heart transplantation had a dramatic and mystical aura about it, but was equally a response to Barnard's youthful good looks and charismatic personality, which naturally drew people's attention to him (Figure 1.i). This life-changing operation ensured not only his place in medical history, but worldwide public recognition for a number of years. Barnard's name has since been inextricably associated with the first heart transplant and with the stunningly beautiful South African city of Cape Town, where the operation was performed at Groote Schuur Hospital, the academic medical centre of the University of Cape Town.

It is unlikely that any physician or surgeon either before or after him has been so widely recognised by the average man in the street. Within days, his face appeared on the covers of *Life*, *Newsweek*, and *Time* magazines (Figure 1.ii). He quickly became in enormous demand as a speaker, both at professional medical congresses and at lay events, and he was soon treated in many ways more as a showbusiness personality—a celebrity—than as a distinguished surgeon. He travelled widely, meeting presidents, popes, and prime ministers, as well as other notables and celebrities. At one time, it was claimed that his name and face were the most recognised in the world, perhaps with the exception of the boxer Muhammad Ali.

However, he had a number of faults, and some of the actions he took in his life were contentious. This charismatic yet complex and controversial character was aptly summed up by heart surgeon, Bob Frater, who had been a colleague of Barnard in Cape Town before moving to New York.

Frater wrote: 'He was then, at once, rough-at-the-edges poor boy and charming sophisticate, democrat and tyrant, selfless healer and boorish egotist, lover and Don Juan, shrewd *parvenu*, and naive acceptor of glitterati adulation—but, above all, surgical visionary and simply the most unforgettable character of the second generation of cardiac surgeons.'

Personally, having first met Barnard in the 1960s, worked with him for several years in South Africa and subsequently in the USA, and maintained contact with him until his death in 2001, I readily admit that he was, without doubt, the 'most unforgettable character' I have met in my relatively long life.

It was when Barnard and Frater were paying a brief visit together to Guy's Hospital in London in the early 1960s to see something of the work of the innovative heart surgeon, Donald Ross, that I first 'met' Barnard, though it can hardly be described as a meeting. I was then a final-year medical student and was acting as the third and lowliest of the assistants helping Mr Ross with an open heart operation. Due to their historically lowly origins as uneducated 'barber-surgeons', surgeons in Britain have the title 'Mr' rather than 'Dr', though many of the public seem to think this places them higher up the professional ladder than their physician counterparts. Barnard and Frater stood with the anaesthetist (anesthesiologist) at the head of the operating table watching the procedure, and made interesting comments on the differences in Ross's surgical technique from their own in Cape Town. I was struck by the energy and enthusiasm of both of these relatively young men (Barnard would have been barely forty at the time) and by their intriguing South African accents.

Donald Ross, a South African himself who had been an exact contemporary of Chris Barnard as a medical student at the University of Cape Town, had been the first surgeon in the world to replace a diseased heart valve with a healthy valve from a deceased human subject (in 1962), which was in some ways a minor precursor to the first heart transplant. In 1968, Ross was to become the first surgeon to perform a heart transplant in the United Kingdom, following Barnard's lead a few months earlier.

I first met Barnard personally a couple of years later—in the summer of 1965—when, having just completed an eighteen-month internship (junior hospital appointments) at Guy's Hospital, I visited Cape Town as a ship's surgeon. My brief sojourn at sea was a means of taking a break to see something of the world before teaching anatomy for a year in the USA. After graduating as a doctor, I had had the privilege of working under Mr Ross at Guy's, and, on learning that I would be visiting South Africa, he recommended that I take the opportunity to visit Barnard's department when my ship docked in Cape Town.

Barnard welcomed me and, to my surprise, seemed as pleased to talk with me as I was with him. Geographically isolated at the southern tip of

Africa, he had little opportunity to discuss cardiac surgical matters with others in this field. Even though I had been only a very junior member of Donald Ross's team, I did know how various surgical problems were dealt with in London, and Barnard was interested to hear what I could tell him. Although I believe at that time there was a cardiac surgical service in Johannesburg, the nearest major centres to Cape Town were several thousand miles away in Europe or North America.

Barnard took me to visit his research laboratories, where his younger brother, Marius, was working, and I also joined him and his staff on a ward round to see the patients under his care. I well remember him discussing one patient with severe heart failure, and was surprised when, after we had moved away from the patient's bedside, Barnard turned to me and said, 'What this patient needs, of course, is a new heart.' I had heard a little about the work that Roy Calne and one or two other pioneering surgeons were carrying out on kidney transplantation in Britain at that time, but I had never heard of anybody considering heart transplantation. Kidney transplantation was still very much in its rudimentary stages and the results were generally poor. I agreed with Barnard's opinion but, so far as I saw this form of treatment as impractical at that time, I thought the remark had been made almost as a joke—as a fantasy for the future rather than the present.

In retrospect, it became clear to me that Barnard's comment had been a serious one and that he had been contemplating heart transplantation as a realistic form of treatment for such patients certainly as early as the summer of 1965. This conclusion was supported by the words of the Cape Town tissue typing expert, Dr Martinus 'M. C.' Botha, who, in 1967, told journalist Peter Hawthorne that two years previously Barnard had approached him 'and said he thought the time had come for us to consider organ transplantation in Cape Town ... He considered it essential that I should go overseas to study the available knowledge and techniques (on tissue typing) there.'

It was little more than two years later that Barnard took the world by surprise with the heart transplant performed on his patient, Louis Washkansky.

Although Barnard was best known to the public for performing the first heart transplant, he made several contributions to medicine. These have been outlined in this book. Suffice it to say that, even without his work in heart transplantation, his reputation in medicine would have been assured, though his name would have been confined to those of us in heart surgery rather than to the public at large.

Like all of us, Christiaan—or Chris as he was known to those who knew him well—had his faults, and his life was filled with controversy and even tragedy. His insatiable desire for beautiful young women contributed to his three divorces. His hedonistic lifestyle alienated many in the medical profession, including several of his close colleagues. It also distracted him from his work, and he lost a golden opportunity to establish a major centre for the study of heart disease and organ transplantation that might have outlived him and been his lasting legacy. His subsequent forays and support for questionable business ventures damaged his reputation among his peers. He held controversial views on such topics as euthanasia. To his credit, he was critical of the political and racial policies that the South African government followed at that time, though with some reservations. These criticisms inevitably alienated some of the country's leading politicians.

My own personal interaction with him continued with a second brief visit to Cape Town in 1973 and then by working under him at Groote Schuur Hospital for several years in the 1980s. Having completed my surgical training in the UK, and being a member of the team at Papworth Hospital in Cambridge that initiated the first permanent heart transplant programme in the UK in 1979, I moved to Cape Town to gain more experience in this field. Working with Chris was like a breath of fresh air. He had an open mind, encouraged me in my research activities, and gave me great responsibility and independence in managing the clinical heart transplant programme in the hospital. I look back and feel that my real career in heart surgery began when I went to Cape Town, and I have Chris Barnard to thank for this.

However, if I had worked under him early in his career, I am sure I would have found life more difficult. In those days, he was much more interested in ensuring that everybody worked in support of him and less willing to allow his juniors some academic independence. He was impatient and intolerant if he considered any of his assistants' actions less than perfect. I may have found working with him then very frustrating, and my memories of him might have been significantly different. By the 1980s, however, he was prepared to delegate responsibility to others as he had never done before. I was fortunate to join him at this time when opportunities opened up for his junior colleagues.

It is not my prime intention here to provide a highly detailed biography of Chris Barnard; he has already done this himself in his first autobiographical volume *One Life* (written with Curtis Bill Pepper) in 1970, which follows his life until the death of the first heart transplant patient at the end of 1967, and his sequel to it, *The Second Life* (edited by Chris Brewer) in 1993, which covers the twenty-five years following the first transplant, in which he steadily became less involved in heart surgery, being lured away by the attractions of being a 'celebrity' and several other interests. The change in the public interest in him is illustrated by the fact that the first autobiography was a great commercial success whereas the second was not.

Both of these memoirs provide interesting and enjoyable reading. *One Life* covers his formative years both in regard to his growing up as a boy and to his training to be, first, a doctor, and, second, a heart surgeon. If not exactly a rags-to-riches tale, it certainly documents a childhood, if not of abject poverty, of limited financial resources, leading ultimately, by dint of very hard work and a flare for the demanding skills of surgery, to his success as one of the world's leading heart surgeons.

The second volume is perhaps of less value to those interested in the world of medical progress or heart surgery because Barnard is defined by his performance of the world's first human-to-human heart transplant and not by his subsequent celebrity status. Nevertheless, it provides an outline of his subsequent innovative and exciting work in heart transplantation as well as details of his later tumultuous personal life—how he reaped the rewards of these earlier preparatory years, rewards that were largely unexpected, certainly beyond his wildest dreams, and probably unequalled by any surgeon before or since.

However, neither volume provides the opinions of others—independent observers of Barnard—or critical assessments of his contributions to heart surgery, his character and personality, his strengths and weaknesses, or his successes and failures as both a surgeon and a man. This is what I have aimed to achieve in this book, which can be considered to be my extended memories of him and his work as well as the personal recollections of many others, most of whom I knew—or continue to know—personally.

How will I remember Chris as a colleague and as a friend? As a colleague, he could be demanding, expecting selfless attention to the patient's care. No amount of effort was too much to bring a patient through an operation successfully. In his younger days, Chris would hover around the patient's bed, checking in and out of the intensive care unit or ward at frequent intervals, phoning his junior doctors every few minutes, never resting or letting his staff rest until the patient was safely on the road to recovery.

As a friend, he could be great fun and immensely entertaining company, and, despite the acclaim and honours he had received the world over, in my opinion, he never allowed himself to become arrogant, pompous, or conceited. He retained a certain humility, which was most noticeable when he was with ordinary people—farm workers, for example, or, especially, children. I never detected a hint of superiority or of condescension when watching him in their company, or in the company of doctors.

Can we summarise Chris Barnard? Not very easily. He was a first-class doctor: skilled, knowledgeable, compassionate, conscientious, concerned, decisive, and wise. He was an inquiring and innovative surgeon with a vision of the future developments in his chosen field and the ability, judgment, and courage to play a part in contributing to those developments. The 'brilliant' surgeon is commonplace in the jargon of the media men and in the worlds of literature, television, and film, yet I believe Chris Barnard was one of the relatively few surgeons who may justify this adjective. He was an informative and highly entertaining speaker and raconteur, a competent writer of work aimed at the layperson (including being a modest novelist), farmer, restaurateur, an unofficial ambassador for his country, and a good friend.

He was, however, a womaniser whose self-centred behaviour impacted the lives of his three wives, some of his children, and several of his medical and surgical colleagues. There are those among his family and contemporaries who were of the opinion that the adulation showered on him after the first heart transplant and the fame that followed led to a change in personality, behaviour, and lifestyle that was to his detriment. I am not so certain that a change took place because, throughout life, he had been attracted to beautiful members of the opposite sex and, in turn, they had been attracted to him. He was at times a difficult person to interact with—in equal parts charming and selfishly demanding; the media brought these personality traits and his behaviour to the public's attention.

Of one thing, we can be certain: Christiaan Barnard lived life to the full. He had an enthusiasm for so many aspects of life—his clinical and research work, writing, public speaking, business ventures, coaching his daughter as a water skier, meeting new people—that one sensed a joy of living in him (a *joie de vivre*) that you do not see in many. This joy was infectious; I almost always enjoyed being in his company. Indeed, I usually felt uplifted just by contact with him. His admirers would surely say that the world would have been a worse place without him, his detractors that it might have been a better place; nevertheless, I am convinced—for me, at least—the world would certainly have been a much less exciting and less enjoyable place without him.

## 2

# Barefoot Boy: Childhood

## Beaufort West and the Great Karoo

Christiaan Neethling Barnard was born on 8 November 1922 into a white family in the small country town of Beaufort West in the Cape Province of South Africa. Beaufort West, about 300 miles or, today, about a six-hour drive north-east from Cape Town, is situated in the Great Karoo, an arid region of scrub grassland where the major activity is sheep farming. Cape Town journalist, Peter Hawthorne, described the Karoo as 'bleak, semi-desert. It is strangely fascinating terrain of wide, sweeping expanses of flat desert and eroded hills, or "*kopjes*" … Balls of windswept scrub bounce across the road and dust devils turn the hot air into whirling threads of sudden wind-power.'

Chris's older daughter, Deirdre, in her entertaining memoir (*Fat, Fame and Life with Father*) describes Beaufort West as being 'in the middle of nowhere'. She remembered that her father likened the Great Karoo 'to the State of Arizona in the USA … It's a vast, seemingly empty scrubland where the sun reflects up off the ground and puts a shimmer on everything in the summer and the winters are so achingly cold the water in the outside troughs freezes over.'

In his later life, after many years away from Beaufort West, when he had accumulated a little money, Chris purchased two sheep farms in the Karoo, stocked them with African animals, and opened them to tourists as a game reserve. Memories of the land and weather of Beaufort West remained with him throughout life. In one of his books on health for the layperson, he explained his love of the sound of thunder.

I grew up amid the endless expanse of South Africa's inland plains … We were frequently plagued by droughts in that part of the Karoo and it often used to happen that sheep died of thirst and you used to find dozens of them lying shrivelled up on the dusty plains. When the rains finally came, they were always preceded by thunder. That thunder used to bring me a feeling of immense relief. Hence my love for this heavenly sound.

Apart from the thunder storms, one of the characteristics of the Karoo is the silence that shrouds you once you have left the confines of a town.

## The Afrikaners

The original settlers in this region were the nomadic San (Bushmen) and Khoi (Hottentots). At the time of Chris's birth in 1922, there were approximately 3,000 white citizens in Beaufort West, and more than double that number of inhabitants of either mixed race or black ethnicity.

Nevertheless, Beaufort West was an 'Afrikaner' town. Afrikaners are the original white South Africans descended from the early, largely Dutch, settlers who migrated into the interior of the country from their original settlement in the Cape of Good Hope, which had been established on the coast by the Dutch East India trading company in 1652. It was planned as a place where their ships, sailing from the Netherlands to the Far East and back, could stop to take on supplies of fresh water, fruit, and vegetables. Indeed, the European 'founder' of Cape Town was Jan van Riebeek (1619–1677), a Dutch East India Company ship's surgeon who was charged with establishing a small community at the Cape. He subsequently became the first governor of what became known as the Cape Province.

Over the next two hundred years or so, the coastal Afrikaners were slowly pushed northwards into the hinterland by British settlers, who followed in large numbers, particularly after diamonds and gold were discovered in regions about 1,000 miles north of the Cape. The Afrikaners held on to their language, Afrikaans (a form of 'old Dutch'), and largely became farmers, to some extent being squeezed out of the much more lucrative mining industries by the British. The Afrikaners became so established and 'tribal' that they have sometimes been called the 'white tribe of Africa'.

Years later, after having travelled abroad, Chris was of the opinion that South Africans, and particularly Afrikaners, had become too provincial: 'too out of touch with the world. It was like the springbok we found in the Karoo after fences had been erected. Unable to run free, the animals inbred and became progressively smaller. We had a similar problem—too enclosed in ourselves. Our fences had to come down.'

Competition for land and minerals resulted in the 'Boer Wars' (1880–1881 and 1889–1902) between the Afrikaners and the British; 'Boers' was another term to describe white South Africans who were not of British descent. The British Army found the Boers difficult to deal with; they were used to hardship and sacrifice and had a legendary tenacity. In his autobiography *Defining Moments*, Chris's younger brother, Marius, states that one of the wars 'was a bloody war that raged for nearly three years, and one that left emotional scars and enduring antagonism between the Afrikaner and the colonial British.'

During the First World War, the white inhabitants of Beaufort West were split in their attitudes to the Germans and the Allies, with the majority of the Afrikaners being hostile to the whites who supported the British. The same split occurred during the Second World War.

Marius Barnard draws attention to the many Nazi sympathisers in Beaufort West during the Second World War. He wrote:

> The community was deeply divided into the anti-war camp of the National Party and the pro-war camp of General Jan Smuts' United Party. As supporters of the latter, we [the Barnard family] were a minority in an overwhelmingly pro-Nationalist community. Among the Afrikaans-speaking people, we were an even smaller minority and were extremely disliked as a result … During the war years, the Nats—from my youthful perspective—were not only anti-English, but very supportive of Nazi Germany. They were, therefore, vehemently against the South Africans fighting on the side of the Allied forces—which included my brother Dodsley.
>
> My feelings were strengthened by my father's strict rule that [the] *Die Burger* newspaper—the Nationalist (Afrikaans language) mouthpiece in the Cape—was not allowed in our house. My father read only the Cape Town [English language] afternoon daily, the *Cape Argus*.

It was in this antagonistic environment that Chris, like his brother, was brought up. Like his father, Chris was staunchly on the side of General Smuts and the 'British', yet, despite joining the cadets at high school, he did not become one of the more than 250,000 South Africans who volunteered to fight for the Allies.

The political rivalry that had developed over decades between the two white groups swung largely in favour of the Afrikaners when the Nationalist government was elected in 1948. Chris later wrote that, as he had been taught racial tolerance by his father, the coming to power of the 'Nats' (the 'apartheid' party) was a 'great disaster'. His father had said to him, 'Son, for some people the mills of God grind slowly but surely.' Chris was to live to see 'Mandela's South Africa' and to realise that the grinding of the mills had indeed been slow.

By this time, the Afrikaners controlled farming and had important stakes in the mining and business worlds. The members of the Afrikaner government that thereafter governed the country consisted generally of well-educated men, but with strong views on race and colour. As exemplified by Chris's father, the Afrikaners placed considerable importance on education, particularly in the fields of law, medicine, and finance.

Marius wrote, 'From the outset, the Nationalist government set about implementing its policy of racial segregation, or apartheid, with a vengeance. Whites were kept separate from blacks, Indians and coloureds [mixed race] in all areas of life, including housing, marriage, schooling, hospitals, transport and entertainment.' Laws were soon brought in that made it a crime to marry or cohabit across the racial divide, and a person could only live in his or her designated and segregated part of town.

Theoretically, development of these various ethnic groups was supposed to be separate but equal. In reality, the opportunities for each group were anything but equal. Facilities for the whites, in education for example, were vastly superior to those of other ethnicities.

During Chris's childhood in Beaufort West, the restrictions on the non-white population imposed by the apartheid regime were very evident. A bell rang in the town at 9 p.m., indicating that all non-whites had to leave the town for the night's curfew. Deirdre reported that her father was never reconciled to the principle of separateness. 'For him, a human being was exactly that and as a doctor, concerned with physical wellbeing, I suppose he saw people often as simply the sum of their component parts. There was no place for colour or creed.'

## The Barnard Family

Born to parents who were identified as Afrikaners, and living in a largely Afrikaner town, Chris Barnard grew up in a local community run predominantly by Afrikaners, though the British retained much wealth and influence elsewhere in South Africa through their mining and business interests. His home and school language was, therefore, Afrikaans. He learned English only as a second language. It was only at university that he began to use English regularly. Marius records how difficult his first year was at university (largely for this reason); it must have been equally difficult for Chris. Despite his later obvious great facility to communicate in English, when I knew him in the 1980s, he would tell me that he occasionally still found it more difficult to express himself in English than in his native language.

Despite his Afrikaner ancestry, however, Chris was very much an Anglophile and admired the accomplishments of the British. He believed that the British authority provided some stability to the country and that royalty, 'being above the ruck of politics and the muck of business, had a kind of magic quality that coloured the whole system. They were the first beautiful people. Corruption never touched them and the system ensured family succession without any grubbing around for votes.' He summed up his opinion as 'Me? I'm an Afrikaner who has been a royalist since birth, like my parents before me.'

The Barnard family's ancestors were not from the Netherlands, the country from which many Afrikaners originated. Chris's forefathers had emigrated in 1708 from Cologne in Germany. In his autobiography, he states that both his mother's family—the De Swardts—and his father's family originated in Germany, but in one of his books on healthcare, he points out that his mother's ancestors were Huguenots, originally from France. The first Barnard in South Africa was Johannes, a soldier employed by the Dutch East India Company, who later became a 'free burgher' of the Cape.

Chris was one of a family of four brothers, the sons of a church pastor and his wife. The family of Chris's father, Adam, had been woodcutters in the Knysna forest about six hours drive east from Cape Town on the south coast of South Africa—the beautiful 'Garden Route'. Adam's family lived in poverty in a primitive brick and mud hut. Born in 1875, Adam's childhood was very tough and he had no opportunity for education. He remained largely uneducated until he learned to read and write at the age of twenty. In his younger adult days (from 1899 to 1903), Adam Barnard was briefly a Salvation Army officer. Marius comments, 'This decision of my father's was to have the greatest influence on his spiritual life, and it is fitting that during the final months of my mother's life she was lovingly nursed in the William Booth Memorial Hospital (a Salvation Army nursing home) in the suburb of Gardens, in Cape Town, where she subsequently died (at the age of ninety-four).'

Poor health, possibly a sequel of typhoid fever, forced Adam Barnard to leave the Salvation Army, after which he took various menial jobs until, in 1903 at the age of twenty-seven, he became a student at the Dutch Reformed Church Missionary Institute in the town of Wellington (in the Western Cape). It was there where he met his future wife, Maria, who had trained at the sister school of the Missionary Institute (the Huguenot Seminary for Women) and, like Adam, was deeply religious. Marius described her as 'a well-educated woman ... well-versed in the skills required of the wife of a future missionary.' In fact, her family of farmers was relatively wealthy compared to Adam's poor family. Adam was ordained in 1909, and married Maria in 1910, with their first child being born in the following year.

In 1911, Adam became minister to the 'coloured' community in the town of Beaufort West in the Dutch Reformed Mission Church (Figure 2.i); as such, he was considered a 'missionary' in South Africa. His congregation consisted only of the non-European (mixed race or 'coloured') inhabitants of the town. The Cape coloured population to whom Adam Barnard devoted his life was descended from south-east Asian nationals who had originally been brought to the Cape as slaves by the Dutch East India Company (the 'Cape Malays'); the population also came from the original inhabitants of the region (the bushmen and Hottentots) as well as by interbreeding between the whites and these other groups. In the tip of southern Africa, therefore, both the white and coloured populations preceded the black groups. The true black African tribes, for example the Xhosa and Zulu, known collectively in South Africa at that time as the 'Bantu', descended into the country from the north at about the same time.

In Chris's 1977 book, *South Africa: Sharp Dissection*, in which he discussed the political situation as it then was in South Africa, he was clearly at pains to stress the important part the Afrikaner had played in the development of the country, and particularly in the area around the Cape. He wrote:

When our ancestors, the pioneers of the White nation of South Africa, planted their civilization in the shadow of Table Mountain in the middle of the seventeenth century, the nearest Black settlements were 800 kilometres away to the north and 1,600 kilometres away to the east, the distance between London and Hamburg and London and Rome respectively. The Whites founded their Mother City (Cape Town) at the tip of the African continent when New York was still a small Dutch settlement called New Amsterdam. At one time there were nearly as many white people in the Cape of Good Hope as in Canada. When the British occupied the Cape in the early nineteenth century, there were twice as many Whites in South Africa as in Australia, and Cape Town was then a large town that could be compared with Sydney.

In *One Life*, Chris wrote about life in Beaufort West:

The two people [the Europeans and the non-Europeans] shared some common ancestors, yet sat in different, untouching churches. Similarly, the two ministers shared a common faith, yet stood in separate, untouching pulpits. Both were ordained pastors of the Dutch Reformed Church. Yet their different assignments in the same town gave them different titles. Mr Rabie was a Dominie, or minister to the Europeans. My father was *eerwaarde*, or Reverend, and a missionary to the coloureds. There were 7,000 of them, against 3,400 whites, living in primitive conditions—suffering from sickness, hunger, and all the inherited ills of social outcasts. My father's mission was therefore immensely more difficult. For this, and for occasionally standing in as minister to the Europeans, he received each month twenty pounds [UK £ sterling], or about fifty dollars [US $] or about forty South African rands—one-third of the sum paid to Dominie Rabie. [It was only when Chris was a boy that his father's salary as a pastor had been increased from £4 to £20 per month.] It did not increase further until his retirement after thirty-seven years' service. Besides this, the minister of the European church socially had little to do with my father, his brother in Christ.

Adam Barnard was a devoted and conscientious pastor, visiting his parishioners in their homes when they were sick or could not attend church. He was also outspoken in his criticism of the official town policy that discriminated against people of colour. In addition, as part of his duties, Adam Barnard was superintendent of both the coloured primary school and the coloured high school. He also augmented his small salary by preaching to the inmates in the local prison every week.

Although the family paid no rent for their small house that adjoined the little church (Figure 2.i), Adam Barnard's salary was barely sufficient to support a family of six. The house, 77 Donkin Street, was connected to the vestry of the church. From the outside, it looks a small house but, according to Marius, as a boy, it appeared as 'a roomy house with large bedrooms and living rooms, set in a sizeable garden.' Chris was born in the house.

Chris's mother, Maria, helped her husband with his work by playing the organ at the church services. She was significantly deaf, and Chris and his brothers, whose duty it was to pump the bellows for the organ, were also expected to ensure that she knew when it was time to strike up the next hymn as she was unable to hear her husband's announcement. Chris later joked that the heart was not the first 'organ' he had been involved with in his life. Years later, when his womanising became well-known, the British satirical magazine, *Private Eye*, drew attention to another 'organ' he was interested in.

Having to attend church services two or three times every Sunday, as well as weddings, baptisms, and funerals, influenced Chris against attending church later in life. His exposure to music as a child, however, 'made an immense impression on me. [Music] can make me sad, soothe me or put me in good spirits.' Throughout life, he appreciated classical music, particularly that of Chopin, Beethoven, and Brahms. He later wrote that one of the most memorable experiences in his life was when he was a guest at the Salzburg Festival. He could never imagine being able to compose a symphony, but thought that perhaps some composers felt the same way about undertaking heart surgery.

As a child, he learned to play the piano, but later gave it up when his hands were afflicted by arthritis. He also 'picked up a rough and ready ability to coax a tune from a concertina,' and it remained 'a lifelong fascination'. As an adult, he would occasionally play the ukulele (which his older brother, Barney, also played), though perhaps not very well (Figure 2.ii). His great friend and father confessor, Father Tom Nicholson, recollected an episode when he and Chris were in Rome together. Chris urged him to hear him play a ukulele that he had just bought, which Tom thought was 'totally out of tune'. Chris sang a favourite Afrikaner song, *'Sarie Marais'*, and strummed his ukulele 'on and on until eventually I told him that it sounded more like a cat in passion than a singer. So, laughing, he packed up the ukulele, and I have never heard him play it since.' However, Chris did play it on occasions, at events held to support various charities.

Later in life, Chris's interests in music steadily widened. Among his favourite songs were 'Take the Ribbon from Your Hair', Billy Joel's 'River of Dreams', and Elton John's 'Nikita'. These songs gave him 'a zest for life'. He developed a particular liking for the music of Elton John, which would immediately affect his mood—from one minute to the next, he would feel happier. Dean Martin was another favourite, his song 'Memories are Made of This', bringing back happy memories of Chris's time (with a girlfriend) in Minneapolis (mentioned in Chapter 4). Indeed, when in the USA as a 'VIP' after the first heart transplant, when asked whom he would like to meet, in addition to President Lyndon Johnson, Chris selected Dean Martin, and the meeting was arranged. The music of The Ink Spots was also close to his heart, and later in life, he would not infrequently play an LP of theirs. He also came to enjoy country and western as well as Dixieland.

Chris Barnard always retained some connection with Beaufort West, though for many years, it was a very strained relationship. Marius, however, more or less permanently severed his ties with the town. The brothers could not excuse the way in which some white Afrikaner inhabitants had treated their father, who was considered by many to be 'beyond the pale'. The Afrikaners in the official 'white' church (the Dutch Reformed Church) looked down on Adam Barnard, even though he was 'a man of the cloth', and Chris and his brothers had often been referred to as 'the Hottentot ('hotnot') preacher's children'. Some of the white citizens would not infrequently refuse to shake their father's hand because he had shaken the hands of coloured people.

What later incensed Chris equally was that, after his father's retirement and move away from the town, the city authorities removed the pews from the church, sold the organ, dismantled the pulpit (in front of which Chris had been baptised many years previously), and converted the hall into a badminton court. When Chris stood before this sacrilegious destruction, I swore vehemently that I would never return to this town until my father's church was restored.' The relationship between the town authorities and the Barnard brothers became worse when Marius openly criticised apartheid and expressed his liberal views on race in South Africa. When Chris defended his brother's opinions, the mayor of Beaufort West stated that he was ashamed that the brothers had been born there. Chris repeated his avowal that he would never set foot in the town again.

Nevertheless, in due course—perhaps seeing the potential business opportunities—the town council decided to establish a museum to Chris. Adam Barnard's church was renovated and restored, as was the adjoining house where Chris had been born, the organ was re-purchased and re-installed, the pulpit replaced, and the baptismal font returned. Both home and church are now museums. Chris decided that this was sufficient for him to abandon his feud with the town, but Marius did not and, indeed, despised Chris's change of heart. 'Chris had the capacity to go back on his word when it suited him,' he wrote. 'Very soon afterwards, he received the Freedom of the Town of Beaufort West and the Chris Barnard Museum was instituted in the old town hall.'

From what Chris wrote and from my conversations with him, his father, Adam, was a 'good Christian man,' dedicated to his religion and to the care of his 'flock'. There is no doubt that Chris admired him immensely for his simple faith and honesty. With his firmly held views on apartheid, it is no wonder that Adam Barnard did not see eye-to-eye with the leaders of the Dutch Reformed Church and the Nationalist government. In one of his later novels, *The Donor*, Chris clearly drew on his own father in his portrayal of the elderly father of the main character, a young heart surgeon (obviously based on Chris himself):

[He was] a religious man [who] could never reconcile apartheid with the teachings of the Bible ... 'How can people who proclaim to be Christians go along with this blatant discrimination?' ... The most important Commandment is that you must love your neighbour as yourself. There is no way that you can obey these laws of the Nationalist Government and pretend that you love your neighbour as yourself.

Marius, whose Christian faith throughout life was arguably stronger than that of his older brother, held an even better opinion of his father. He told journalist Peter Hawthorne, 'I sincerely believe he went straight to heaven when he died. He was a man whose consideration was only for others. He was the kind of person who would give someone in need the last crumb out of his own mouth.'

Marius recalled:

Religion was in our very marrow. Every day at lunch and dinner with our parents we played an active part in devout meditation [on their knees]. As my parents had done in the morning, we too would participate in reading from the Bible and singing and praying in the afternoon and evening … In company and among their children, my parents were the picture of a decorous, upstanding couple. Though they were unquestionably devoted to one another, I don't think I ever witnessed a physical display of love pass between them.

In his book, *Good Life, Good Death,* in which Chris put forward his views on passive and active euthanasia, he also commented on this aspect of his childhood. 'In my youth,' he wrote, 'growing up in the puritanical culture of South Africa in the 1930s, death was regarded as no more a fit subject for discussion than the other realities of life such as love, sex, and bodily functions.'

At one stage of Chris's childhood, his father was in the habit of taking him for walks in the surrounding countryside on a Saturday or Sunday afternoon between church services. They sometimes hunted together.

My father taught me not just racial tolerance but the kindness of life, the love of nature. He would take me walking in the veldt [open country or 'bush', in some ways the equivalent of the Australian 'outback'], and he'd point out the plants and the creatures there and we'd look at the stars like a glittering blanket above us. From him I developed my love for the veldt and the wildness of the Karoo and many years later I was able to return and buy a farm outside of Beaufort West. That's where my roots are.

During some of these walks, father and son would discuss the family's precarious financial situation. To some extent, although in his early career he was not driven by a desire to make money, worries about his financial status remained with Chris much of his life, and may have been a factor in his later enthusiasm for financial transactions when the opportunities arose after he carried out the first heart transplant.

It was during one of these Sunday strolls that 'my father explained to me the meaning of death, leaving me perhaps more puzzled than ever,' Chris wrote.

> It taught me that in times of crisis, such as a serious illness of a family member, religion played an important role. I saw that people who had faith in a higher power, those who believed in an afterlife, had it much easier than those who had no religious beliefs to support them in the face of death. Yet, even against this background, I do not see myself as basically a religious man. That is, I do not embrace a specific religion. But I do admire the personal discipline that religious belief instils in its adherents, particularly the demands of exacting faiths such as Roman Catholicism and Judaism.

This is an interesting comment because Adam Barnard was strongly antagonistic to the Roman Catholic Church. He once told Chris that if he (Chris) became a Catholic, he would disinherit him, not that he had much material wealth to pass on to Chris, but the threat of displeasing his father so much—in effect, alienating him—must have weighed on Chris's mind. Long after his father's death, Chris was to marry Roman Catholics as his second and third wives, and even contemplated becoming a Catholic himself. His father would not have been pleased.

The fact that Adam Barnard was not a very worldly man to some extent accounts for the family's relative poverty. However, apart from the example he set his sons through his high moral standards and firmly held principles, he was not the major influence in their lives. It was their mother who influenced them more. She was the power who set the rules at home, who pushed them in their studies and other activities but, despite success, insisted they remain humble and ensured they 'toed the line. Chris later wrote:

> If my father taught me tolerance, my mother taught me ambition. You must always be the first, she used to say. But she also tempered that with humility. When the plum tree is full of ripe fruit, she said, its branches hang low to the ground. Achievement doesn't mean having a high opinion of yourself. I think that helped me later in life. Whatever happened to me I always tried to find time for everybody, not just the notable people but the man-in-the-street. Some people say I'm abrupt and arrogant. But I've always been straightforward and honest even though sometimes that honesty has been detrimental to me.

Marius remembered that, 'although she was a devoted mother, she was driven by a burning ambition for her boys. She was also the family disciplinarian. Once, while in high school, I slipped from the top position in the class. This made her terribly angry—I received a hiding I never forgot.' She 'had such a forceful nature that I always felt predisposed to please her, to be the dutiful son. It was indoctrination of a kind that is hard to explain.' Maria Barnard was not a 'warm' person, but was known for her sudden changes of mood; she sometimes flew into rages that frightened her young children. It was only the frequent intervention of her husband that prevented their sons from receiving even more beatings, often delivered with a large hairbrush. Chris attributed some of his ambition to succeed in life due to the pressure put on him as a child by her.

The brothers consisted of Johannes (Barney) (who had had a stillborn female twin), the eldest, who was twelve years older than Chris; Dodsley, five years older than Chris; and Marius, five years younger than Chris. There had, in fact, been a fifth brother, Abraham, who was older than Chris, who sadly died of heart disease as a young child. Abraham's death left life-long emotional scars in his parents, particularly in his mother. When looking at his photograph, Maria would sometimes openly weep, and Adam cherished the last biscuit his little son had sucked on just before he died. Maria left instructions that she was to be buried with her son, Abraham, rather than with her husband. Seeing his mother's anguish may possibly have influenced Chris's decision to study medicine. Ironically, the skills Chris developed as a surgeon would almost certainly have saved Abraham's life.

## Everyday Life

The Barnard house in Beaufort West had no flushing toilet, but only an outhouse equipped with a bucket at the far end of the garden. For Marius at least, and I suspect for Chris also, a walk in the dark in the middle of the night to attend to the call of nature 'was a scary experience'. There was no hot water and so a weekly cold bath sufficed. In the hot summers, there was no air-conditioner, and in the bitterly cold winters, there was only a small wood-burning fireplace that was rarely used as the smoke aggravated Adam Barnard's asthma (a condition from which Chris was later to suffer). In the summer nights, the mosquitoes were unbearable. They had no telephone or radio, and so communicated by telegram or the postal service, and acquired news by reading the *Cape Argus*.

The family existed on a financial shoe-string, and had no luxuries. They evidently could rarely afford to eat meat and were indeed just grateful to have food on the table. In *The Second Life*, Chris recalled:

In those days my evening meal consisted of a few slices of homemade brown bread on which I spread dripping-fat, sprinkled with salt and pepper. On special occasions, we had golden syrup which we mixed with the lard before spreading it on the bread. I had a choice of drinks then too—either black coffee with sugar or black coffee without sugar and it was the best coffee I've ever tasted—made by my mother from coffee beans that she roasted in an iron pot on the Dover stove ... The coffee was percolated by placing the coffee grounds in a sock made by my mother [from the same material that she used to make our pyjamas] which was suspended on the neck of the black kettle with a wire ring.

Their meagre diet was in part a result of their limited financial resources, but also because of their mother's puritan beliefs; in her mind, poverty was close to godliness. She also ensured that her sons had chores at home, which she insisted were carried out meticulously.

Nearly all of Chris's clothes at one time had belonged to Dodsley and some even to Barney before him. Outside of school, where shoes were compulsory, the boys went barefoot almost all of the time, though this was not uncommon in Beaufort West in those days.

In a later newspaper article, Chris recollected:

[Khaki clothing was] standard dress for me as a youngster. In fact, I have a feeling that if it hadn't been for the invention of khaki I'd probably have gone to school naked. Not that the Barnard khaki shorts weren't a very exclusive article. In fact, they were designer shorts. Today, it is very fashionable to wear designer clothes, but I have to admit that the Barnards were first with the idea. The designer was my mother. She was also the seamstress. The cloth was donated by my father—after he had put in a good few seasons wearing it in the form of khaki trousers. My mother could put together a pair of *kortbroek* [shorts] from second-hand material faster than anybody I know. She had plenty of practice. She'd been doing it for years. If you were lucky, as I was sometimes, you got a pair of shorts that were only second-hand. There were times when they were third- and fourth-hand, as was the case when passed on by my brothers. The pocket was big enough to hold a catapult and a tennis ball, with enough space left for catty ammo or perhaps a few marbles. You could also keep a tennis ball and a frog, or a catapult and a frog, but not all three together. I know because I tried it. The frog got a bit squashed between the ball and the handle of the catty.

As a child, Chris and his friends got up to all the mischief common to most young boys. Passages in his autobiography (and that of Marius) read like excerpts from one of Mark Twain's novels, such as *The Adventures of Tom Sawyer* or *The Adventures of Huckleberry Finn*. They 'stole' fruit from their neighbour's gardens (yards), swam in the local pond, raced used tires down the hills, and built boats from corrugated tin sheets. They caught scorpions in the veldt, and watched them fight each other in a shoebox. They took every opportunity to make a little money; this included catching rats and mice, for which the local authority paid a small sum for each one caught or killed. They sold fruit from their own garden and collected items of refuse to sell to the local dealer (at times actually 'stealing' from the dealer's yard and 'innocently' selling the items back to him again).

The father of one of Chris's friends was manager of the only department store in the town. The two boys would spend time in the gramophone record department, listening to the records that were played. They particularly enjoyed music from faraway places as this gave them a glimpse of the world outside the confinement of the Karoo.

Although I feel quite sure it was a prohibited activity in the Barnard household, Chris did surreptitiously develop an intermittent habit of smoking, which later, when he realised the health implications, he shook off. He began at the tender age of eight or nine. 'In those days, and at that age,' he recollected, 'smoking a cigarette seemed a terribly manly and grown up thing to do. Not having the necessary finances, we were forced to go for a home-made version. We collected dried-out donkey manure, rolled it into pieces of old newspaper and lit it. These were our first cigarettes.'

He claimed he was never 'a serious smoker', which I believe was true, but 'a few times when I had problems I smoked cigarettes.' The cigarette he liked best was 'the one after an operation. That cigarette seemed to relax me.' He smoked most during his divorce to his second wife, Barbara, when he became very stressed and depressed. Perhaps he did not consider himself a 'serious smoker' because he had a reputation for cadging a cigarette from his colleagues at the hospital; his research technicians would often mention this to me. He wondered why smoking is so attractive to so many people, and suggested that perhaps it is 'just a subliminal memory of time when we were babies and totally focused on our mother's breast.' All three of his wives were smokers, which perhaps made it more difficult for him to break the habit, which he eventually did 'cold turkey' more than twenty years before he died. Subsequently, he admitted he became irritated when people smoked around him as it gave him 'difficulty in breathing', possibly by aggravating the asthma he developed later in life.

The young Chris befriended a local man and would follow him through the surrounding veldt, having the 'privilege' of carrying his hunting bag as he shot hares for the dining table. Chris later wrote, 'That way I picked up an amazing amount of veldt lore. He showed me how the morning sun reflected the passage of small animals through the dew, taught me to walk face down so that bird panic did not alarm the game and pointed out how the lie of the hare's ears would indicate the direction of his next jump.' Years later, in Chris's first novel, *The Unwanted*, the main character (clearly based on Chris himself) recounts exploring the veldt with the son of a coloured farm worker.

The veldt was also a place to which Chris could retire when under stress. He recollected that, as a child, he would run away into the bush at times 'when there was something I didn't want to face.' He would occasionally also do this later in life when pressures mounted.

Marius pointed out that his 'first playmates were mostly black (coloured) children from my father's congregation. They made very good friends because, since I was white, I was always the leader and always allowed to win. My playmates were simply following the example set by their elders.'

The Barnard family always had pets at home but, surprisingly, as a boy, Chris never liked dogs. His love was for bantam chickens, cats, and scorpions. 'I don't know what attracted me to these dangerous creatures,' he later wrote about the scorpions, 'They could be found under every stone in our neighbourhood. Baboons love to eat them, but I never tried one.' Unlike many budding doctors, he did not dissect them. What fascinated him about scorpions 'was that after they mated, the female killed the male.' Looking back on his own very 'active' sex life, he commented that 'I'm glad that isn't the case in human terms, otherwise I would have been dead many times already.'

As an adult, however, he came to dote on dogs, who he called man's 'faithful friend. Its unbelievable, unconditional faithfulness always moves me. I know that for my dog, I will always be a miserable scoundrel because before we did the first human transplants, we experimented with dogs, but what other choice did we have?' When working as a young surgeon in Cape Town, he would sometimes take home dogs from the experimental laboratory. 'Out of pity we accepted Sixpence, a mongrel, from the laboratory; Ringo was a gift from a patient. From beginning to end it was an extraordinary experience in faithfulness, loyalty, and affection, which we were given in return for their daily meal.'

As boys in Beaufort West, there were occasional visits to the town by a funfair or circus. As they could not afford to buy tickets for the circus, they found surreptitious ways of getting inside the big top. They could occasionally afford to buy tickets for the Saturday matinee movie at the 'Bioscope' but were rarely able to attend the plays that were performed in the local cinema, which were generally based on Afrikaner history.

Perhaps surprisingly, in view of their impecunious state, the family owned a holiday 'house'—though a very basic one—at the Wilderness, a naturally beautiful little town situated on the south coast of South Africa. Equally surprisingly, Adam was able to run a Model 'T' Ford, which enabled him to visit far-flung members of his church, and which the family used to drive to the south coast for their annual holiday (Figure 2.iii). This two-week holiday that began on New Year's Day was the only time that Adam and Maria were free of their responsibilities to the members of their congregation. In the Wilderness, the boys would caddie at the local golf course to make extra pocket money.

Only the relatively wealthy could afford the luxuries of a 'holiday home' and a car in those days, and it is surprising that Adam Barnard could maintain them. Although there is no hard evidence, it could be that they were made possible by some financial help from Maria's family. However, Adam would sometimes receive gifts of food from his parishioners, which clearly may have allowed some money to be directed towards upkeep of the cottage and car. In addition, for many years (1916–1929), the family income was augmented by a lodger who boarded with them. Miss Dodsley-Flamstead was an English woman who was headmistress of a Beaufort West school for girls; she clearly influenced the Barnard boys' education.

## Sexual Awakening

Their parents' extremely conservative attitude to life resulted in Chris and Marius gaining little experience with girls. Marius claims he only discovered that girls menstruated when taking biology classes during his first year at university. Their mother thought dancing was a sin, and their father, although he would allow the occasional 'social' event for the young people of his church, would immediately draw it to a close if it became in any way frivolous.

From the age of thirteen, Chris attended the whites-only high school in the town, to which both boys and girls were admitted. According to author Chris Logan, the girls at the school thought he was good-looking, fun company, and romantic. His girlfriends of that era observed his admiration for celebrities, such as Hollywood film stars, and those who had made it to the top in life.

Chris felt that his ability to attract girlfriends was limited by his inability to 'wine and dine' them, or at least take them to the bioscope, as he rarely had any money. He wore khaki shirts and patched shorts, even when dating at the age of seventeen; some of his friends felt sorry for him. Nevertheless, the Beaufort West girls found him attractive. His lack of money evidently became something of an obsession to him, and may well have been the psychological basis for his efforts to improve his financial situation later in life.

Chris wrote about these adolescent sexual awakenings on several occasions in his later columns in the *Cape Times* newspaper. In one column, he commented on his first experience (as a young teenager) in the company of a member of the opposite sex. 'Until then I had thought of women as a drag, if I thought of them at all. I didn't know that an arm around the waist could feel like a million-volt charge, that conversation could bubble like champagne, that a kiss on the mouth could be more than a greeting, that it could be a return to Eden.'

In another article, Chris wrote:

Friday night experience as a skinny sixteen-year-old … My problem was that I wasn't allowed to go to the Friday night dance in the local hall. Dancing, my mother believed, was the quickest way to Hell. For me, it was the only way to teenage popularity. No girl would look twice at anybody who couldn't dance or, worse still, wasn't allowed to go to dances. So, I solved it by doing the whole Cinderella thing. At 7 p.m. I'd slip out of the house without a tie, do a primp and brush up at a friend's place, meet my best girl at the hall and dance away the evening until the clock showed ten. Then it was hell for leather back home and hope that my excuse didn't turn into a pumpkin before I got there … Leaving the party to be home by 10 o'clock wasn't in the least funny, more so when everybody else stayed behind enjoying themselves.

Remembering an early girl 'acquaintance' during his family's annual vacation to the south coast, with whom he had his first real kiss, he later wrote:

It was all so naïve and innocent that it seems a bit simple-minded compared to today's situation where teenage sex is the norm and the idea of celebrating New Year's Eve by walking on a beach is enough to cause hoots of mirth. Regardless, it wrecked my childhood world and firmly separated the girls from the boys. I remember that time as if everything was shrouded in pink mist. Much later I realised that it was Cloud Nine, but by then she had passed out of my life and we had gone our separate ways.

Later, as a medical student in Cape Town, Chris had continued to date her, but found that he could only afford to take her out about once a month.

# School

At the local school, Chris was always near the top of his class. Chris Logan reported that Chris passed his final school examination 'first class', enabling him to be admitted to university. It is likely he did well if only because his mother threatened to 'whip' any of her sons who failed to measure up to her expectations. The fact that he went on to university is an indicator that his performance must have been good. However, according to Marius, who excelled academically and in sport, he (Marius) was the only one of the four brothers 'to be placed top of my class academically, and the only one to be voted head boy.' Chris's leading role in the class, however, is illustrated by the fact that he was selected by his peers to give the 'address' at the time of their graduation from high school.

Chris's long-time friend, Tom Nicholson, told me that Chris had expressed regret that his education had been limited and that he did not know much about literature and poetry. Personally, I was sometimes surprised at the literary knowledge that Chris displayed in some of his newspaper columns written many years later, but possibly this reflected the knowledge of his 'editor', Bob Molloy, more than his own.

Being above average height and naturally athletic, Chris was active in school sport, such as tennis (becoming school champion), rugby (becoming captain of one of the school teams), and swimming, and seems to have been more than competent, if not outstanding. In his autobiography, he placed emphasis on his running ability. In the mile race at school, which he ran barefoot, he was beaten by a former school friend who was by then at college. The friend, Daantjie, was the son of Dominie Rabie—the 'superior' counterpart to Adam Barnard in the Beaufort West Dutch Reformed Church—which perhaps increased the competition that Chris felt. As Danntjie was four years older than Chris, he gave Chris a 150-yard head-start. The defeat had a big psychological impact on Chris, and he frequently looked back on it when faced with possible 'defeats' later in life. Perhaps because of his mother's influence and the scar left by his running defeat, he developed a strong desire to be successful in whatever he attempted. Chris also later wrote that people with a 'Type A [personality] are driving, ambitious, even obsessive types [of which I am undoubtedly a good example], while Type Bs are laid back, unhurried, and easy-going.'

His attitude to sport may have been summed up in a statement he made in a book he wrote many years later on how to maintain a healthy heart. His opinion was that, 'If you always lose at sport, you will lose your enthusiasm and enjoyment in the activity.' This is probably true of almost any activity that an ambitious person undertakes. I once asked the American surgeon, Norman Shumway, the other great pioneer of heart transplantation, whether, when progress was very slow, he had ever contemplated giving up his research. He replied, 'Not really. There was always just enough success—just enough gratification, if you will—that you could see that it probably would ultimately work.'

Chris never expanded on what drew him to a career in medicine, though he claimed that he had 'always wanted to be a doctor because I wanted to help people,' but he realised that his ambition 'could certainly not be taken for granted since we were not very well off.' Attending university required some financial support. It seems that his parents, particularly his mother, encouraged him (and Marius) to become doctors, as to have sons as members of the medical profession signified to them that their boys had achieved academic and professional success. Chris may also have been influenced by his oldest brother, Barney, who told him that doctors made a good deal of money.

It is perhaps remarkable that Adam Barnard found the financial resources to put three of his four sons successfully through university; Dodsley was the odd one out as he dropped out of college before completing a degree. It is also of interest that Chris and Marius attended an English-speaking university rather than one where the teaching was in Afrikaans, but this was because Stellenbosch University, the major Afrikaans university in the country, did not have a medical school at that time, although Adam Barnard's dislike for the Afrikaner attitudes to life may have been a factor in directing some of his sons to an English-speaking university.

Barney took a degree in mechanical engineering at the University of Stellenbosch and worked his way up to become a safety inspector of the South African railway system, a position of responsibility and some authority. Dodsley, after several years fighting in the South African army in the Second World War—and becoming a prisoner of war after being captured by the Germans in the battle of Tobruk—dropped out of college, moved north to the Transvaal, became a bookkeeper and accountant, and undertook several business ventures. After his move north, he thereafter played little part in family activities.

Although Marius was to become Chris's supporter in his professional life during the key period of his career at Groote Schuur Hospital, their relationship as children was competitive and strained. Marius comments in his own autobiography that as children, they were always fighting, and it is no secret that they did not often see eye-to-eye as adults. Indeed, throughout life, their relationship was rarely amicable. 'Though separated by only five years, Chris and I never got on with one another. We fought incessantly all our lives. As youngsters, we used our fists; later words and other means were our weapons of choice.' In other words, 'brotherly love' was in short supply.

In his surgical career, Marius became a recognised and well-regarded cardiac surgeon in his own right. In addition to his activities at Groote Schuur Hospital, he did much charitable work to establish heart surgery in Romania; in 2002, at a ceremony in Bucharest, he was awarded the Order of the Gold Cross by the president of that country.

In large part because he found it so difficult to work with Chris, in 1980, Marius resigned from his position at Groote Schuur Hospital and entered South African politics as a Member of Parliament for the liberal opposition, the anti-apartheid Progressive Federal Party. He later went on to make significant innovative contributions to the world of health insurance, of which he was clearly proud.

There is no doubt that living in Beaufort West in a very conservative, 'Calvinist' society—particularly in the home of two old-fashioned, narrow-minded parents—must have been frustrating to the brothers as teenagers. Both Chris and Marius were pleased to leave their home and the town to move to Cape Town as students. Marius's view was that, 'if I never saw this town again, it would be too soon.' Although I do not believe Chris felt so alienated, to some extent I know he felt similarly.

# 3

# Learning His Trade:
# Medical School and Junior Doctor

Having done well enough at the local school in Beaufort West, Chris progressed in 1941 to medical school at the University of Cape Town (UCT) and its major teaching hospital, Groote Schuur Hospital (GSH, sometimes known colloquially as 'Grotties'). In South Africa, as in the United Kingdom, after high school, students move directly to medical school, although their course of study is rather longer than the four years of US medical schools, where the student has already studied for an undergraduate degree.

If Chris had not visited Cape Town previously, he was in for an immensely pleasant surprise as the setting for the city is one of the most spectacular and beautiful in the world (Figure 3.i). The environment—both geographic and social—and climate must have proved a significant improvement on Beaufort West.

The University of Cape Town began life as the South African College in 1829, becoming the University of Cape Town in 1918. In 1928, it moved to the grounds of a large estate bequeathed to the nation by the British mining magnate, Cecil Rhodes (Figure 3.ii). Eventually, Groote Schuur Hospital was built on the same Rhodes estate (*Groote Schuur* is Afrikaans for 'Big Barn') and was opened in 1938. For many years, a house built by Rhodes on the estate became the official residence of the prime minister or president of South Africa, though the house is now a museum.

When I first visited Cape Town in 1965 and again when I lived there in the 1980s, GSH was a large attractive building on the slopes of Devil's Peak, just east of the famous Table Mountain, which overlooks the city of Cape Town. There can hardly be any more attractive site for such a building in the world, and the original GSH is one of the most elegant hospital buildings I have ever seen (Figures 3.iii and 3.iv). As have many architecturally beautiful hospitals worldwide, it has since been replaced by a far less attractive building, although fortunately the original building is still in use. It is a government-funded hospital. The original GSH was constructed with the aid of public subscription and government funds, construction beginning in 1932. To build the present new hospital, which was opened in the late 1980s, numerous small houses in the vicinity of the original hospital were bulldozed, including a boarding-house in Clee Road where Chris and Marius shared a room for two years. Today, GSH remains the major academic teaching hospital of the University of Cape Town.

## Medical School

Chris enrolled as a student at the university, but most of the preclinical science lecturing and laboratory activities were carried out in the medical school, which is close to the hospital, with the clinical teaching taking place at GSH or at several other specialist hospitals in Cape Town. At the time, the university had taken in a larger number of medical students than usual as applications had risen from those who wished to avoid conscription into South Africa's war effort, which was opposed by many of the Afrikaans population. Possibly as a result of this, relations between the Afrikaner students and those of British origin were not always good. There were almost 200 students in Chris's first year class, though this number would be significantly eroded over the years as some would fail the demanding examinations or drop out for other reasons. Of interest, another student who enrolled at the same time as Chris was Rodney Hewitson, who was later to become a valued surgical colleague in Chris's heart transplant team at GSH and Chris's chief assistant at the first heart transplant operation.

When Chris became a medical student (Figure 3.v), although UCT was liberal by the South African standards of the day, there were considerable restrictions on non-white students. Marius records:

Coloured and (East) Indian students (of which there were very few) were permitted in the 'non-European' wards from 1943, on condition that they had absolutely no contact with white patients, even when conducting *post-mortems*. Such racism persisted, and in 1944 there was a public outcry about the presence of black students at an operation on a white child ... At the time of my enrolment at UCT's Faculty of Medicine in 1945, there were four non-white medical students in my class. They were required to leave the lecture theatre when a white patient was demonstrated on, they were not given access to the white wards, and they were not permitted to examine white patients.

There was, therefore, considerable discrimination. Many years later, Chris used this discrimination as a basis for his first novel, *The Unwanted*.

Later, when a surgical trainee, Marius Barnard was quoted in the newspapers stating that he believed apartheid was being practiced in the hospital.

> The university's professors at Groote Schuur always started their ward rounds on white patients and conducted the rounds in the blacks ward afterwards. Operations would take place on white patients first, and only then would blacks be operated on. Furthermore, surgery on black patients would often be assigned to junior staff.

Following his complaint, it appears that this discrimination was corrected.

The first-year classes included chemistry, physics, zoology, and botany. As lectures were delivered in English, the first year proved difficult for Afrikaners. Even a few years later, by which time Chris was a clinical student, one of his surgical mentors commented on his difficulty with English. Chris found the first-year physics course particularly difficult as he had little background in this subject. After failure in one of the preliminary examinations, followed by a great deal of hard work and some extra tuition from Barney, who had graduated with a degree in engineering, Chris passed the course with flying colours.

In the second year, the students progressed to a study of anatomy, physiology, pathology, and pharmacology. Chris once told me that he was particularly impressed by the professor who taught anatomy as he could draw anatomical structures on the blackboard in coloured chalks using both hands simultaneously. Chris steadily worked his way through *Gray's Anatomy*, the 'bible' of medical students in those days.

London surgeon, Donald Ross, whose parents had emigrated from Scotland and was a contemporary of Chris at UCT, told me that 'at that time, education in South Africa was probably as good as any in the world, if not better. It was excellent. The teachers were mainly from the old Scottish schools. The anatomy teaching was superb, the pathology excellent. In fact, all the basic sciences were wonderfully taught, and the clinical teaching was equally good.' He added that, among the students, 'the English-speakers tended to be a jolly, drinking lot, and the Afrikaners were—I think to their credit—more hard-working.'

Marius, who became a medical student at UCT five years after Chris, writes:

> The total annual cost per student in those years [was] £60 [UK pounds sterling]. Both Chris and I had been awarded bursaries of £20 a year each

from the Bolus Scholarship and the same amount from the Helpmekaar [Fund]. The remaining £20 required for each of us was provided by my parents.

Chris estimated that he lived on scholarships of 140 South African rands [R140] a year. Due to this very limited budget, at first, he lived at the modest home of his brother, Barney, who generously provided him with a small 'spending money' allowance, which Chris spent largely on dating girlfriends. He frequently walked several miles from Barney's home in Rondebosch to the university and back each day. He did not have enough money to buy a raincoat, and on rainy days, he would sit in bus shelters, shivering in wet clothes, waiting for it to stop pouring. As he could not afford to purchase lunch at the medical school cafeteria, he took homemade sandwiches with him.

As continued support from his major scholarship depended on his continuing academic success and his passing the examinations, it appears Chris had little time for other activities, such as sport. In any case, although he had been a good rugby player at high school, the standard was much higher at UCT. When he did occasionally play, it was for one of the lower teams. Marius, however, found time (and money) to play rugby for the university's first team, and so must have been a very good player.

Early in his medical student career, Chris was influenced by a friend to take an interest in communism, but found he could not fully embrace it because of its emphasis on atheism. At the other end of the political spectrum, he avoided contact with the more conservative Afrikaans students.

Chris admitted that he studied medicine 'with a certain feeling of panic. I was always afraid of failing one of my exams, as my family could hardly afford the expensive tuition. I will never forget the day my eldest brother failed an exam. It was a virtual tragedy for the family; for days we all reacted as though we had lost a good friend.' Evidently, Barney was so ashamed that he did not come out of his bedroom for two days. This episode clearly made a big impression on the young Chris and was his motivation to give up sport and women. He realised that every day he studied was a financial burden on his family. Chris also admitted to always being 'very goal-oriented and ambitious. I never thought of these as bad qualities. I put great effort into my studies.'

However, Chris was distracted for a brief period of time by the lure of playing poker with his contemporaries, but it was relatively short-lived. He later philosophised:

Poker-playing medical students, I found, are a contradiction in terms. You are either a successful student or a poker player, never both. But when I set out to become the terror of the gaming tables, the biggest drawback was not my medical studies but my puritan background. All the Barnard ancestors as far back as the family Bible recorded them believed that nothing worthwhile could be gained without hard work. Anything short of this ideal was sinful. Gambling was one of the more lurid sins. Anybody who sits down at a poker table with that in mind was bound to lose. As I did, often. I suppose my psychological motivation was that if I were losing money I couldn't possibly be a sinner. My venture into the card sessions at medical residence probably lasted about six weeks, long enough to convince me that there might be easier ways of throwing money away but certainly no faster one.

When Marius arrived in Cape Town in 1945, he shared a room with Chris in a house near to the hospital. Chris, who was then close to graduating as a doctor, had moved out of Barney's house as relations between him and Barney's wife had deteriorated. It would appear that Chris was not an easy person to live with. Marius recollected that 'we had nothing in common and I don't think either of us enjoyed the experience.' Marius believed that he did not receive the support and generosity from Chris that he hoped for, but admits that 'perhaps I wasn't particularly generous towards him either … Problems in our relationship stemmed back to the sibling rivalry of our youth. Chris and I had often fought like cat and dog in fist-fights when he had returned home during university vacations. He was older and taller, but I was stockier.'

A fellow student of Chris was Lourens A. P. A. Munnik (always known as 'LAPA' Munnik), who was later to become a member of the Executive Committee in charge of Hospital and Health Affairs in the Cape Provincial Administration (which is similar to a state government in the USA or a county council in the UK). In this capacity, he was to play a significant role in supporting the heart transplant programme at GSH in the late 1960s. He remembers Chris as a student as always being 'cheerful and his laugh was infectious—he was never in dull company as his heartiness lifted everybody's depression and one conveniently forgot about one's studies.' I believe Chris retained the ability to lift the spirits of those around him until very late in life.

Enthusiasm, energy, and optimism would appear to have been Chris's trademark characteristics as a student as they were throughout most of his life. His great interest in all of his studies was perhaps illustrated by his reputation among his peers for asking many questions of all of his mentors. He had the confidence to 'pin down' the lecturers to clarify any points they had made that he considered doubtful or unclear.

When visiting his parents in Beaufort West, Chris would sometimes travel there by train with another medical student from the town, Percy

Helman. Evidently, according to Deirdre Barnard, when the train pulled into the Beaufort West station, where both sets of proud parents would be waiting to welcome their sons, Helman would take out a bottle of ether and dab it over himself like perfume. 'My mother has to smell that I'm studying to be a doctor,' he would explain. Evidently, Chris did not need to resort to such ploys for his parents.

The first thing Chris would see, wrote Deirdre, was his parents' 'high expectations of him just shining out of their eyes. After all, they were spending money they could ill afford on his training, hoping that in the future it would not turn out to be money wasted.' It certainly was not. During the periods he spent in Beaufort West, he would 'shadow' one of the local general practitioners to learn more about medical practice. On one occasion, he was allowed to watch the doctor perform a minor operation—the first Chris had seen—but the sight of blood proved too much for him and he had to sit down to avoid fainting. Back at medical school, his first experience of attending a *post-mortem* examination (an autopsy) was equally upsetting, and he had to leave the room. These unsettling early experiences, however, are not unusual for medical students the world over.

As is the case with many medical students, Chris was much happier when he began to see 'real' patients during the final three 'clinical' years of study. He was particularly influenced by the charismatic professor of obstetrics and gynaecology, with whom he built a special relationship. For some time, he felt that this specialty might be his chosen career.

On his own admission, Chris was not one of the truly outstanding students in his class—it was Donald Ross who took most of the prizes—but he worked very hard and passed all of his examinations, some with honours. On 13 December 1946, he graduated as a doctor with the MB, BCh (bachelor of medicine and bachelor of surgery) degrees, the equivalent of the 'MD' in the USA.

In the one month he had free before he took up junior appointments at GSH, he carried out a 'locum' job, standing in for a general practitioner in South West Africa (now Namibia).


## Junior Doctor

One of the surgical staff, Professor Jan (Jannie) Louw, who was later to become the head of the department of surgery, took a special interest in Chris as a student and fledgling doctor, and subsequently became his major mentor throughout his early career. Some years after Louw had retired, at my request, he described his impressions of Chris at that early stage of his career.

Soon I discovered that Chris [when a medical student] had a great asset, namely an ability to win friends and influence people, which has stood him in such good stead for the rest of his career. He was bright at his work and conscientious … I was so impressed with his intelligence and performance that I made up my mind that he should be one of our interns [junior resident doctors] after qualification … So, at the end of the year, Chris was appointed as one of the interns at Groote Schuur for 1947— the first six months in obstetrics and gynaecology, then six months in surgery on the professorial firm … He was, therefore, given the lion's share of the operative work allotted to interns, which he handled with remarkable expertise. He was also an excellent assistant and I therefore often invited him to assist me in my private practice … He demonstrated another characteristic which stood him in good stead through the years, namely that he knew his limitations and how to act when a crisis arose.

As an aside, Louw recounted an occasion when he had invited Chris to his home for lunch. Louw's wife, who had not been warned to expect a guest.

[She] apologised to Chris for the frugality of the meal and asked him whether he would like some blancmange. He obviously did not know what it was, but when he saw the apricot jam his eyes lit up and he accepted with alacrity. On tasting the dessert, he smacked his lips and then proceeded to gobble up the whole dishful.

Thereafter, Louw and his wife always referred to blancmange with apricot jam as 'Chris's pudding'.

At the Peninsular Maternity Home, he was responsible for delivering babies in the homes of coloured patients in one of the poorest districts of Cape Town. His experiences there are reminiscent of those of students and junior staff at the great London teaching hospitals not many years previously, who delivered the babies of their patients in the surrounding slums. At times, the poverty and squalor had to be seen to be believed. Writer Somerset Maugham, who many do not realise trained as a doctor at St. Thomas's Hospital in London, called on this experience when writing his first successful novel, *Lisa of Lambeth*, published in 1897. Unusually for an Afrikaner, Chris was at ease when interacting with his coloured patients, no doubt a result of his close contact with this community at his father's church in Beaufort West.

As a junior doctor, Chris was impacted by the suffering of some of his patients. He was particularly affected by one young patient, Maria.

She lay apart, alone in her private room, her cell of pain and sorrow, with its view of a green lawn and one white ionic column. In a way, it was our room, our cell, for I went there often, to hold her hand. I had never seen anyone suffer so much pain and found myself drawn with increasing frequency to her bedside, where I did whatever was possible to relieve the increasing agony of her inevitable crucifixion ... Duty called for a cure by using all means. If no cure was possible, the doctor was required to alleviate as much pain and suffering as possible. And for the supreme relief of the supreme sufferer, there was only one lasting answer.

Even at that early stage of his career, he began to consider euthanasia, which he was later to support—theoretically, at least. In Maria's case, he progressed as far as drawing up an excessive dose of morphine into a syringe, which he intended to inject into her to relieve her pain permanently, but then had second thoughts.

I squirted the morphine into the sink and started to leave—just as Maria awakened ... The next day she seemed to be better and six weeks later she left the hospital—free of pain with her disease arrested for a few more years. I watched her go wondering how I had come so close to committing a tragedy.

## Marriage

During his days as a medical student, Chris had met Aletta Louw (nicknamed 'Louwtjie', pronounced 'Lowkey')—no relation to Professor Jannie Louw—an attractive nurse whom he began to date regularly. Her family home was a farm in South West Africa, where the climate was not greatly different from that in the Karoo. Financially, Louwtjie's Afrikaans family was much better off than Chris's. According to Marius, their romance was very stormy: 'I witnessed many arguments and tears.' Although there seems little doubt that Chris was not an easy person with whom to live, my understanding is that perhaps neither was Louwtjie.

They were engaged to be married for almost two years—Chris had sold his little second-hand car (purchased from his income from various part-time jobs as a student) to buy the engagement ring—before they set a definite date for their marriage, the delay being mainly because their financial state was so insecure. It was only when Chris had decided on a period in private practice as a general practitioner that they felt able to be married.

It seems that almost everybody who knew Chris wrote a book of their memoirs, including Louwtjie. In her brief autobiography, *Heartbreak,* written after the first few heart transplants when her marriage had broken up, she remembered him at the time of their marriage as 'an ordinary, personable young man. He was ambitious, had a zest for living and a determination to succeed. We were simply two small-town people who had met accidentally, were attracted to each other and gradually fell in love. This was no whirlwind romance, it just happened slowly and surely.' However, she also remembered that he possessed 'an irresistible charm for women and I was no exception.'

They were married in the Groote Kerk (literally the 'large' or 'great' church, also called the 'Mother Church' of the Dutch Reformed Church in South Africa) in Adderley Street in Cape Town on 6 November 1948 (Figure 3.vi). This had been the first Christian place of worship erected in the Cape, following the arrival of Jan van Riebeek in 1652. The building's cornerstone was laid in 1700. Marius acted as his best man. The newlyweds spent their honeymoon at the Wilderness, the seaside resort where Chris had spent so many childhood vacations with his family.

Of interest, in his book, *50 Ways to a Healthy Heart*, published more than fifty years later (in 2001), Chris claimed that he 'did not have sex until I was twenty-five—older than most of my contemporaries—and that was with my first wife. I was part of a generation that still placed a certain value on waiting until marriage before having sex.' Even though his generation was far more disciplined morally than those of my own generation less than twenty years later, I must say I was surprised to read this statement, particularly as sex became such an important part of Chris's life. My doubts about the veracity of his claim were increased when, in the same book, he also claimed that 'as a student I had no fear of sex.' What does this mean? Was he not afraid to have sex (but chose not to 'put a toe in the water'), or was he having sex fearlessly? However, the virtual 'indoctrination' he had been exposed to throughout childhood by his very conservative parents may have influenced his attitude to sex before marriage.

In her memoirs, Louwtjie wrote that their wedding night was 'exactly the way I had imagined … It was the most beautiful night of my marriage.' She added that 'our sex life was always perfect.'

## Family Practice

Chris accepted an opportunity to become a family physician in Ceres, an attractive little town in the centre of a fruit-farming area about 80 miles inland from Cape Town. Dr Tim O'Maloney, who practiced in Ceres, had taken leave for a year, and one of Chris's fellow interns at GSH, Dr Erhard 'Pikkie' Joubert, took over the practice for this period. Dr Joubert soon found there would be enough work for two, and invited Chris to join him. Although Chris had some deep feelings that his long-term future was more in the field of hospital practice, possibly in obstetrics and gynaecology, he and Louwtjie were planning to marry and he was attracted by the increased security and financial rewards of a family practitioner compared with those of a junior hospital doctor. Chris therefore joined Pikkie Joubert and, during his sojourn in Ceres, he and Louwtjie settled into married life. Their first child, Deirdre, was born at a maternity home in Cape Town in 1950.

According to Chris, he enjoyed family practice immensely, though there were occasions when he felt inadequately prepared for the rigors of such a practice in a rural community. The doctor frequently stood alone, and the patient might live or die on the single doctor's knowledge, decisions, and skill. Very sensibly for a young and inexperienced doctor, he would on occasion telephone his former mentors at GSH to ask for their advice.

During what Chris referred to as 'his eager-young-man phase,' he treated every patient as a challenge to be overcome. Every time he went out to do 'battle with pain and illness', he was 'mentally astride a white charger … That was how I lived my life then—fights to be fought and obstacle courses to be taken at a run.' This eagerness to accept a challenge, particularly a medical one, was to remain with him for most of his life. The two young doctors were allowed to carry out minor surgical procedures in the small local hospital. Chris gained something of a reputation for wanting to take on almost any surgical challenge, which his colleague, Pikkie Joubert, felt at times verged on recklessness.

Chris and Joubert worked hard and were popular in the town. The practice rapidly expanded and, by the time Dr O'Maloney returned, it was clear that it could support all three of them. For a while, their partnership progressed well, but friction gradually developed between Chris and Dr O'Maloney. When patients, who had formerly been those of the senior physician, asked to be seen by Chris, who had attended to them during Dr O'Maloney's year of absence, the older physician's feelings and pride were clearly hurt. Similarly, there were occasions when Chris would be disappointed when a patient with whom he had developed a close relationship, and to whom he had given considerable service, requested to be seen by Dr O'Maloney. It may be that the young Dr Barnard did not handle the situation with the tact that was required to smooth over this transitional period. Eventually, Dr O'Maloney could no longer tolerate Chris's continuing presence and he asked his junior partner to leave the practice.

Chris was naturally very aggrieved by this request, even though he had already been considering returning to hospital practice to train as a surgeon, particularly when he learned that his friend, Pikkie Joubert, was in agreement with Dr O'Maloney. Dr Joubert was of the opinion that Chris had been too aggressive in competing for patients and, as a result, had 'humiliated' Dr O'Maloney. As the two young doctors had worked closely together to build up the practice and, indeed, Dr Joubert had boarded in the same house as the Barnards, Chris was upset to find his friend was not supporting him against the senior physician.

At first, Chris's response was to consider establishing a rival practice in the town and, with this in mind, he set about sounding out several of his most grateful patients as to whether they would continue to use his services if he opened his own office. To his great disappointment and chagrin, he found that none of them was prepared to make such a commitment. They were clearly loath to show any disloyalty to the established medical figure in the town, Dr O'Maloney. Although many of them readily agreed that they preferred to have Chris attend them, they could not bring themselves to sever their ties with Dr O'Maloney. Chris felt deeply hurt and, indeed, humiliated by the attitude of people he had believed to be his friends. The enmity between him and his two colleagues increased further.

Chris then turned to the local Dutch Reformed Missioner, the Reverend Ernst Holtzapfel, whom he refers to in his autobiography not only as a 'constant source of strength and wise counsel' but also, significantly, as 'one more in an endless chain of substitutes for the living reality of my father.' Reverend Holtzapfel was as loyal as ever and promised that he and his family would remain Chris's patients if he stayed in Ceres, but he advised Chris against setting up in practice in opposition to his former colleagues. The pastor's counsel prevailed and Chris and Louwtjie departed from Ceres under a cloud, moving back to the Cape Town area.

Later, however, Chris listed this event as one of the luckiest of his life. If he had not been forced to leave general practice, which he enjoyed, he might have remained a general practitioner for life and missed all the excitement of heart surgery and, particularly, heart transplantation.

Chris had no job to go to, even though his former bosses at GSH were keeping an eye open for an appointment for him on the junior staff. However, the family was not homeless. His wife's parents lent them their holiday home in the Strand, a seaside town about 30 miles from Cape Town.

Due to his subsequent several changes of jobs, the family was to lead an itinerant lifestyle for many years. Years later, Deirdre, in her memoirs, likens Chris's family to 'camp followers. My father was the important one. Wherever he went for his work, we went along like a gypsy troupe tagging behind.' Louwtjie even wondered if Chris had married her 'because he knew I would be his slave'. Although the need to move from job to job is today less than it was in the 1950s and 1960s, it is still not unusual for wives and families to follow young surgeons and physicians from place to place during their training years.

## Postgraduate Training in Cape Town

This was clearly a most depressing time for the young doctor and his wife. Their second child, André, was born (in 1951) while Chris remained unemployed. Chris filled the time by studying for his higher surgical examinations, planning to travel to London to sit the onerous and challenging examinations for the Fellowship of the Royal College of Surgeons of England.

Before he could do so, however, a junior post became vacant at the City Hospital for Infectious Diseases in Cape Town and, after a competitive interview, Chris was offered the job. He had responsibility for patients in five wards—those with diphtheria, measles, typhoid fever, pulmonary tuberculosis, and tuberculous meningitis. He became especially interested in children suffering from tuberculous meningitis (tuberculosis affecting the lining of the brain and spinal cord), for whom there was little or no effective treatment, and a majority of them died. In his autobiography, *One Life*, Chris described his little patients in graphic terms.

> Behind the bars of each bed was a coloured baby or child in some stage of deformity. Many of them had little bodies with heads as big as basketballs. They could not easily carry such a load and lay on their backs, eyes blinking from massed flesh—vacant stares as if they had seen an abyss of such frightening horror that it had left them mute with awe and fear.

They were suffering from hydrocephalus, a massive accumulation of fluid around the brain, thus stretching and enlarging the skull. Their major problem was that the tuberculosis prevented the fluid that surrounds the brain and spinal cord (the cerebrospinal fluid) from flowing normally, and so the fluid would build up and cause pressure on the brain, ultimately causing death. Chris clearly had great compassion and empathy for his little patients; this compassion and empathy for children stayed with him throughout his career.

Chris threw himself energetically into finding an effective treatment, working long hours, often through the night. His aim was to prevent or reduce the blockage caused by the disease. He first tried injecting cortisone, an anti-inflammatory agent, into the space around the spinal cord, together with anti-tuberculous drugs. When this was not sufficiently effective, he tried injecting trypsin, an enzyme that would dissolve the exudate that was causing the blockage, thus reducing the pressure on the brain by allowing the fluid to flow again. Much of what he attempted was new, and he had no idea of the effect that his treatment would have. He justified this daring—some might say reckless—approach by pointing out that there was no other therapy, and his patients would undoubtedly die if he did nothing. His enthusiasm for his research sometimes led him to neglect some of the more routine aspects of his job, but his seniors seemed to accept this as they could see his passion and, I believe, his potential.

Although some patients improved significantly and their lives were extended, unfortunately no treatment was entirely successful (as is often the case with new approaches in medicine). Eventually, Chris had treated 259 patients (between March 1951 and March 1953), the largest investigation of this dreadful disease that had been carried out to that date. Using data he had accumulated, he wrote a dissertation for which he was awarded the Doctor of Medicine (MD) degree, the highest medical research degree that can be obtained in South Africa. This was perhaps the first sign that he had a definite aptitude for medical research.

It was during this period that his wife claims that, in a letter she had 'the misfortune to read', she found evidence of Chris's affair with a nurse. Louwtjie challenged him with the 'proof', but he soon convinced her otherwise. 'I do not believe that there is another man in the world who has the ability to charm a woman like Chris,' she later wrote. 'In fact, he charmed me so well that in the end, I was the one who apologised, ashamed at having thought him capable of such a thing as infidelity.' Whether this was his first extramarital affair is uncertain, but it certainly was not his last.

In *One Life,* Chris wrote about drawing cerebrospinal fluid samples from his unfortunate little patients, but his description provides a clue to his amorous activities at the hospital. 'Gene [the nurse] did it beautifully, holding Flavia [the patient] against her magnificent thighs as I drew out the fluid'—hardly an innocuous medical description.

He also states that, because he was studying for examinations and his enthusiasm for research, 'I often studied through the night in the doctors' bungalow (residence) without returning to Louwtjie in our apartment.' He records times when he would call a nurse (living in the nurses' residence) at night to demonstrate to her some aspect of his research, and end by taking her to a café for a social snack or meal.

In my personal experience, many a young (or even older) doctor has attributed his absence from home to the demands of his work. Often, this is absolutely true, of course, but sometimes it has been used as an excuse to continue an extramarital affair. For a young man looking to have an affair (or, frequently, affairs) junior doctors are in a particularly enviable position. They usually have access to a bedroom in the hospital, making it easy to rendezvous with nurses and other female staff (who in Chris's days often also lived on site). All of the requirements for an affair (or one-night stand) were easily available.

## Return to Groote Schuur Hospital

Chris was then offered a junior position as a registrar (a training position equivalent to a resident in the USA) in the department of medicine (not surgery) at GSH. He was delighted as this gave him the opportunity of completing his study of (internal) medicine before moving on to his real love, surgery. He was also relieved to be able to leave the City Hospital, which he saw as 'a bottomless cradle of suffering and sorrow, a frightful realm ruled by an unconquered disease.'

For Chris, returning to GSH was like 'coming home from a long trip.' Robert 'Bob' Frater, a medical student at UCT at the time (and later an eminent heart surgeon in New York City), remembered Barnard during this early phase of his career. 'I first met him when I was a student in Cape Town and he was teaching medicine. He impressed us students immensely. He was so dynamic, so energetic—a funny guy with a squeaky voice, and a dynamic approach to everything. Everything was done at top speed and with maximum emphasis.'

Chris records an event from his days in training that impacted him to the point that he wrote about it more than twenty years later in one of his newspaper columns. A patient of his had died early one morning just as his boss at the time, physician Sam Berman, was beginning his ward round.

> Sleepless, bleary-eyed, and depressed, I gave Sam a play-by-play account of my efforts to keep the poor man alive, ending with an abject, self-pitying, 'Sorry, sir, I did my best.' Sam heard me out attentively, his lips pursed and his manner, as always, impeccable and thoughtful. When I had finished, he indicated that he did not like his staff to appear on duty unshaven. 'Moreover, Barnard,' he added coolly, 'let us not be too pious. Let us rather recognize that your best was simply not good enough!'
>
> Had anyone else made the remark, I would probably have struck him or muttered something obscene. But, coming from this superb doctor, it was a revelation. An affirmation of belief. 'You're right, Sam,' I thought, 'you clever bastard. You're absolutely right. There are innumerable instances when our best just isn't good enough!'

Perhaps this is why Chris always demanded the highest possible standards both from his juniors and from himself.

Chris was almost overwhelmed by the huge number of very sick patients who were being admitted to the hospital—patients with diabetes, heart disease, and so on. He again worked very long hours, often studying throughout the night at the hospital rather than returning home. Eventually, he was ready to take the examination for the postgraduate degree of Master of Medicine (M. Med.) of the University of Cape Town. Like many examinations in medicine and surgery, it involved passing written papers and also oral examinations (known as 'vivas').

His mentor in surgery, Professor Louw, recollected that, 'during the long-drawn-out orals of this examination, he (Chris) became so frustrated (by the endless questions) that he rose and said (to the examiners), 'Gentlemen, you know enough about me by this time to either plug me or pass me. I leave it to you,' and walked out. The point is that his ultimate objective was not internal medicine but surgery, and he was anxious to begin with surgical research.'

I have never heard of any other examination candidate taking this dramatic (and highly risky) step during an oral examination. Remarkably, Chris passed the examination.

## Surgery at Last

It was not long (in 1953) before Chris was able to transfer to the department of surgery. Chris's enthusiasm to learn his craft was unbounded. In one of his later newspaper articles, he wrote of always being the first surgeon of the operating room team to be gowned and gloved, having 'spent half the night poring over the surgery list and reading about the problems that might come up. By the time I reached the (operating) theatre I was so hyped-up and eager to go that it was a problem to pretend to be as nonchalant as the others.'

Here, he again came under the influence of Professor Louw, by this time the head of the department of surgery at the UCT Medical School. During this period, Chris not only gained considerable clinical and operative experience in general surgery, but also, under Professor Louw's guidance, performed some ingenious and technically highly skilful research relating to the cause of intestinal atresia (bowel obstruction present at birth) in infants.

Louw suggested that they should try to find the cause of this congenital abnormality (birth defect) to help in solving the problem of the high mortality with which it was associated. Louw had carried out some

research in London in 1951 that suggested that the abnormality was due
to a 'vascular accident' in the foetus, resulting in critical ischemia (loss
of blood supply) of segments of the bowel. The resulting damage to the
bowel wall might lead to obstruction of the bowel. Louw stated:

> Chris immediately offered to 'try the experiment' by operating on
> bitches in the late phase of pregnancy. At first there were many problems
> in finding suitable bitches and also many failures, but once again he
> demonstrated his grim determination, and success was achieved. He
> produced lesions in puppies identical to those in infants. It cost forty-
> three experiments and a year of sleepless nights, but his drive and hunger
> for victory enabled him eventually to succeed in 80 per cent of the
> experiments. This work, which was widely acclaimed, had far-reaching
> effects.

This research, carried out on dogs in the experimental laboratory, was
squeezed into whatever time could be found, frequently in the evenings
and nights after a long day in the operating room and wards. In fact,
during this period of time, Chris was literally working day and night—
carrying out his clinical duties as a trainee surgeon during the day and
often covering emergencies at night, yet pursuing a demanding research
programme in the evenings whenever he was free. Many years later, he
once told me that, when he was a young man, he could never remember
feeling tired. He certainly must have been tired frequently, but the
excitement, stimulus, and enjoyment of working in fields where he had a
passion must have prevented the fatigue from becoming obvious.

Indeed, in his autobiography, Chris described how his 'real life' began
in the evenings when he could go to the animal house to begin his
experiments.

> How can I begin to describe the excitement with which I first entered
> the little animal building, stuck in between the medical school and the
> graveyard? [The medical school today is still flanked by an extensive
> cemetery!] It smelled of guinea pigs, rabbits and hundreds of mice. Yet it
> was like heaven, and even today those odours excite me with memories
> of our first days, so filled with hope and dreams—and bitter anguish.

He worked with little support and only basic facilities, being assisted
by two 'boys' (using the common term then for coloured and black
men, which is now considered derogatory but not necessarily intended
to be so in those days) and occasional help from volunteer nurses and
doctors. Research and innovative surgery clearly excited him like nothing

else, acting almost as a prequel to his later innovative work in heart transplantation. In my opinion, you either have this attraction to research or not, and Chris certainly had it.

The studies on intestinal atresia are worthy of further comment as the skill involved in the performance of this work was of a high order. The experiments involved opening first the abdomen and second the womb of an anesthetised pregnant bitch, removing one of her developing puppies, opening its abdomen, and performing a surgical procedure on the puppy (tying off a blood vessel), closing the abdomen of the puppy, replacing the puppy in the womb, closing the womb, and finally closing the abdomen of the bitch. Hopefully, the bitch recovered without aborting her litter, and later gave birth to a puppy with a blockage of the gut, which had resulted from the surgical procedure performed on it when in the womb. As someone with fifty years of surgical research behind me, I recognise that this experimental study must have been exceedingly difficult to perform successfully. He then went on to demonstrate that the blocked section of gut could be excised (cut out) and the bowel joined up again, thus curing the condition.

According to Louw, Chris's research led 'to modifications in the operative treatment of intestinal atresia [in human babies] which converted a 90 per cent mortality rate into a 90 per cent survival rate ... The experimental work was repeated by others in many parts of the world and opened up the whole field of intrauterine surgery [surgery performed on the developing baby in the womb].'

Although surgical procedures on foetuses in the womb are well-established (though still relatively unusual) today, this was certainly not the case when Chris was carrying out his research. In the early 1950s, this was an extremely ambitious research programme for such an inexperienced young surgeon, and he can certainly be considered something of a pioneer. There are surgeons who have expressed their opinion to me that this was the best research work that Barnard ever did. Chris was later to submit this research in the form of a dissertation to the University of Minnesota, for which he was awarded the degree of Doctor of Philosophy (PhD).

Although Professor Jannie Louw was Chris's main surgical mentor at GSH and influenced his career over many years, their relationship was not always a completely happy one. Chris was clearly not the easiest young staff member to work with, and it would seem that his competitive nature and desire to excel and progress in his career at times irritated his senior colleague (just as it had irritated Dr O'Maloney in Ceres). On one occasion, Chris actually walked out of the operating room in the middle of an operation at which he was assisting Professor Louw. Chris described this act as 'unethical and unforgivable', and believed his career was finished, at least at GSH; however, after he had apologised to his senior colleague, Louw magnanimously took him back.

Later, Professor Louw was to record this event. Chris was evidently exhausted from working on a dog all night, 'but had to hurry away to assist me in the operating theatre. I immediately noticed that his assistance was not of the usual high quality, but not realising that he had been up all night, I became short-tempered and said, 'If you don't feel like helping me, then get out of the operating room.' With this, I pushed his hand aside, and he took off his gloves and walked out of the [operating] theatre.' Having initially refused to apologise for his walk-out, 'he then came to say 'I'm sorry,' and we shook hands.'

Some years later, when Marius Barnard was also working under Professor Louw, he certainly felt that Louw's prior difficulties with Chris influenced the way he was being treated, which he thought was poorly and sometimes unreasonably. Marius believed that there was clearly some friction between Chris and Louw. Marius admittedly did not appear to like either Chris or Louw; he stated:

> They both enjoyed the limelight but, even though Professor Louw was his senior, Chris for the most part overshadowed him. As a result, the two had a very uneasy relationship and, from that time on, watched each other like hawks ... [Chris's] work [on intestinal atresia] was well received internationally, but a dispute arose between Chris and Professor Louw as to who had originally conceived the idea. I have no doubt in my mind that it was Chris, and he therefore deserved all the praise for this research.

Whether Marius is correct is certainly debatable. If Louw had been interested in this topic previously when in London, it seems highly likely he suggested it to Chris as a research project.

Marius claimed that 'Professor Louw remained extremely jealous of Chris and tried to take this out on him, but Chris was equal, if not superior, in fighting back. Consequently, I became Professor Jannie Louw's lightning conductor, and he would often vent his spleen on me in the most childish and ridiculous manner.'

Like Chris, however, my understanding was that Marius was not the easiest person to work with, and his problems with Louw could have been of his own making. Although I accept that Louw and Chris did not always see eye-to-eye and occasionally clashed, from a personal perspective, I can only report that when I first visited Chris in Cape Town in 1965, he took pains to introduce me to Professor Louw, and their relationship seemed amicable, collaborative, and respectful.

# Invitation to Gain Experience in the USA

It was while at GSH that Chris was approached by Professor John Brock, the professor of medicine, who asked him whether he would be interested in furthering his surgical experience at the University of Minnesota in the USA, where a vacancy for a young surgical resident or research fellow existed. Professor Brock had been approached by Professor Owen Wangensteen, the well-known (indeed, legendary) chairman of the department of surgery in Minneapolis, who had been impressed by a previous South African, Alan Thal, who had worked in his department.

Chris immediately accepted the offer and his young wife reluctantly but generously agreed to let him go. By this time, they had two little children, and they felt it would be disruptive to the family if they accompanied him. In any case, the scholarship he was offered would possibly not cover their living expenses in the USA, whereas it might if his wife and children remained in Cape Town, where the cost of living was significantly less and where Louwtjie had obtained a job as a nurse in a department store. Even though they decided that the family might follow him later, initially this move would involve prolonged separation.

It is interesting to note that Chris immediately accepted the offer of spending time in Minneapolis, almost certainly realising that it would necessitate separation from his family. The decision was primarily selfish, but this is by no means unusual in ambitious young men in almost any field of endeavour.

In his autobiography, Chris expressed his admiration and gratitude for the 'splendid way Louwtjie accepted my sudden departure and the courage with which she set about to hold our family together.' In the event, as we shall see, he perhaps did not repay her 'courage' as well as he should.

Soon, he found himself, at the age of thirty-three, *en route* to the USA, the first time he had been out of southern Africa.

## 4

# The New World:
# Surgical Training in Minneapolis

Chris's arrival in Minnesota in January 1956 was in the winter, a climatic condition almost unknown to the young man from the sunny climes of South Africa. When the plane landed in Minneapolis, the bewildered young Chris saw what appeared to be 'mountains of white' on either side. He had never been close to snow before, and had never owned an overcoat; in South Africa, it generally only snows in the high mountains. A further shock was to come when he exited the plane and the Minnesota winter cold hit him. It was not an auspicious, or comfortable, start to his sojourn in Minneapolis.

There was nobody at the airport to meet him, and it took him sometime to contact Professor Wangensteen, who eventually sent someone to collect him. The small-town boy from Beaufort West wrote, 'I was so lost because the world was just too big for me, and I was not able to cope with all this.'

His first few months in Minnesota were disappointing and frustrating for him because Wangensteen put him to work in the experimental laboratory, whereas Chris wanted to obtain clinical surgical experience—operating on patients. In the relative isolation of the laboratory, and away from his family and many friends in Cape Town, he felt desperately lonely. He stayed in the laboratory late in the evening just to be able to speak to the janitorial staff. When he returned to his lodgings, he was faced with the loneliness of his small bedroom. 'That's the one thing that's outstanding,' he wrote, 'the tremendous loneliness.' Chris was a gregarious person, and so it must have been particularly difficult for him to deal with the solitude he experienced.

Another young surgical trainee there at the time was John Perry, Jr, a Texan, who befriended Chris and later recorded for me his recollections of him in those early days.

My first meeting with Chris Barnard occurred when he appeared at the surgical research laboratory in which I was working at that time. He was a tall young man with prominent ears and was not particularly impressive in appearance. He was dressed in a nondescript sports coat, tie, slacks and a nylon wash-and-wear shirt. Those nylon shirts aged after repeated washings and they soon became a uniform grey in colour. Later he told me that this was his best suit and most practical 'costume' for travel since one could be away from home for long periods with little luggage. After a long day, Chris was able to take a shower—still wearing his shirt, undershorts, and socks. He washed them as he bathed, and then removed them and hung them up to dry to be ready for the next morning.

Others have told me that Chris would sometimes decline invitations to parties at his senior colleague's homes because he felt he would be inappropriately dressed as he did not have a decent suit to wear.

Chris had an easy smile, and talked in an accent I had come to associate with white South Africans. He completely lacked the imperious air I had hitherto come to associate with some of his countrymen and instead was an easy-going and friendly person with a dry wit. His overall dress and manner was that of a person expecting to receive no particular favours from life. His affability was infectious and he readily made friends with all the surgeons and technicians working in the laboratory. It was readily apparent from conversation that he was well-informed and up-to-date in surgery.

Chris fitted readily into the mould. He asked many questions about what we were doing, why, and how we were doing it, and what it would lead to. Scepticism greeted many of our answers. He was not sure all the efforts we were expending on experiments day after day were really leading anywhere. However, after an initial period to familiarise himself with the laboratory, its people and its surroundings, he dutifully began the experiments Professor Wangensteen had assigned him.

One of the research projects being investigated in Wangensteen's laboratory was trying to heal stomach ulcers by cooling the inside of the stomach. Many years later, the young 'heroes' of Chris's first two novels were said to be carrying out this same research.

Chris's frustration at being confined to the experimental laboratory increased, particularly when he heard rumours of previous fellows from abroad who had been 'forgotten', surfacing from the laboratory only after several years. He pestered Wangensteen so frequently that eventually the senior surgeon allowed him to participate in the work of his clinical surgical service. From then on, Chris's life became almost overwhelmingly busy.

After that, John Perry remembered:

[Chris] received Dr Wangensteen's approval to pursue a doctorate degree [a PhD] and to study cardiovascular surgery, Chris Barnard assigned to himself a series of near impossible tasks and seemed to be busy day and night. He was simultaneously working on his experiments on intestinal atresia, learning surgical pathology, and learning to read French and German, the latter to fulfil the requirements for proficiency in languages for his advanced degree. (This requirement dated back to pre-World War Two when it was expected of budding American surgeons to spend time studying at one or more of the great European hospitals, or at least read the European surgical literature.) Simultaneously, he was often working on the ward services. He seemed like a man driven to accomplish in two or three years that which for most others was requiring seven years.

In order to accomplish all the tasks required of him—a feat Wangensteen thought 'impossible'—Chris drew on his experience in Cape Town. For example, his experience in performing autopsies on patients with tuberculous meningitis proved invaluable for his study of pathology, and his surgical studies on intestinal atresia would form the basis of his research dissertation.

Chris's opinion of the medical and surgical teams at the University of Minnesota was mixed. Many years later, he told me:

I immediately recognised that clinically they were far behind South Africa, although in special investigations they had more facilities than we had. But as far as handling and diagnosing patients, South African medicine was way ahead of them. When I looked at the results of operations like gastrectomies that we also did in South Africa, I had never experienced complications like these in my life. Everybody had to have re-exploration for abscesses, and they were on drips and suction, and things like that. I had never seen anything like that before. I was not impressed at all.

It is sometimes the case that the staff of a department that places immense importance on research, as Wangensteen's department did at that time, may not be as skilled and efficient at caring for the average patient as those at some other centres. Indeed, in my personal experience, it is unusual for a department to excel in both aspects of surgery (clinical care and research) unless the two are closely related.

Bob Frater, who studied medicine at UCT but trained in surgery at the Mayo Clinic in Rochester, Minnesota (a major medical centre approximately 80 miles from Minneapolis) when Chris was in Minneapolis, also reported that, as a result of his medical education in Cape Town, he knew far more cardiology than any of the attending physicians at the Mayo Clinic. It seems as if clinical medicine and surgery were of a very high standard at UCT in that era as they still were when I was on the staff in the 1980s.

Chris continued, 'I can't talk about cardiac surgery because we were not doing cardiac surgery in South Africa, but in general surgery, they were way behind us. To be honest with you, I must tell you that I didn't think very much of the Minneapolis school of surgery. However, I'm very grateful to that institution [the University of Minnesota] for the opportunity it gave me. If it was not for those people, I would never have been able to do the first heart transplant.'

While working in the field of general surgery, Chris's introduction to heart surgery was to some extent by chance.

One day during that period [in 1956] I walked past a laboratory where a colleague, Vince Gott [Vincent Gott, later to become cardiac surgeon-in-chief at Johns Hopkins Hospital in Baltimore] was working on the heart-lung machine. I knew they were doing heart surgery, but I hadn't paid much attention to it until that day. He asked me to give him a hand. When I saw this work with the heart-lung machine, I was fascinated by it, so I told Wangensteen I would very much like to switch to cardiac surgery. He wasn't very keen on this because he wanted me to go into general surgery, but he relented and I became chief resident on [Richard] Varco's service [a highly regarded colleague of Walt Lillehei, the major pioneer in this field]. I would think I had been there for about a year by this time.

Thus, Chris was exposed for the first time to heart surgery in Minneapolis, even though this was very much in its infancy. In this respect, Chris was very fortunate to be in the right place at the right time. Minneapolis was the place where it was 'all happening' in heart surgery at that time. This initial experience was a revelation to Chris, who immediately grasped the immense potential of open heart surgery offered by the heart-lung machine.

Before we follow Chris's career in Minneapolis further, let us see how heart surgery had developed before he arrived there in 1956. Which surgeons had pioneered the field before his Minneapolis mentors, Lillehei and Varco? What role had his mentors played in its development? How was it developing during his stay in Minneapolis?

## Heart Surgery before Barnard

Arguably, the two greatest advances in surgery (as opposed to medicine) in the twentieth century were the developments of heart surgery and organ transplantation. Chris Barnard drew on both of these new branches of surgery, then both in their relative infancy, to carry out the first human-to-human heart transplant in 1967.

How far had these two surgical specialties progressed before he trained as a heart surgeon? Having been introduced tentatively in the late 1930s and 1940s, heart surgery had advanced rather more rapidly than organ transplantation, which did not get underway until the 1950s and 1960s. It was on these two relative newcomers to the surgical armamentarium that Barnard had to build if he were eventually to perform a heart transplant successfully.

The development of heart surgery is an immensely exciting story full of interesting and eccentric characters (which I have recounted in full in a previous book, *Open Heart*). In the mid-1950s, it culminated in the development of the heart-lung machine (or pump-oxygenator, as it is sometimes known), a prerequisite if a surgeon were to attempt to carry out heart transplantation. Without a means of supporting the circulation of the patient, and in particular supplying oxygen and blood to the patient's brain, heart transplantation would not have been possible. The heart-lung machine fulfilled this role. It had, however, taken many years to achieve this goal.

## 'Closed' Heart Surgery

Early attempts at what we loosely call heart surgery were, in fact, related to surgery of the major blood vessels close to the heart. The first of these (in 1938) involved tying off (ligating) a blood vessel that remained open after birth (when it should normally close down). If the ductus remained open, the lungs would be flooded with blood, creating difficulties in breathing. Remarkably, the first ductus operation was carried out by Robert Gross, who was then only a trainee (chief surgical resident) at Boston Children's Hospital; he did this when his boss was out of town.

Surgery on the heart itself as an elective procedure (other than under highly risky emergency conditions, such as suturing a stab wound of the heart) had to wait a few more years until 1948. In the intervening time, however, another Boston surgeon, Dwight Harken, working at a US Army hospital in the UK during the Second World War, had removed seventy-eight bullets or fragments of shrapnel within or in relation to the great blood vessels in the chest, and a further fifty-six in or in relation to the heart—a total of 134 operations, remarkably, without a single death. Given the relatively primitive suture materials and post-operative care facilities available at that time, these outcomes say much for Harken's skills.

Harken's operations contributed the first major series that demonstrated that the heart would withstand considerable manipulation. This was an immensely important learning experience for the surgeons, including Harken himself, who would soon after the war begin their tentative efforts to conquer heart disease.

Like Gross's operation for patent ductus, the next major step towards heart surgery also involved blood vessels near to the heart (rather than the heart itself), but in this case, the surgery partially corrected a problem that was inside the heart. Without going into details, in children with a condition known as Fallot's tetralogy (named after the French physician who described it), there is both a hole between the two pumping chambers of the heart (the left and right ventricles) and a narrowing (stenosis) of the valve that leads from the heart to the lungs (the pulmonary valve) (Figure 4.i). The end result is that there is a reduced blood flow to the lungs. As a result of the poor oxygenation of the blood and other factors, babies with this condition have become known as 'blue babies'. Their lips, fingers, and toes look blue to the eye.

A paediatric cardiologist at the Johns Hopkins Hospital in Baltimore, Helen Taussig, suggested to the chief surgeon, Alfred Blalock, that the creation of a ductus would improve patients with Fallot's tetralogy—the very reverse of Gross's operation. Although it would not be curative, it would, at least, provide more blood to the lungs. Blalock and his chief technician, a remarkably innovative and technically skilled African-American named Vivien Thomas, designed such an operation in dogs. Nevertheless, under the circumstances of the very sick children with Fallot's tetralogy, the operation was technically very difficult and extremely risky.

However, at Blalock's first attempt in 1944 (with Thomas standing behind him and giving him advice every now and then), it was carried out successfully. The patient made a splendid recovery and, when further patients did equally well, Blalock and his team became world famous (though nowhere near as well-known to the public as Barnard would become), and surgeons from around the globe came to Baltimore to learn how to do the operation. A movie based on their experience, *Something the Lord Made*, was released in 2004.

A few years later, in 1948, an alternative approach was designed by an early mentor of mine, Russell Brock, at Guy's Hospital in London. Brock took an even bolder approach for patients with Fallot's tetralogy or pulmonary valve stenosis by expanding the restricted opening in the pulmonary valve directly, which required inserting a knife into the right ventricle of the heart (while it was still beating) and pushing it up through the narrowed valve into the pulmonary artery. This was an extremely risky approach in those days (and still would be today), but Brock achieved it successfully. As with Harken's work during the Second World War, the fact that patients would tolerate an incision being made in the muscle of the right ventricle was a significant stimulus to further heart surgery since it demonstrated the heart's tolerance to manipulation and direct surgical intervention.

Furthermore, it also provided experience for a similar approach to the mitral valve (another valve within the heart), which was frequently narrowed as a result of rheumatic fever. Brock was one of three surgeons to carry out an operation to expand the mitral valve (mitral valvotomy) in 1948, the other two being Charles Bailey of Philadelphia and Dwight Harken of Boston. 'Mitral valvotomy' was achieved by inserting a finger (or instrument) into the heart and forcibly opening the narrowed valve.

In those early days, the mortality associated with this so-called 'closed' heart surgery (indicating that the inside of the heart was not actually visualised as it is in 'open' heart surgery) remained frighteningly high. Patients referred for these operations were inevitably at death's door and, like the first patients who were later to undergo heart transplantation, were aware that this was their one chance of surviving more than perhaps a few days or weeks. Russell Brock wrote that 'the great pressure to aid the development of mitral valve surgery came not from the doctors, but from the patients'. The patients were well-prepared to take the risk, but it must have required surgeons with nerves of steel to attempt these procedures.

An example of how patients were prepared to take this risk (and indeed grateful to be offered it) was a young woman who was subjected to mitral valvotomy by Harken, unfortunately unsuccessfully. She died on the operating table, always a shattering experience for the surgical team (as well as for the patient's family, of course). Harken went home as depressed as always. Within a few hours, a messenger came to the door with a handwritten letter from this very patient, obviously written before she went into the operating room. The letter simply said, 'Thanks for the chance'. Such a message, though intended to raise Harken's spirits, must have brought tears to his eyes—I know it would have done to mine. Even today, whenever I recount this tragic story to others, I inevitably choke back tears.

In the early days, these three surgeons found themselves in a catch-22 situation. It would not be justified to attempt an unproven operation of this magnitude and nature except on a very sick, dying patient, yet the debilitated condition of the patient greatly increased the risk of the operation. The surgical technique could be practiced in healthy dogs, but they did not have mitral stenosis or all of its debilitating sequelae. It was not only the surgical technique that needed to be developed and proven; the anaesthetists were on an equally steep learning curve, as were those who cared for the patient after the operation—if the patient survived that long. Some twenty years later, these same ethical dilemmas faced Chris Barnard and the other pioneering surgeons in the field of heart transplantation. Indeed, these surgeons were to face similar emotional stresses.

With increasing experience, however, the results of the operation of mitral valvotomy slowly improved, and the surgeons began to be referred patients in whom the disease was less advanced. These patients could better tolerate the operation, and so the results improved further.

## 'Open' Heart Surgery: Hypothermia

There were, however, a very limited number of operations that could be performed without opening the heart and visualising the problem that needed to be corrected. If heart surgery were to become really useful and widespread, it was essential that a means be developed by which the heart could be stopped from beating, opened, and the defect or pathologic condition could be dealt with, with the surgeon able to see what he was doing.

The first advance towards this aim was introduced in an experimental laboratory by a Toronto surgeon, Wilfred 'Bill' Bigelow. He had realised that, if the body were cooled, the heart could be stopped for a longer period of time than if the body was at normal temperature. This was because the brain required less oxygen at 30°C than at the normal body temperature of 37°C, just as meat can be preserved longer in a refrigerator. At normal body temperature, without oxygen the brain may suffer irreversible damage after four minutes. At 30°C, this period was extended by a mere two minutes, but six minutes gave the surgeon the opportunity of correcting very simple defects, such as holes between the two collecting chambers of the heart (an atrial septal defect or 'ASD').

Bigelow therefore developed a method of cooling anesthetised animals down to 30°C by placing them in a cold water bath or by placing electrical cooling devices around them. When the temperature approached 30°C (a state of 'hypothermia'), he would rapidly open the chest, clamp the vessels entering and leaving the heart, and open the heart to operate inside it. Within the next six minutes, he had to complete the operation, close the heart, and get it to beat again. The operation—a cut-and-thrust procedure, if ever there was one—clearly carried significant risk, but it was the first real approach that allowed access to the inside of the heart.

However, Bigelow was not the first to carry out an operation under hypothermia in a patient. That laurel went to Minneapolis surgeon, John Lewis, who was the first of the Minnesota surgeons to enter the world of heart surgery. His operation on 2 September 1952, when he was a mere thirty-six years old, was the true beginning of open heart surgery and initiated the rapid development that took place over the next twenty-five to thirty years. At this historic first operation, in which Lewis closed an ASD, he was assisted, among others, by Walt Lillehei, who was subsequently to become an even greater pioneer in heart surgery and the most important mentor of Chris Barnard. That first patient was known to be alive and well forty-two years after the operation.

Remarkably, in great contrast to Walt Lillehei and, particularly, Chris Barnard, Lewis never received any honours (honorary degrees or other formal recognition) for his contributions to cardiac surgery. When he told me this, it shocked me that the surgeon who had taken this monumental step forward, even though the concept of hypothermia was not his own, had not received some public or academic recognition, or at least some recognition by the medical community—how different from what was to happen to Chris Barnard.

## 'Open' Heart Surgery: The Heart-Lung Machine

Hypothermia, however, was cumbersome and provided too little time to repair complicated defects, such as a hole between the two pumping chambers of the heart (a ventricular septal defect or 'VSD') or full and definitive correction of Fallot's tetralogy. Something further was needed that would allow the surgeon a longer period of time to operate inside the heart; that something was a heart-lung machine.

Construction of a heart-lung machine had been the goal of Philadelphia surgeon, John Gibbon, Jr, since 1930. With the exception of the Second

World War years, which he spent as a surgeon in the Pacific, he worked on developing a heart-lung machine from 1930 until it came to fruition in 1953. He made slow progress, but, eventually with the help of engineers from International Business Machines (IBM), he was successful in developing a machine that could support the circulation of experimental animals.

In 1952, he attempted the first operation on a patient unsuccessfully. However, in the following year (on 6 May 1953), he operated successfully on a teenage girl, Cecelia Bavolek, with an atrial septal defect. This is a simple condition that could have been dealt with successfully under hypothermia, but this first success with a heart-lung machine is rightly considered a major event in the history of surgery. Although this patient survived, his next two patients died, at which point Gibbon took the quite amazing decision not to involve himself in open heart surgery further. Many surgeons at that time, and subsequently, were shocked that Gibbon should 'chicken-out' so early, particularly after the twenty years he had put into developing the machine. However, it is believed he found it difficult to accept the high mortality that was clearly associated with heart surgery in those early days.

The Gibbon heart-lung machine was subsequently taken over by John Kirklin and his colleagues at the Mayo Clinic, who used it to slowly develop a successful open heart surgery program. When Chris later visited the Mayo Clinic, he was impressed by the work of Kirklin's group. 'They were better organised, and you could see that they really knew what they were doing.' Importantly, Kirklin's group was less innovative, a quality that was clearly needed if progress were to be made in this new field of heart surgery.

## 'Open' Heart Surgery: Cross-Circulation

As Chris Barnard, who arrived in Minneapolis (at the beginning of 1956) only a couple of years after Lillehei's first open heart operation, soon realised, an atmosphere conducive to innovation had been introduced into the department of surgery at the University of Minnesota by the chairman, Professor Wangensteen. It was his *protégé*, Walt Lillehei, and his several colleagues who, like their predecessor, John Lewis, took full advantage of this environment. There was a competitive spirit among the younger members of the staff, which Wangensteen did nothing to discourage. Without doubt, the five or six years in Minneapolis from 1951 through 1956 were among the most exciting and important ever experienced in the long history of medicine. Chris was immensely fortunate to arrive there towards the end of this epoch-making period, when open heart surgery was still very much an experimental field. These were men he would come to know well.

Walt Lillehei (Figure 4.ii) first approached the problem in a very innovative but risky way. One of his research fellows, Morley Cohen, a Canadian, realised that his pregnant wife was supporting the life of their developing baby by pumping oxygenated blood to it as an extension of her own circulation. He suggested to Lillehei that possibly an adult could supply oxygenated blood to a child on the operating table and maintain the life of the child, including supplying the brain, while the child's heart was stopped and operated on. They explored this approach (which they called 'cross-circulation') in the animal laboratory, using large dogs as the 'heart-lung machine' and small dogs as the 'patients', with considerable success.

They then proposed to use the method in the correction of heart defects in young children that they would not be able to correct within the six minutes allowed by hypothermia. By joining the two circulations, a parent's heart and lungs could pump and oxygenate the blood for both parent and child—at least for a limited period of time. In other words, the parent would be the heart-lung machine for the child. This was a highly controversial and risky approach, in large part because this would be an operation with a potential 200 per cent mortality (if both the parent and child should die). If you planned such an operation today, more than sixty years later, even with our vast experience of heart surgery, it would remain a risky procedure. It took a surgeon of great courage to pursue this approach.

Nevertheless, Lillehei and his colleagues were given permission to go ahead, and they carried out their first cross-circulation operation on 26 March 1954, on a thirteen-year-old boy, Gregory Gidden, whose father provided the circulatory support—in other words, was the 'heart-lung machine'. A young surgical resident, Norman Shumway (later to become, like Chris, a major pioneer in heart transplantation) assisted at this first operation. Lillehei was only thirty-five years old. In total, they performed forty-five such procedures, with a patient survival rate of more than 50 per cent, which was good for that era; fortunately, there were no deaths of the human heart-lung machine (the parents), although one did suffer a brain injury from which she never fully recovered. This, however, was a result of human error rather than an inherent failure of the technique.

# 'Open' Heart Surgery: The DeWall Oxygenator

Lillehei then set another of his young research fellows, Richard DeWall, the task of designing and making a new heart-lung machine, one that he insisted should be much simpler and cheaper than the complex and expensive Gibbon machine. In 1955, DeWall successfully achieved this goal, developing a very simple 'bubble' oxygenator (similar to those devices that bubble air in fish tanks), which enabled Lillehei to discontinue cross-circulation as a means of performing open heart surgery and replace it with the DeWall heart-lung machine. Lillehei was impressed that the system was so simple, believing that the less complicated it was, the more likely it would be successful.

The other significant point that was important in popularising the DeWall oxygenator was the fact that it was so inexpensive to make—in the order of $50 (in comparison with an estimated $50,000 for a Gibbon-IBM heart-lung machine) This gave it one more advantage: because it was so simple and so cheap, it was disposable. After use, you simply threw it out and built another, whereas the Gibbon oxygenator was taken apart and laboriously cleaned for its next use. No matter how well the various parts were cleaned in those days, some 'toxins' (foreign proteins) remained, and could cause significant complications in the patient on whom it was next used, such as fever and low blood pressure. It was safer to use a completely new and sterile oxygenator each time, as in DeWall's design.

The first patient on whom the bubble oxygenator was used underwent surgery on 13 May 1955, only a few months before Chris Barnard arrived in Minneapolis (in January 1956). There was again a learning curve, with the first patient dying, the next seven surviving, but the next six being unsuccessful. The DeWall oxygenator is considered a landmark development in the advance of heart surgery as it enabled surgeons in quite small hospitals with limited resources to embark upon open heart surgery. Thus, open heart surgery was developed successfully. Remarkably, for some months (apart from Stockholm in Sweden), the only places in the world where a patient could undergo open heart surgery were two centres in Minnesota approximately eighty miles apart—namely, the University of Minnesota and the Mayo Clinic.

It was into this exciting milieu that Chris was thrust when he persuaded Wangensteen to let him train with Lillehei and Varco.

# Chris's First Experience in Heart Surgery

Chris, therefore, became a small but integral part of the pioneering team of surgeons who did much to put open heart surgery on the medical map. He worked immensely hard, learning the fundamentals of the heart-lung machine and how it was used in open heart surgery. He explained to me how the Lillehei-Varco team worked at that time.

> [Richard] Varco had his own service and [Walt] Lillehei had his service, but when Lillehei did open heart procedures, Varco would help him. They helped each other. Varco did open heart surgery, but not as often. Varco was technically very brilliant. He was a fat man with fat fingers, but very good. Lillehei was not a very good technical surgeon, but he was a great thinker. He had ideas. His main strength was his courage—tremendous courage to go on and on.
>
> The chief resident would do rounds about six in the morning. Then we had some breakfast, and were in the operating room by seven o'clock. During that period, I also did three months of running the heart-lung machine. In those days, you had to put the whole thing together, piece by piece. I must say it was excellent experience because I got to know the heart-lung machine very well.
>
> We did one case a day. Often, when you had the chest opened already, Lillehei wouldn't be there. He wouldn't even be in the hospital. You had to wait until he came along. The patient was heparinised [to anti-coagulate the blood to prevent clotting as it circulated through the heart-lung machine], connected to the heart-lung machine, and we would do the surgery and close the chest. The patient would go back to the recovery room, and you had to stay the night with the patient—unless the patient died during operation or died before the night. We lost a lot of patients.

There were occasional weeks when they would operate on five patients, but none of them survived. It must have taken absolute faith and immense commitment by Lillehei and his team to persevere under such setbacks. As one of today's heart surgeons commented, 'Can you imagine going to work and having somebody die on you every third day? I think it takes a very extraordinary person who can withstand that and make something positive of it.'

I once pointed out to Dr Lillehei that one of the qualities that Chris Barnard admired most about him and his colleagues at the time they were developing open heart surgery was the courage they had to keep going when they were having a 'bad run'. My understanding was that even when they were experiencing a series of operative or post-operative deaths, Dr Lillehei persisted because he knew what he was doing was right, just like Brock (and others before him) and Barnard (and others after him). I asked him how he had coped with the deaths at the time.

> That is a good observation because persistence was an important consideration, but it wasn't always easy. At times, after a particularly frustrating experience, I was almost ready to quit. After a good night's sleep, and maybe a few belts in the local bar, the next morning you felt much better. And I had a great group of colleagues. Usually, we could come up with a solution—perhaps not always the right solution, but something we should have done or should not have done, or could do differently in the next case. Then we went on. One success, of course, rejuvenated you, so to speak, and you could go on. I must say persistence was an important quality. I never understood how a guy like Gibbon could start working in the 1930s and make a lot of progress, and then suddenly quit because of failures. But he did. I later read that, at one time before going into medicine, he wanted to be a poet. Poets are maybe more sensitive than surgeons.

Lillehei's mention of 'a few belts in the local bar may not be as facetious as it may sound. His powers to "party" were legendary among the staff in Minneapolis. According to one of his erstwhile surgical residents, Aldo Castañeda, Lillehei worked very hard, partied very hard, almost every day, and had the constitution of an ox. He would end rounds about 10 p.m. every day, and then he would usually go with some of the guys and have some drinks. The next day, the guy was just there. Amazing! How he did it, I don't know.'

Others felt, as perhaps did Lillehei himself, that his fairly regular alcohol intake helped him cope emotionally with the deaths of his patients. Castañeda believed that a surgeon in that era had to be totally convinced that the ultimate goal (of making open heart surgery safe and routine) justified the deaths. He described it as requiring 'a certain touch of "immorality" ... You had to be absolutely convinced internally that you were right and that everybody else was wrong. Walt had that, but he was not a person to discuss this kind of personal stuff. Those guys were tough. They kept it to themselves, very close.'

Several surgeons from that era told me that keeping as busy as possible—operating again the very next day, and the next—helped them forget the failure and death, not because they were callous, but because their minds were occupied by the new task in hand. Too much brooding could mean the end of their careers.

Chris Barnard, who clearly had to have the same conviction when he later introduced heart transplantation, also commented on this aspect of the work at Minneapolis. 'I honestly believe,' he told me, 'that human beings were just experimental animals at that stage. You operated on them because you wanted to see what happened. We had a very high mortality. The deaths were probably from 'metabolic disturbances' [abnormalities in the body chemistry] because we didn't test for these.' However, it was only through this 'learning experience' that the nature of the 'metabolic disturbance' slowly became understood and then could be corrected or prevented.

Throughout this time, Chris was also continuing his research in the experimental laboratory, while still augmenting his small stipend with various other part-time jobs. Having finalised his dissertation on intestinal atresia (much of which he had carried out in Cape Town) to be awarded a PhD at the University of Minnesota, he also had to pass examinations in two foreign languages. He chose Dutch (not French as John Perry remembered) and German, in both of which his fluency in Afrikaans was a major help. Chris then also switched his research towards heart surgery. He was again productive, carrying out interesting and valuable studies on the heart-lung machine and on the dynamics of one of the heart valves, the aortic valve (Figure 4.i), for which he was designing a replacement mechanical valve.

'I worked with a professor in mechanical engineering,' he told me. 'I never gave this guy any credit, but he was a fantastic man. He helped me a lot. In fact, some of the things that I was working on experimentally we used in patients. Some of them worked and some didn't very well.'

The leaflets of all of the heart's valves open and close approximately seventy times a minute (depending on whether the subject is exercising or not), which is more than 100,000 times a day, or thirty-six million times in a year. To develop any form of mechanical or artificial valve that would function satisfactorily for many years therefore required an innovative design and careful production. By working very hard—including on Sundays, of which Wangensteen strongly disapproved—Chris came up with an artificial valve (a prosthesis) that seemed to have all of the necessary qualities.

For a dissertation on some of this work (particularly on the development of an artificial heart valve) submitted to the University of Minnesota, he was awarded the degree of Master of Science in Surgery (MS), yet another degree for his research. Once again, he had shown that he was not afraid of hard work, a quality that remained with him throughout his career. He told me:

I was in Minneapolis for two and a half years. I must tell you that during my time in Minneapolis, the maximum salary I ever had was two hundred dollars a month. That's why I did jobs like washing cars, mowing lawns, and nursing. I would work the whole day and, at night, I would stay nursing a patient. We got five or ten dollars for nursing a patient all through the night. I was sending money home. I can't say that I enjoyed it there [in Minneapolis]. I would like to have the same medical experience, but I wouldn't like to repeat the personal life. It was really very, very tough.

## A Mentor's Opinion of his Trainee: Walt Lillehei on Chris

Lillehei's opinion of Chris during these months is worth recording.

I always considered him a reliable technician whom I trusted completely. He was certainly very capable. He probably wasn't as smooth as a Denton Cooley [the Texas heart surgeon with exceptional technical ability], who is obviously unusual. But as you well know as a surgeon, it's unlikely that anybody, with a few exceptions, is ever born a surgeon—they have to learn. He was a quick learner, there is no doubt about that. One of the things that is frequently expressed is how quickly he caught on to things. He was an excellent student. He wanted to research technique and read the literature and find out what was known about the subject and talk with experts, and so on. He became an excellent technical surgeon through hard work.

I remind you of the famous case he wrote about in his autobiography. Chris was opening the chest of a patient for me, and circling the inferior vena cava [the largest vein in the body that drains blood directly into the heart] he accidentally made a hole in the heart. He sort of panicked and, instead of putting his finger over the hole and calling for senior assistance, he tried to connect the patient to the heart-lung machine. The heart began to fail, and he started to massage it. And every time he massaged it, of course, blood poured out. The patient died on the operating table. He related this story quite poignantly in his book, *One Life*.

Chris also pointed out that the little patient's father was watching the proceedings from the observation dome above the operating room; I cannot imagine a worse experience for either a father or a young surgeon.

After the incident, I talked to him, and said, 'We all make mistakes. I hope you have learned from this one. Don't panic. Put your finger down there, and call for help. Don't try to repair the hole.' I think he learned a lesson; he said he did.

In those days—and I don't think he's changed a lot either—he had intense personal drive. In those two and a half years he accomplished what normally takes about five or six years. In other words, he went completely through our residency in general surgery and thoracic and cardiovascular surgery and yet was still able to spend half the time—maybe more—in the experimental laboratory. He was an excellent researcher—very productive. For six months, he was my senior resident. He probably had another four or five months on my service as a junior resident.

I think everybody who knew him in those days was struck by his intense ambition and ability to work—certainly I was. It has often been related, I think, to his early life. He always presents himself—and I assume it is true—as someone who grew up under considerable poverty and hardship.

He was very innovative and his research projects bear that out. However, I would mention that he was one of a group of surgical residents that subsequently became internationally successful. This was certainly a pretty high-level residency group. The younger ones were attracted to come to Minneapolis like a magnet. I didn't know it at the time, but some of the best brains in the world came here. At that time, they seemed like ordinary surgical residents—the 'John Hunter type' [referring to the great eighteenth century British surgeon-scientist, who was from a simple, rural Scottish family]—loud and profane, addicted to drink and low company, especially female, but as you look back in the records, they were outstanding individuals. All we did was give them the opportunity and encouragement.

In that high-level group, I think the outstanding thing that most of us noticed about Chris was his intensity and seriousness. He was not a playboy at that time. When he went out in the evening I had to track him down sometimes because I wanted to talk to him. I found him at a couple of different addresses, but he was taking calls. He was intensely hard-working and ambitious. But Chris Barnard stood out in that group. I think one of the reasons was his intense ability to work hard. But he was also very intelligent.

He had a prodigious memory. I recall one incident which I have never forgotten. When he first became my senior resident we were making rounds, and in those days we had at least thirty-five, sometimes forty, patients on our service. Some of them were being worked-up preoperatively. The work-up wasn't left to the cardiologists in those days. Anyway, we had a large number of patients, and we used to make rounds. The residents would make rounds twice a day, and I would make afternoon rounds—though they often became evening rounds because they took place after surgery was completed for the day. We would see all these patients. All of my senior residents before and after Barnard carried a pocket-sized notebook, and took down all the blood tests and X-rays I suggested should be done. On the first day that Chris was with me, I noticed that he never took down a single note, but I didn't comment on it. On the second day, probably I did mention it. I said, 'Chris, get a notebook and take down these things. It's important.' He said, 'Yes.' I think the next day he still didn't have a notebook, so I was kind of sharp to him and said, 'Get a notebook.' He said, 'Listen, Dr Lillehei [he was always very polite, of course. As a matter of fact, I have never got him to call me by my first name] ... Dr Lillehei, have I to date forgotten anything that you have suggested?' He hadn't, so I said, 'No.' He said, 'Well, I can remember these things.' And he did. I thought it was very unusual, since there were dozens of shopping list type things to be done. He had a superb memory for detail as well as excellent intellectual ability.

His ego did not appear, as you say, bigger than any other cardiac surgeon's (ego). One thing that was quite noticeable, even in the early days, was that he could be very charming but, on the other hand, he could provoke a rather intense dislike among some people—colleagues and staff—because he was always outspoken and often had unconventional ideas. This was good, of course, but not necessarily a way to win friends sometimes. He had a somewhat abrasive personality in the sense that he was not only outspoken but very self-confident. As a matter of fact, if I was hiring somebody, those are all good qualities, but they are not necessarily ones to run for office on.

But the independent sort, such as Chris was, often does make a good researcher. Chris certainly was stubborn, possibly a result of his Dutch upbringing, or I should say his Afrikaner upbringing. Obviously, nobody is perfect. I think he was somewhat selfish, and I say that because some of the people who later worked under him were very critical. Now I don't know whether there is an element of jealousy in this criticism, but one of Chris's previous assistants [probably Bob Frater], whom I admire and is an excellent person, felt that Chris could be very self-centred and arrogant. Some people feel that Chris wanted everything to be perfect for himself, so that his own results were good, and didn't always give others the opportunities they felt they deserved. According to these people, he didn't necessarily lean over backwards to give credit where credit was due. But, by and large, that's about Chris's only detrimental characteristic, as far as I am aware.

It should be added, however, that some of Chris's colleagues in Minneapolis considered him to be too aggressive and self-centred.

## The Most Exciting Period of Chris's Professional Life

Chris spent a highly productive year under the tutelage of Drs Lillehei and Varco, and had the opportunity to learn the surgical techniques of correction of many congenital heart defects (structural abnormalities of the heart with which babies may be born). He remembered:

> The medical side was very exciting. We were in a new era. I sometimes felt a little frustrated because they didn't allow me to do things [operations]. I always just assisted. They never allowed me even to ligate a patent ductus [which had become a relatively simple operation since Robert Gross's first attempt in 1938]. When I returned to South Africa was the first time that I was alone and did the operation myself.

Although it may come as a surprise to the reader, Chris has often admitted that his two-and-a-half years in Minneapolis, together with the next few years after his return to Cape Town where he set up a busy heart surgery program, were the most exciting of his life, even more stimulating and exciting than the late 1960s, when he planned and initiated the world's first heart transplant program. He was not alone in holding this opinion.

As Dr Lillehei had mentioned, among the other young men in training at the University of Minnesota at that time were several who were later to make their marks in the world of heart surgery. Indeed, as we shall see, one of them, Norman Shumway, became the major pioneer in the field of heart transplantation, contributing more to its development than Barnard even though Chris carried out the first transplant in a patient before him. Indeed, Shumway had preceded Chris as Lillehei's chief assistant. Christian Cabrol was another Lillehei trainee, and later established the leading early heart transplant centre in France.

Both Shumway and Cabrol also told me how exciting their time was in Minneapolis. Cabrol pointed out that, when open heart surgery was successful, it provided instant success—the patient walked out of hospital completely cured. After heart transplantation, however, the operation was just one step in the treatment of the patient. Continuing care of the patient was needed and, despite a successful operation, the graft could be lost from rejection. Heart transplantation, therefore, did not offer 'instant' success.

Cabrol remembered Chris from that period as being 'not a very bright operator, but a hard worker, working all the time, and not paying too much attention to other things except work ... Like all of us during those years, Chris wore his hair very short; this was the "crew cut", and it did little for his looks.' I have sadly been unable to find a photo of Chris with a crew cut.

One young surgeon with whom Chris built up a special bond was Gil Campbell, who was experimenting with dog lungs to oxygenate a patient's blood during open heart surgery. The technique never became established successfully (as the lungs were soon 'rejected' by the human blood), but his efforts illustrate the great range of innovative research continuing in Wangensteen's department at that time. For a period of time, Chris and Campbell would meet most mornings at 6 a.m. for an early breakfast, after which they would work on their pathology studies together.

Wangensteen was very supportive of his junior staff. For example, he arranged for Chris to visit Houston in Texas to see some of the work of the two famous cardiovascular surgeons there—the irascible, many would say unpleasant, Michael DeBakey, who almost threw Chris out of his operating room because he felt Chris was leaning over too much to see the operation and was 'contaminating my operating area,' and the relaxed and friendly Denton Cooley, whose technical mastery impressed Chris very much.

## Rheumatoid Arthritis

It was during his stay in Minneapolis (1956) that Chris first developed a deep-seated and persistent ache in some of his joints, beginning in his feet, but then particularly affecting his fingers. In *Chris Barnard's Program for Living with Arthritis*, a book that Chris later wrote to advise the lay person on what he or she could do to improve the quality of life if afflicted by rheumatoid arthritis, Chris recollected this worrying episode in his life.

> I had got interested in ice skating, but as I earned only two hundred dollars a month, I couldn't afford to buy skates, so I borrowed a pair from a friend, John Perry, who worked with me. The skates were rather narrow for my feet, and I remember that after going out skating one day, next morning I woke up with tremendous pain and soreness in my right foot.

Chris's friends suggested he had sustained a fracture of a bone in the foot from the skating, but then the foot became very swollen, and at the same time, he developed pain in his hands, which also became swollen. He sought medical advice and was devastated to be given the diagnosis of rheumatoid arthritis, a disease that had the potential to cripple him. As a doctor, he was more aware than most patients that the disease could hinder or even totally prevent his career as a surgeon. One can only imagine the anguish and frustration this knowledge must have caused.

Chris's first reaction to the diagnosis was 'to feel bitter—the world was unfair and it owed me a living. I could have wallowed in self-pity for ever if I hadn't been lucky. I was forced to meet a hectic research schedule and find my bread and butter in a strange country where people were remarkably unresponsive to the problems of sensitive young doctors, particularly those who thought the earth had a special place for them.'

Chris feared that, because of his arthritis, he would never make it to the top in surgery. This fear of not being able to pursue a career in surgery caused him many sleepless nights. He fought a battle every morning against pain and stiffness in the joints of his hands, and experienced difficulty in extending his fingers to pull on his surgical gloves.

'I found that the evening or morning after a difficult operation in which I had to use my hands in awkward positions, there would be an exacerbation of the arthritis in my fingers. Similarly, whenever I was under above-average emotional stress, the arthritis would light up.'

Fortunately, the disease never progressed to the point where it totally disabled him from carrying out surgical operations, but long operations—and most open heart operations were very long in those days—could accentuate the pain in his fingers. The almost constant dull pain he felt in his hands, and later in other joints, must have made operations—and so many other aspects of life—much more difficult to complete than they should have been.

He gave great credit to his physician in Minneapolis who, without withholding any facts from him, convinced him that, although rheumatoid arthritis would undoubtedly handicap him, on the basis of his blood tests, it was unlikely he would become totally incapacitated. It was then that Chris fully appreciated how important it is 'to have some light at the end of the tunnel.' Chris later told his daughter, Deirdre, that he learned an important lesson from that physician which proved of great value to him in his interactions with his own patients in his subsequent career, and that is that you always need to leave the patient with hope. 'He gave me hope,' he told her. 'Nothing is more important than that.' She later wrote:

It was something he incorporated into his own attitude to life ... something he passed on to his children. No matter how bad things seem to be, there is always the undeniable possibility that eventually they will improve. To abandon hope just doesn't make sense ... He was a man who saw possibilities in even the most daunting medical prognosis, and outside the medical environment, he was a man who was positive about life. He was always excited about what the future might hold and he was particularly enthralled by the progress being made in his own field (of medicine) and those fields adjacent to it, and liked to keep himself up to date.

Nevertheless, arthritis—and, many years later, asthma—troubled him for the rest of his life.

His right foot developed a deformity. Chris wrote that since that time, he had always been very shy about showing people his feet, especially his right foot. 'Conversely, I always admired beautiful feet, especially women's.' In order to ease the pain while standing in the operating room, he wore special shoes to take the weight off the metatarsal joints, which helped a little. But his appetite for work was 'voracious, pain or no pain. Could I have subconsciously thought that I might have a limited life span and thus developed the tremendous drive and determination to achieve as much as I did in those gruelling two and a half years?' Although he was never consciously aware that the thought of having limited time to practice surgery drove him to work harder, he felt sure that subconsciously this had been a stimulus.

However, Chris learned from his experience with rheumatoid arthritis. He later wrote:

When I'd thought it through, suddenly the concept of the old and the aged came into focus. Where before they were only wheezing and often-misshapen caricatures of life—cantankerous and boring—I found real people. By real people I mean wives and husbands, sons and daughters, lovers and loners, winners and losers, each with a history, beginning with a success formula and ending in the backwaters of life, often as helpless as the day they arrived on earth and sometimes as comprehending. The missing factor, of course, was youth. Take it away and success goes flat, while wealth only eases the pain. Take away that wound-up feeling in the gut, that eager panting after the next quarry—whether it be a person, place or thing—and suddenly there is no need to show enthusiasm, to open the gift, to walk that extra mile.

Chris would hold this theme of the attractions and advantages of youth close to his heart, and comment on it throughout life—until old age caught up with him personally.

Fortunately, as his physician had predicted, rheumatoid arthritis never crippled him. Despite almost constant pain, he was able to continue with his life and, especially, his career in surgery.

## Personal Life

Due to his very limited financial status, Chris lived very frugally in Minneapolis. However, he later received a bursary from the university which, together with the money he made from a variety of other jobs—usually filling his weekends—allowed him to consider arranging for his wife and two small children to join him. Some of his colleagues in Minneapolis were of the opinion that it was beneath the dignity of a doctor to be carrying out these other menial jobs, but Chris placed the necessity of providing for his family above his pride and dignity. His landlady and some neighbours, however, understood his need and donated furniture or household items to him. Even the manager of the bank he used bent the rules to provide him with a loan to buy a small car. He made enough money to put together a home that had the comforts he thought his family required: toys for the children, even a television (which had not yet been introduced in South Africa, and would not be available there until 1976).

Chris had several girlfriends in Minneapolis, failing to tell at least one of them that he was married with a family. However, after about six months, Chris's wife and two small children, now aged about five and six years old, set out to join him. It began badly for Louwtjie. She and the children had booked a passage on a cargo ship—the cheapest way to travel—from South Africa to Boston. When they landed, they had missed their flight to Minneapolis, and had something of a nightmare overnight journey getting there via New York and Chicago. By the time they arrived, Louwtjie was exhausted.

After that, she never seemed to really enjoy the US. Their rented apartment was close to the airport, and Louwtjie was irritated by the 'constant noise' of the airplanes. It did not help her equanimity when a plane crashed, wiping out a few houses close to their home. She wanted to find a job to help with the family's expenses, but she could not obtain a work visa. She led a rather secluded life, making very few friends. Chris undoubtedly did not help matters by working (or 'socialising') until late in the evening before going home. Louwtjie seemed unduly irritated by some Americans' lack of knowledge of South Africa; for example, when she spoke to the children in Afrikaans, she was asked whether she was speaking Zulu. In view of the obvious racial discrimination she found in Minneapolis, she resented the Americans' criticism of apartheid in South Africa.

Chris believed that his children really enjoyed living in America, and it was an experience that they never forgot (Figure 4.iii). He remembered showing them the sights of Minneapolis, 'acting as if I had created it myself.' Little André 'was as proud of me as if I had. He became a Wild West fan when I gave him a toy fort full of soldiers and cowboys.' Chris's friend, John Perry, remembered this time:

> Chris anticipated the arrival of his wife, Louwtjie, and his children, Deirdre and 'Boetie' [André]. America was strange and new but I believe the children enjoyed living here; Mrs Barnard seemed homesick and unhappy from the beginning. Given a more auspicious introduction to America, things may have been different. Her family and old friends were far away, she made few new acquaintances, and she saw little of Chris who was working at the hospital day and night.
>
> The family was in America about a year. One day Chris told me that his son's teacher in school had instructed the children to draw their country's flag and Boetie had drawn the Stars and Stripes. Chris had decided, he said, based on this that it was time for the children to return to their homeland. His friends, however, sensed that the reasons were deeper than those expressed and that Chris and Louwtjie no longer shared common goals and interests. The family did return to South Africa shortly after this.

According to Louwtjie, it was her decision to return with her children to South Africa. Chris drove them to New York and they returned to Cape Town by ship. Chris was left with a feeling he had failed his family. He immediately sold all of the furniture and other items he had collected together, or gave them away, and moved into a rented room. He had expected to be home in Cape Town within about four to six months but, in the event, his work and surgical training in Minneapolis extended longer than anticipated. In fact, he stayed a further fourteen months after his family had left.

John Perry noted:

> In his autobiography *One Life*, Christiaan Barnard makes no secret of his lifelong attraction to beautiful women. Whether this propensity for the opposite sex had any influence on the abbreviated stay of his family in America I am not prepared to say. I do recall that following the departure of his family he did develop some relationships. He later recalled to me that one of these culminated in the disappearance of a joint

bank account that he and the young lady in question had established together. He concluded this had been an interesting but brief and costly experience.

During this fourteen-month-period, Louwtjie noticed that Chris's letters became less frequent, eventually dwindling 'to about one a month—sometimes none. They had become more and more like notes from a stranger: cold, sometimes not even inquiring about Deirdre and André. All my instincts told me there must be another woman.'

She was right. After his family had returned to Cape Town, Chris developed a strong friendship with at least one particular young lady in Minneapolis, Sharon Jorgensen, with whom he may have been continuing a covert relationship even when Louwtjie was in the US. When Bob Frater, who was training under John Kirklin at the nearby Mayo Clinic at the time, and Chris crossed paths at this stage of their careers, according to Frater, Barnard was 'still a bright, smart, energetic guy, (but) a bit screwed up—a hopeless womaniser already; it was already very obvious and evident.'

Frater remembered that, when Chris visited him at the Mayo Clinic 'he made a significant impression. Some of our guests objected to the rather overt way he approached the females in the room. Others were impressed with the enthusiasm and energy which he displayed. No one was indifferent.' Eventually, Chris felt ready to return home.

## America's Generous Gift

When I decided I would go back to South Africa [in 1958], I went to see Wangensteen. He said, 'Are you sure?' And I said, 'I'm positive I want to go back there.' He offered me a job in Minneapolis, and said he would like to have me on the staff as a surgeon anytime. But I was terribly lonely. I loved the work yet I wanted to go back to South Africa to the medical school where I had trained, where I knew the people, and where I would have opportunities to go ahead with my work. [I am not sure if it is significant that he did not include his family among these reasons.] If I had stayed in Minneapolis, I don't think they would have given me the opportunities to really explore my capabilities because I would have been working with Lillehei and Varco and all these other people. I would never have done the first heart transplant.

Wangensteen then very generously arranged for the major research funding organization of the United States, the National Institutes of Health

(NIH), to provide Chris with a heart-lung machine and some financial research support so that he could develop open heart surgery in South Africa, for which Chris was immensely grateful. In those halcyon days, a well-known and influential surgeon, such as Wangensteen, could just pick up the phone and arrange a grant like this within minutes. Today, it is very different.

Chris personally 'packed the heart-lung machine with great care, crated it for dispatch, and fussed over it all the way through the customs.' He therefore returned to Cape Town with a grant-purchased heart-lung machine and a further $2,000 a year for three years to help him establish his new heart surgery program—an example of the US's generosity at a time when the country was booming economically.

Chris officially left Minneapolis on 30 June 1958. He had thus been there for two and a half years. Some months later—typical of Lillehei's inability (or lack of enthusiasm) to cope with the 'paperwork' that distracted him from his clinical responsibilities—Lillehei wrote a letter to Professor Jannie Louw to update him on his trainee's progress while in Minneapolis. An abbreviated version of his letter, dated 13 February 1959, is here reproduced.

Dear Professor Louw:

I fully anticipated getting this letter off to you some months ago, but a number of factors have conspired with the result that I am many months behind in some of my important correspondence.

This is in regard to Doctor Christiaan Barnard who spent the period 1 January 1956 to 30 June 1958 at the University of Minnesota taking graduate training in the Department of Surgery. During the latter part of Dr Barnard's tenure here, approximating almost two years, he worked virtually full time on cardiovascular problems ...

Following his experience in the laboratory, Dr Barnard worked upon our clinical service and was my Senior Resident for a period of six months. During the period that Dr Barnard was on the clinical service, he participated in more than 300 open heart operations utilising the heart-lung machine. These were carried out for a variety of congenital or acquired cardiac conditions. In addition, Dr Barnard spent a period of approximately three months running the heart-lung machine in the operating room daily for open heart surgical cases. [i.e. being responsibility for setting it up and ensuring that it worked well throughout the operative procedure. Today, a technician would carry out these responsibilities.]

During this period of time I got to know Dr Barnard very well and have been continually impressed by his abilities and devotion to duty. As

I have already mentioned, Dr Barnard has shown an excellent aptitude for experimental and clinical investigative work.

His preoperative and post-operative evaluation and care of our patients was excellent due in no small part to his thoroughness as well as his previous training in internal medicine. As a result, he was afforded full responsibility in these areas.

I am fully convinced that, given the opportunity, and even a modest budget for equipment and facilities, Dr Barnard will soon have open heart surgery thriving in your area and doubtless will be a stimulus to many others in that area.

It has been a real pleasure as well as fruitful to us to have a man like Dr Barnard with us for a period of time.

Most sincerely yours,

C. Walton Lillehei, MD

Professor of Surgery

By the time Lillehei found time to write this letter, Chris was well ahead in establishing an open heart surgery programme at Groote Schuur Hospital.

# 5

# Mentor and Maverick: Walt Lillehei

In regard to the specific story of heart transplantation, it is important to note that it was largely Lillehei and his colleagues who trained Chris Barnard in the use of the heart-lung machine and in the fundamental techniques of open heart surgery. Due to his highly influential position in regard to Barnard, it is worth considering Lillehei's career and personality in some detail.

Clarence Walton Lillehei (Figure 4.ii) is, in my opinion and in that of many past and present surgeons, including Chris Barnard, the major figure in the development of open heart surgery. He was certainly the boldest of the surgeons involved in this branch of surgery. The other important heart transplant pioneer, Norman Shumway, agreed that Lillehei was the dominant figure in the development of heart surgery. 'Yes, by far,' he told me. 'He was the great innovator and driving force. I had the greatest respect for him. At that time [the 1950s], he was the greatest surgeon in the world. He was a great student and scholar with tremendous mental aptitude, but he also had fantastic perseverance, and was a very hard worker.'

Like several innovative surgeons before him, Walt Lillehei was something of a maverick, and possibly the most colourful character among the surgeons involved in the development of heart surgery. As a young man, he cheated potential death from a malignant tumour. For the rest of his life, he had a slight but obvious deformity of his neck that resulted from the major surgery to which he was subjected in order to remove it; this may have contributed to his living somewhat dangerously throughout most of the rest of his life. Not only did he live dangerously as a surgeon, taking risks that most others balked at, but his personal life was also one of risk-taking, some would say recklessness. His lifestyle eventually led to the total collapse of his career, from which he never fully recovered, although by the time of his death he had regained much of the professional respect he indubitably deserved. His life was a veritable rollercoaster of triumphant highs and humiliating lows—in some ways even more so than Chris Barnard's life.

Bob Frater, who knew Lillehei well, though not as one of his trainees, remembers that he 'was a man with a great fertility of ideas. Ideas came pouring out of him, and he was absolutely open in his discussion of those ideas. He had a willingness to pass these ideas on to somebody else to try and develop them ... Lillehei was an absolutely marvellous fellow.'

With regard to Lillehei's influence over Chris, Frater's opinion was that 'Lillehei was a remarkable man for encouraging younger surgeons in their investigative efforts. He did not need to light a fire in Chris, but I am sure he fanned it.'

However, Frater described Lillehei's sartorial taste as 'quite bizarre; colour schemes were all wrong, and very flashy. Half the time, he looked like a bookie from a racetrack.'

In my personal experience, Dr Lillehei was always warm, affable, and friendly, with a nice sense of humor. In an after-dinner speech at a function in 1987 in Oklahoma City to celebrate the twentieth anniversary of the first heart transplant performed by Chris Barnard, Lillehei said that 'Chris readily admits that I taught him everything he knows about heart surgery.' He paused, and then, much to Chris's amusement, slyly added, 'But I didn't teach him everything I know.'

Walt Lillehei was born in 1918 and grew up in Minneapolis. His father was a dentist, and he had two brothers who followed him into medicine. The youngest, Richard, developed an international reputation as a surgeon, particularly by carrying out the world's first pancreas transplant in Minneapolis (in 1966), before tragically dying at a relatively young age. All of Walt Lillehei's education was in Minnesota—grade school, high school, undergraduate, and medical school. Having completed his schooling very quickly, he graduated as a doctor at age twenty-one (instead of the usual twenty-six), and joined the US Army in June 1942. He was soon shipped to the United Kingdom, and was later involved in the North African, Sicilian, and Italian campaigns in the Second World War. In North Africa, he commanded a Mobile Army Surgical Hospital (MASH) unit in the campaign against German Field-Marshal Rommel's Afrika Corps. From Africa, in 1944, Lillehei participated in the landing and bitter fighting at Anzio, south of Rome. After forty-six months in the army, he was a lieutenant-colonel and had been awarded a Bronze Star, a Bronze Arrowhead, and a European Theater Ribbon with five battle stars.

In October 1945, still only twenty-seven, he returned to Minneapolis for formal surgical training, which for all Wangensteen's trainees, as Chris was to find out, included a substantial period in the research laboratory.

It was during the last few months of his surgical residency in 1950 that Lillehei developed a lymphosarcoma (a notoriously malignant condition) in the glands in his neck. On the day after he completed his residency, Lillehei underwent more than ten hours of radical surgery to his neck and chest to remove all of the lymphatic tissue, and he subsequently received radiation therapy to this area. John Lewis (Lillehei's close friend) and Wangensteen were members of the team of surgeons who performed the long operation. Norman Shumway donated a pint of blood that was transfused into Lillehei during the operation. Lillehei was forced to take four months off from his work to recover from this therapy, after which Wangensteen appointed him to his staff.

When Wangensteen retired in 1967, Lillehei was disappointed not to be appointed to the job of chief of surgery, and so he accepted a position at Cornell University Medical Center in New York City. To put it mildly, Lillehei's time in New York did not work out well. Shumway later wrote that Lillehei's tenure of his professorship there 'made the French Revolution look like a church ice cream social.'

Lillehei, always a man who enjoyed a few drinks and a good party, went wild in the 'Big Apple'. His personal situation was probably not helped by the fact that his wife and children did not accompany him to New York, as it was felt wise for the children to continue their education in Minneapolis. He hung out in bars, and drank even more heavily than usual. To make his job at New York Hospital easier, he had been given the use of a penthouse apartment, in which he threw lavish parties for hospital staff and other 'friends' (often female) he accumulated in New York City. His wife was quoted as remarking, 'I don't mind the fact that he had lady friends there, it was the class of the lady friends I objected to.'

By July 1970, after a mix-up when Lillehei should have been in the operating room in New York but, through inadequate planning, found himself in Chicago, Lillehei was removed from his role as department chairman and chief of surgery. He was only fifty-one. However, worse was still to come.

In 1972, a grand jury in St. Paul, Minnesota, indicted Lillehei on charges of evading $125,100 in income taxes, a very considerable amount of money at that time. If he were found guilty, he could have faced up to twenty-five years in prison. Lillehei, who his biographer, Wayne Miller, called the 'legendary procrastinator', had for many years been late (often years late) in filing his income tax returns to the Internal Revenue Service (IRS). A special agent was put onto his case who, by delving into Lillehei's personal affairs, found that he had been 'leading something of a secret life—a life that included mistresses and even a Las Vegas call girl.'

His trial began in January 1973. He was accused of not reporting his income from many different sources, and of claiming parties, gifts to girlfriends, and a call girl as tax-deductible expenses. Veterinary bills for his pets, dance lessons, and tuition were also billed as tax-deductible expenses. Some 164 witnesses were called by the prosecution, including girlfriends to whom he had given expensive gifts, and sixteen by the defence. More than 6,000 exhibits were entered into evidence. According to Bob Frater, 'a check for "secretarial duties" was made out to a person who appeared on the stand; she was an obvious tart. It was a sad, sad tale.'

In his defence, Lillehei admitted that his billing system had been lamentable and his filing system had been one of index cards in a shoe box; in other words, his financial affairs were in chaos through his own neglect, bad judgment, carelessness, and procrastination, but not, his lawyer claimed, from fraud. However, some of his index cards were found to have been altered, for which Lillehei was unable to provide any explanation.

The chaos of Lillehei's financial affairs was confirmed to me years later by Bob Frater. 'When he died, there were a couple of rooms in his house totally filled with papers. The people from the St. Jude company [a medical device company for whom Lillehei had consulted after leaving surgical practice] helped his wife, Kaye, sort the stuff. They allegedly came across $100,000 in cash in one place or another.'

In court, Wangensteen, Shumway, and several other colleagues testified on Lillehei's behalf. His lawyer attempted to paint a picture of a man overwhelmed by his surgical work and without the time to spend on his personal affairs. The trial took twenty-one days. The jury found him guilty on all counts. The judge, however, could not bring himself to imprison Lillehei, stating that he recognised, 'You have this great talent that should be of use to society.' The judge felt that imprisonment would either destroy that ability or render it useless for a period of time. He therefore fined Lillehei the maximum $50,000 and ordered him to serve six months' community service.

New York Hospital/Cornell Medical Center ordered him to leave by the end of the year, even though they honoured his contract through the end of 1974. Sadly, despite the judge's hope and intention, after December 1973, Lillehei never performed another open heart operation. According to Frater, Lillehei's appointment to New York Hospital had been 'a total disaster. Lillehei's personal life sort of collapsed, although his wife stuck with him until he died; she is a marvellous woman.'

In his mid-fifties, Lillehei found himself in the surgical wilderness, an outcast in a field to which he had contributed so much. For more than ten years, he remained a pariah to many in surgery. It was the distinguished heart surgeon, John Kirklin, who, in 1979 in an address as president of the American Association for Thoracic Surgery, began Lillehei's rehabilitation in the eyes of his colleagues. It took some ten to fifteen years before his reputation was fully re-established.

Ultimately, in addition to the money he had earned as a busy surgeon, Lillehei made a great deal of money through royalties on St. Jude prosthetic heart valves in whose design he had been involved, and from investing in the stock market in the 1940s and 1950s. According to Frater, 'When he died, he left $15 million.' After his death in 1999, Lillehei's widow donated $10 million from his estate to the department of cardiothoracic surgery at the University of Minnesota.

Despite his checkered personal life, Walt Lillehei was unquestionably the greatest innovator in the development of heart surgery, and Chris Barnard was inordinately fortunate to have him as his chief mentor.

# 6

# Proving Himself: Establishing Heart Surgery in Cape Town

Chris Barnard returned to Cape Town to a medical school that was humming with activity and innovation. Bob Frater remembered:

> The University of Cape Town Medical School in 1959 was an extraordinarily exciting place. There was a concentration of bright energetic people working in a free atmosphere at a time when the tools of advancement in clinical medical science were not particularly complex. The Scottish pedagogic tradition that had founded the school was very much alive. It was combined with a humility that made it automatic to seek whatever good there was to be found elsewhere and put it to good use locally.
>
> All of this was exemplified in the Cardiology Department. There were [Robert] Goetz, [Louis] Vogelpoel, [Maurice] Nellen and [Velva] Schrire [all internationally well-known cardiologists]. They had done one hundred cardiac catheterizations [i.e. inserting a long tube into a vein or artery and guiding it up into the heart to take pressure and oxygen saturation measurements]. They had angiography [X-ray pictures of the chambers of the heart] as good as that of the Karolinska Institute in Stockholm, phonocardiography [a means of recording heart murmurs] of the calibre of the National Heart Hospital in London, and dye dilution curve analysis [to measure the heart output] on a par with that at the Mayo Clinic in Rochester, Minnesota. As students, we found cardiology enormously exciting.

Within a few weeks of arriving back in Cape Town in the middle of 1958, Chris had initiated the first successful open heart surgery programme in Africa.

Chris told me that his original suggestion was that he would assist Professor Louw, the chief of surgery, and teach him the techniques he had learned in Minneapolis. 'He would be the cardiac surgeon, and I would be his assistant. But he [Louw] decided that I was going to be the cardiac surgeon because I had been trained in cardiac surgery. He really helped me a lot to establish the unit there, and supported me very, very much.'

As the Minneapolis surgeons, who to some extent were learning the techniques themselves, had not allowed Chris to carry out any heart operations himself, but had restricted him to being an assistant, establishing a successful programme in Cape Town cannot have been easy. Every surgical trainee knows that it is one thing to watch the senior surgeon perform an operation, but it is quite a different matter when faced with the responsibility oneself.

There is a joke among surgeons that, with regard to doing operations, under less than ideal training conditions, the surgeon has to 'see one, do one, teach one'. Chris at least had the advantage of seeing many open heart operations before actually doing one, but the development of his surgical skills was not ideal.

The ideal way to learn, of course, is to assist an experienced surgeon on several occasions, then to have him assist you several times, then carry out the operation alone (but with the senior colleague available, if required), before moving on to full independence. In Chris's case, this stepwise learning curve was not possible. Isolated at the southern tip of Africa, he had only himself to rely on. There was no one to call if he found himself in difficulties. Imagine a new pilot flying a jet plane for the first time having never once flown it with an instructor on board.

Chris personally went to the Cape Town docks to fetch the heart-lung machine, unwilling to trust anyone else to deliver this new treasured item. The machine component parts arrived in rather fine cardboard boxes. Victor Pick, a coloured man who was one of the senior assistants in the animal laboratory, requested permission to take the boxes home with him as he realised their potential as pieces of furniture.

Chris trained a technician, an excellent person named Carl Goosen, in the use of the heart-lung machine. Chris and Goosen, who was to prove invaluable to Barnard during the initiation of his program, set up the heart-lung machine in the operating theatre. Chris remembered that several other laboratory technicians 'jostled around breathing down each other's necks' to take a look at it, and colleagues came in from time to time to inspect what became known as 'Chris's gadget'. The first successful open heart surgical programme on the African continent was initiated at Groote Schuur Hospital on 28 July 1958, only a few weeks after Chris had left Minneapolis.

The anaesthetist, Dr Joseph 'Ozzie' Ozinsky—another invaluable colleague who later was to anesthetise the first patient to undergo a heart transplant—kept the patient asleep. Professor Louw watched from the operating room viewing dome, which was full of interested hospital staff. Although Chris was extremely nervous, the first operation, a relatively simple operation—coincidentally carried out on Victor Pick's young niece, Joan—went without complication.

Chris hovered over the patient for the next several hours until convinced she was doing well, thus beginning a habit of meticulous post-operative care of his patients that was to remain with him until close to his retirement from surgery more than twenty years later. Much to Chris's satisfaction, on the following day, this historic operation made the front page of the South African newspapers, the government taking the opportunity to draw attention to the fact that the patient was a coloured girl. Joan Pick later married, had a family, and died more than forty years later from stomach cancer.

This good result gave Chris and his team confidence to take on patients with more complicated conditions. For the first few patients, Chris was asked to work with one of the senior chest surgeons, Dr Walter Phillips, who was experienced in lung and 'closed' heart surgery; however, he had no real experience of open heart surgery, so Chris soon took over himself.

## Influence of the Cardiologist, Velva (Val) Schrire

The success of the heart surgery team at GSH at this time was in no small part due to the vision and support of Professor Velva (Val) Schrire (Figure 6.i), the professor of cardiology, a quite outstanding clinical physician who acted as Chris's mentor for many years and would play a major role in the first heart transplant a few years hence. Schrire had had a stellar academic career as a student at UCT, graduating with numerous gold medals and scholarships. In 1949, he had been awarded a fellowship from a British medical foundation to spend time in London at the National Heart Hospital, one of the major centres of cardiology in the British Commonwealth. He had returned to GSH to establish the specialised Cardiac Clinic. Bob Frater thought:

> Val was important because he understood that surgery was going to be the crucial spur to the development of cardiology; otherwise, cardiology would just be like neurology [at that time] with only the diagnosis and elegant discussion of what was wrong, without any way to make patients better. When Chris went back to Cape Town, Val Schrire realised that Barnard, because of his two years in Minneapolis, knew a hell of a lot more than Walter Phillips, the current thoracic surgeon at Groote Schuur

who wasn't about to relinquish his throne. And so the idea was that Schrire would feed cases to Chris and to the other surgeon on an equal basis. Schrire told me that he called in from the waiting list twenty ASDs, twenty pulmonary stenoses, twenty VSDs—all straightforward cases— and then [after this learning experience] gave Chris his first tetralogy [a more complicated condition to correct surgically]. For Phillips, Schrire selected only difficult cases. Then Schrire said to Phillips, 'I'm sorry. Barnard's cases are living, and your patients are dying, and so I'm going to give the cases to Barnard.'

Dealt this dreadful pack of cards, Phillips remained in Cape Town for a while as Barnard's assistant, but eventually left to start a surgical practice in the USA. To his great credit, when news of the first transplant crossed the world, Phillips was one of the first to write to congratulate Barnard. On Phillips's departure, Chris was made head of cardiothoracic surgery at GSH.

Chris had immense respect for Schrire (another 'father figure') and hardly a day passed when he would not visit the cardiologist in his office to discuss a patient or some other topic of mutual interest. A few years later, Schrire was to support the initiation of the transplant programme wholeheartedly, selecting suitable patients and playing a major role in their medical—rather than surgical—care, though later he relatively quickly became disenchanted with Chris's celebrity lifestyle. The experience Chris gained under Schrire's wise mentorship, and his own obsession with attaining perfection in his surgical practice, led him to develop superb clinical judgment.

Very sensibly, Chris explored and practiced new operative techniques in the animal laboratory before attempting them in patients. Each time a technique was perfected in the laboratory, it was applied in the operating room. With increasing experience, he and his team were able to deal with very difficult operations, which remained very challenging throughout the 1960s. Schrire's wisdom, sometimes clearly quite ruthless, in nurturing the heart surgery programme at GSH is exemplified by another of Dr Frater's recollections.

I came back [from the USA, where he had trained under John Kirklin at the Mayo Clinic] to Cape Town as Chris's assistant [at the end of 1961]. He needed somebody who had been trained in cardiac surgery. Chris was operating with two 'attendings' [trained staff surgeons, which is a great advantage for any surgeon, particularly if carrying out a new or difficult operation] and one trainee. The trainee registrar [resident] stood by the toes [of the patient], scrubbed all through the case, but doing nothing, and the other attending and I did the assisting. He never did a case with just a raw registrar helping him; he always wanted somebody with a bit more experience than a completely raw trainee. He [Barnard] wasn't a comfortable operator. He needed, or at least wanted, that kind of [experienced] person to help him.

Chris was fine about that, but he didn't want me to be an independent surgeon. That was the problem. He didn't give me the cases. There was no way that Chris wanted to have another surgeon. It was at Val Schrire's insistence, you see [that I had been invited back]. Anyway, Chris got hepatitis and was sick. [Hepatitis was not an uncommon occupational hazard for surgeons in those days if they pricked a finger on a surgical needle during an operation on a patient carrying this virus.] He announced from his sick bed that there would be no more cardiac surgery until he recovered. Val went to see him, and said that this was nonsense. 'You asked for Frater to come back. I encouraged you to do that. I want to have two cardiac surgeons here, and we're going to continue operating. And you're too sick to argue with me.'

There was a chap with a pulsating aortic aneurysm [weakening of the wall of the main blood vessel of the body] bulging through the sternum [i.e. the chest wall, an extremely high-risk condition that to this day remains difficult to operate on]. With great excitement, I went to Val because now I was going to do an independent case. He said, 'You're not going to do that case tomorrow.' I said, 'The chap is going to die.' He said, 'Yes, and if you operate on him tomorrow, he's going to die tomorrow. I've got a case for you. It's an ASD [a simple case], and you're going to do the ASD tomorrow.' So I did. Just the way Val brought Chris along, he did the same with me while Chris was sick.

As an aside, Chris did not prove to be a compliant patient himself. His physician, Stuart Saunders, later to become chairman of the department of medicine at UCT, wrote:

[I] had the privilege of being his [Chris's] personal physician from time to time when he was ill. In particular, I remember his chagrin when a quite severe bout of viral hepatitis interfered with his travels overseas. He dealt with the interns and residents in a pre-emptory manner and I was forced, as was always the case with him as a patient, to be firm and direct in order to be sure that his exuberant personality would not interfere with his recovery and convalescence. The words I am using give only an inkling of the scene.

It says much for Chris's skills and organization that he set up a first-class cardiac surgical programme at GSH (Figure 6.ii), and an equally good, if not even better, programme in the surgery of congenital heart disease (birth defects) at the nearby Red Cross War Memorial Children's Hospital, which was established by the Cape Region of the South African Red Cross Society as a memorial to the 'sacrifice, suffering, and service' of South Africans in the Second World War.

During this critical period of development, Chris consulted Dr Lillehei in Minneapolis by telephone or letter on a number of occasions when faced with problems, just as he had consulted his former teachers when in general practice in Ceres. Lillehei recorded:

[Chris] wrote at least twenty-five or thirty letters to me between the time he left us in 1958 up to 1961. All of them were about the patients he was seeing and operating on in Cape Town. He asked questions about various types of surgical techniques. I was well aware that he was making superb progress, and that was confirmed later by the excellent results he obtained in difficult cases like [Fallot's] tetralogy. In particular, he took on some very sick babies early in his career—which was difficult surgery. He was making a name for himself, and not solely because he was the first surgeon to do successful open heart surgery on the African continent. In the numerous letters he wrote to me, he said, 'It is so distant here in South Africa.' News was so hard to come by. The medical journals arrived three or six months late.

This was still the case when I worked in Cape Town in the 1980s.

As a heart surgeon, Chris soon had almost unequalled range; there was no operation he could not perform, including valve replacement (which became common by the mid-1960s), the correction of a complex birth defect, and repairing an aortic aneurysm. He proved himself to be, if not the most naturally dexterous of surgeons, one with excellent judgment and the ability to obtain the result he desired. Bob Frater remembered:

Barnard had a surgical intuition that helped him throughout his career [including with the later heart transplant patients]. Chris would say, 'I don't like the look of this heart.' I'd say, 'What's wrong with it?' 'I don't like the look of it, man.' I'd say, 'Chris, the blood pressure is okay.' 'No, no, there's something wrong with this heart.' Sure enough, about two seconds later it would fibrillate [i.e. fail to pump out blood effectively]. He was functioning from gut feelings, but the gut feelings were based on something he had seen with his eye. He had detected some change—perhaps the heart wasn't 'squeezing' [contracting] quite the way it was before. There was a subtle difference. He was integrating this information, and relating it to his previous experience. And he was right.

Chris was completely uninterested in really going through the hard slog of a series of experiments to prove something. He very much worked out of instinct, and on ideas and impressions. He had plenty of them.

By the time I arrived [to become Chris's colleague at GSH], Chris was in complete control. However, it was soon obvious that he was not a natural surgeon. The technical manipulations standard to surgery did not come easily to him and when he operated there was clearly both a significant effort of will to perform manoeuvres successfully and a significant element of anxiety while doing so. To counter this, there was a high level of determination, tenacity and resilience. There was no question of not achieving the tasks at the best possible level of surgical execution.

This tendency to inductive rather than deductive reasoning, to instinctive rather than planned thinking and acting, was carried through to the post-operative period. Although obviously there can never be any reasonable proof of anything more than coincidence in these happenings, it was notable that he would often arrive at a patient's bedside, without being called, at precisely the moment when the patient's condition changed for the worse.

However, like all of us, Chris was by no means infallible. Dr Frater remembered occasions when Chris's judgment, and even his responsibility to his patient, would fail him.

There was one case in which air embolism occurred [air bubbles got into the blood and went to the brain—a potentially lethal condition], and Chris, extremely upset, left the operating room, certain that the patient had no chance of survival. The senior surgeon who was assisting Chris [Walter Phillips], stayed scrubbed, got rid of the air and had a live, awake patient to show for it.

## Behaviour in the Operating Room

Chris maintained that his greatest need in the operating room was silence. Some surgeons choose to operate with the soft sounds of music in the background, although this does not always succeed in providing the calming effect that is intended. Chris's contemporary in London, Donald Ross, would often request soothing music but, oddly, if he ran into difficulties with the operative procedure, he would shout, 'Turn that damn music off.' Chris, however, desired only to be surrounded by peace and quiet so that he could concentrate completely on the patient lying in front of him, something he believed he owed the patient.

However, despite the peaceful atmosphere, Chris was perhaps more likely than most surgeons to 'lose his cool' when under stress. Indeed, he was prone to vitriolic outbursts of temper and frustration at times when the procedure was not progressing as well as he would have liked, and he would verbally abuse his surgical assistants or the heart-lung machine technicians, blaming anybody and everybody but himself.

British cardiac surgeon, Sir Terence English, born and brought up in South Africa, though he studied medicine at Guy's in London, remembers visiting Barnard in Cape Town in the early 1960s.

I had two shocks. One was that, after the operation, his registrar [surgical resident or assistant] had to sit with the patient all night, taking the blood pressure, because Barnard wouldn't trust the nurses. This seemed to me to be quite extraordinary. The other thing I noticed was how uncontrolled he was at the operating table. But there was no doubt that the result of his work was quite extraordinarily good. It was a reflection of his obsession with getting things right despite making it very difficult for everyone around him.

As Terence English had observed, Chris was notoriously difficult to work with in the operating room, particularly when he found himself in technical difficulties or when he perceived he was not receiving the help he should be; he frequently shouted and screamed, or even swore, at his assistants and the operating room staff. From visits to GSH, Sir Brian Barratt-Boyes, the great New Zealand heart surgeon (who in my experience was critical of most other surgeons) remembered Chris as 'an average technician—competent, but a messy operator—but very difficult to get on with in the operating room'.

Bob Frater commented on Chris's behaviour in the operating room:

[He could be] absolutely outrageous. I don't particularly like confrontation, and I never really stood up for my colleagues or for the residents he abused. It made me feel uncomfortable because I was standing by while he behaved outrageously. For example, he opened a patient with mitral valve disease, and found calcified leaflets [i.e. the valve had deteriorated to the point that 'bone' deposits had developed in it, making any corrective surgery very difficult]. He said, 'Send for Professor Schrire'. Val came in, and Chris said, 'Val, look at this shit you gave me to operate on.' Val would just look at it and say, 'I'm sure you can do something about that. Why don't you see what you can do?' He [Schrire] would 'nurse' him, you see.

On occasion, Schrire, to whom in Frater's opinion Chris owed more than
any other single individual, would be called into the operating theatre and
asked why he sent such 'rubbish' for surgery, and why he could not make
a more accurate diagnosis rather than give the surgeon unanticipated and
unexpected difficulties in the operating room. Frater elaborated on Chris's
behaviour.

> We had a perfusionist [who ran the heart-lung machine] and general
> master of all trades, Mr Carl Goosen, who also absorbed enormous
> abuse. He was, in fact, one of the very best cardiopulmonary bypass
> technicians there has ever been and he was a critical component in the
> success of cardiac surgery in the early days in Cape Town. Sometimes
> when Chris would have a problem, he would say to the heart-lung pump
> technician, 'I can always trust you to kill my patient.' He would say to
> an assistant, 'Why are you so f---ing useless?' This was a weird world we
> lived in. It really was.
>
> 'But Barnard couldn't possibly suggest that people weren't trying to
> help him achieve the success he wanted. In fact, the culture in Cape
> Town was a very obedient culture. In the schools we went to, we had
> been brought up to 'serve'. Service was something we were supposed to
> do. We were not supposed to argue with the captain. So it was a free
> atmosphere in terms of the interchange of ideas in cardiology, but it was
> also a hierarchical atmosphere in terms of the chiefs of service. The boss
> of surgery was clearly the boss of surgery. You don't hear the stories
> of instrument-throwing surgeons anymore, but they were real enough
> thirty to forty years ago. Despite all that I am describing, there was great
> loyalty to Chris and to the whole enterprise.

Indeed, despite his at times outrageous behaviour, Chris developed a loyal
group around him who were committed to the same aims as he was. For
example, Dene Friedmann, one of Chris's heart-lung machine technicians
and the daughter of one of his best friends, wrote:

> Once you had worked for Chris, it was so exciting that working for
> anyone else was dull in comparison. He had the power to make you
> want to please him and strive for a word of praise. Because of his
> mercurial temperament, you had to know when to tell him or ask him
> certain things. If you did this at the right time he was quite easy to
> manage. He could not tolerate inefficiency and would speedily get rid of
> his secretaries if they were not up to scratch. This happened very often.
> [But] I've never known anyone who inspired so much confidence and
> trust. It seemed as if as long as Chris was there, everything was alright. If

Chris said to you, 'jump off a large building and I promise you nothing will happen to you,' you would almost agree to do it.

Dene thought his strengths were 'the ability to instil you with confidence ... He was always very positive about things, and also very charming, and always had time to listen to you. He was dynamic, interesting, fun, and he liked young people.'

Senior heart-lung pump technician, Carl Goosen, who had been such a valuable member of Chris's team, was not so enamoured with working with Chris and, in 1966, left to take up an appointment at the Medical College of Virginia in the USA, where he became a successful inventor and entrepreneur.

Johan van Heerden, the heart-lung technician who took over from Goosen and was the senior technician at the first heart transplant (with Dene), admitted initially developing 'an uncomfortable stomach ache whenever he would be working with Chris. However, he also remembered that occasionally Chris's 'outbursts could be tinged with humour. On one occasion when he scolded one of my colleagues, the perfusionist tried to explain his problems and, hoping to gain some understanding and sympathy, added, "and my wife is pregnant as well." Immediately, Professor Barnard retorted, "Well, that's not my fault."'

Amelia Rautenbach (always known by her nickname, 'Pittie'), who was for many years one of Chris's leading operating room nurses who scrubbed to assist at his operations (including the first heart transplant) recollected that he 'knew very well that his impatience with lesser beings caused dissatisfaction, but outwardly it did not seem to upset him very much. One day he walked into the staff tea room [lounge] and, laughing, said, "Oh well, I have been reported again to the Director of Hospital Services. They want me to stop shouting at the staff." He shrugged his shoulders, gave a smile all around, and sat down to have some tea.'

In my personal experience as a surgeon, 'losing one's cool' in the operating room is often a sign of insecurity—for example, when an operation is proving too difficult for one's abilities or experience, or when unexpected problems arise. During these early years of Chris's career as a heart surgeon, Chris's relative lack of experience might excuse some of his outbursts. There is also no doubt that he always felt a very high degree of responsibility towards the patient, which may well have increased his 'fear' of failure. However, I have worked with a few conscientious surgeons who seemingly never let their insecurities control them.

To some extent, Chris maintained his staff's loyalty by his behaviour outside of the operating room. For example, when Pittie Rautenbach was involved in 'a car accident—nothing serious, just minor abrasions,

Professor Barnard came to see me in the trauma unit. He always made time for us. When he saw that I was fine, he laughed and said, 'And here I thought I could use your liver for my waiting liver transplant, Pittie'.

As Bob Frater had pointed out, in all of Chris's operations, he wanted to be assisted by experienced surgeons. One of these was former medical school classmate, Rodney Hewitson (who worked with Chris from 1960), an excellent surgeon who was in some respects a calming influence in the operating room. Another of Chris's erstwhile colleagues, Terry O'Donovan, remembered Hewitson's contributions to the work of the department.

> One of the people who stand out most clearly in my mind is Dr Rodney Hewitson. I think that he was justly described as Chris's right-hand man. Not only did he act as a stabilising influence on Chris when he was inclined to make rather emotional decisions and get 'uptight', but he was also a very sensible, skilled cardiac surgeon, who frequently made sensible suggestions and would often, technically, keep Chris out of trouble when he was maybe not doing things exactly correctly. Knowing Rodney Hewitson to be the quiet, retiring, self-effacing individual that he was, I think that in many ways he lost out on the acclaim that he should have had for being the sheet anchor of the department. He was much more than Chris's right-hand man, being a very helpful influence on him altogether.

Yet even his most senior and valued surgical colleagues, such as Rodney Hewitson, received their share of abuse. Bob Frater told me:

> During the few short years that I worked in Cape Town, Chris continued to insist on being assisted only by 'attending' surgeons [i.e. fully trained staff]. One, a Christian gentleman, if ever that epitaph can appropriately be applied [who I am sure was Rodney Hewitson], took enormous abuse from Chris without demur, feeling that his job was to see that the patient got good care above all.

Chris's younger brother, Marius, spent a year in Houston, Texas, working with the well-known surgeons, Michael DeBakey and Denton Cooley, planning to become a vascular surgeon (operating on blood vessels rather than the heart). On his return to Cape Town, no position in vascular surgery was available to him at GSH, and so—reluctantly, in view of his life-long poor relationship with Chris—he accepted an appointment in Chris's group as a heart surgeon (in which field he had gained some experience in Houston). In view of their volatile relationship, Chris probably offered Marius the position with some misgiving, and was likely motivated by a desire to help his sibling find a job. Both were later to regret this move. Marius remembered:

> In Chris's presence, there was … a degree of tension, even fear. He operated very slowly but his work was meticulous. He handled the tissues with the greatest of care, making sure that the heart muscle was protected against rough handling and making doubly sure that the risk of post-operative bleeding was reduced. Although he appeared to struggle—and he often did—his results were excellent and world-class due to his great knowledge and understanding of cardiac surgery. His uncanny knack for spotting complications, before we could, was amazing—I always said he would have made an excellent detective. No criminal would ever have escaped his ability to find any clue at the scene of the crime.

Marius remembered occasions when Chris's tirades against his junior staff produced some humorous moments. One morning, Chris arrived in the Intensive Care Unit to examine the post-operative patients with the trainees who had been on call overnight.

> [Chris was] in a foul mood. A registrar from Portugal, whose English was very poor, was on duty. Chris immediately observed signs of possible complications, which had been missed by the registrar. If not responded to, they could lead to the patient's death. Chris exploded, giving the registrar not only a lengthy lecture on the mistakes he'd made, but also a vivid description of his stupidity and his lack of responsibility. He told the registrar that if the patient died it would be due to him, and him alone.
>
> When, after more than ten minutes of ranting, Chris finally stopped to take a deep breath, the registrar had a chance to get a word in. In broken English and with a blank face, he said, 'Please repeat, Professor. I did not understand.' This reply stopped Chris in his tracks. He gaped at the registrar and stormed out of the ward without saying another word.

However, 'most importantly', wrote Marius, although Chris's staff and the hospital authorities sometimes grumbled about his behaviour, 'the patients never complained about him'.

Although by no means as vitriolic as Chris, at times Marius could be overly critical of his assistants in the operating room. I was told by a colleague that on one occasion he was particularly critical of a burly Eastern European surgical fellow (I believe from Serbia) who, after much goading, decided he had taken enough abuse and left the operating table, telling Marius he would 'wait for him outside'. He took off his gloves and gown and walked through the door, folded his arms in front of him, and stood waiting. Marius could see him through the window in the door. The large, muscular young man looked angry and formidable. Whereas, like Chris and the other senior surgeons, Marius would usually leave his junior colleagues to close the chest, on this occasion, he completed the entire operation himself, even stitching the skin—an almost unheard event for a senior surgeon. Every few seconds, he would glance at the door to see if the young man was still waiting for him. Ultimately, he had no choice but to leave the operating room, where he was accosted by his large adversary. Unfortunately, I never heard the end of the story.

## Management of Patients After the Operation

One of the major achievements of his career, Chris believes, was the introduction of the practice of intensive care of patients at GSH (and also at the Red Cross Children's Hospital), creating what was probably the first intensive care unit in Africa. Although commonplace today, intensive care was virtually unknown before the introduction of open heart surgery. It involves continuous, second-by-second care of the patient by a team of highly trained and skilled nurses and doctors and is essential for the success of a major heart operation. Almost every pioneering heart surgeon I have ever met has been proud of initiating intensive care in his home institution.

Chris demanded perfection in the post-operative care of his patients. According to Professor Louw, outside of the operating room, Chris 'drove his registrars to work like Trojans, which accounted for a great deal of his success'. There is no doubt that the trainees in Chris's department were expected to be available at all times day or night, a situation that would not be acceptable today (2017). Dimitri Novitzky, who trained in cardiac surgery at GSH late in Barnard's career, felt:

This aggressive attitude made coexistence between colleagues extremely tense in many aspects, and probably some of them quit the department due to the stress of the training. For example, he always demanded to have two residents on call, and for one to be awake at all times. Therefore, the night should be shared by two. On occasion, a resident would be sick. Therefore, due to the shortage we had, it was necessary to work two or three days in a row before getting some rest. I think he enjoyed this sort of game with his staff, but, on the other hand, those who managed to pass this endurance test had all the benefit in the future.

The main reward was participation in the performance of surgery, or being incorporated into the transplant team.

When Chris was overseas, he would always phone the intensive care unit to ask how the patients were doing. He and the registrar would discuss details of the progress of each and every patient over the phone.

John Terblanche, who as a young man spent time with Chris in the research laboratory and the operating room, but later became chairman of surgery and therefore officially Chris's boss, wrote that Chris 'was determined to do well. Patients whom he had operated on had to do well. He expected his junior staff to work as long as required and continuously, for days on end, if needed in the interest of his patients. A weakness was that he was not really interested in patients in the unit operated on by other surgeons'.

However, in the period 1965 to 1967, when Terblanche was working in the United Kingdom (where his three sons were born), he was clear who would operate on them had they been unfortunate enough to have a heart defect. 'Only Barnard would have been good enough. Fortunately, this was not put to the test'. Terblanche also commented on Chris's unreasonable demands and accusations.

One often felt personally to blame if one of his patients developed a complication or unfortunately died. One of the best runs of four letter words I have ever heard occurred when I was responsible for the heart-lung machine with one of the technicians in the early hypothermia days. We had a water cooler associated with our homemade hypothermia machine which required a modified garden pump which pumped twelve gallons of cooled water per minute. This unfortunately became disconnected in the middle of an operation and the large swinging hose pipe sprayed iced water around the operating theatre at twelve gallons per minute. Barnard's reaction was probably predictable.

Terblanche also emphasised how intensely loyal Barnard's technical staff were because they could clearly see the exciting way in which cardiac surgery was developing. Nevertheless, his demands on them were excessive.

Barnard's demands on his staff were not only for patient care. When his family's young tomcat needed spaying, this was presented to us in the laboratory. Being used to somewhat larger dogs, we unfortunately overdosed it with anaesthetic and more than one of us spent many hours nursing the cat until it had fully recovered before returning it to

Barnard. In 1960 he acquired a small ocean-going fishing boat. When this broke down we were loaded into his car on a weekday and taken out to Simonstown harbour to assist with its repair and maintenance.

At the end of my full-time year with him in 1960 he gave me a cooking dish as a Christmas gift which my wife and I still possess. This was a very unusual gesture on his part as he was not particularly demonstrative and this probably meant that we got on reasonably well during that time.

Terblanche added that 'in these early years before 1961 Barnard had not yet developed his taste for expensive tailor-made clothes. His appearance was often scruffy. I well remember an occasion when he came into the hospital for a Sunday round in his tweed coat with patched elbows and was taken for a hospital porter by one of the nursing staff'. 'Scruffy' may be too strong a word, because Chris was always well-groomed, but he certainly had no interest in fashionable clothes in those days.

Despite his growing reputation and stature as a heart surgeon, Chris remained touched by simple gestures of thanks from his patients or their family members. He recorded one such example.

I once found a gift on my desk that made my entire day. It was a box of apples. A closer look showed they were fly-specked, bruised and certainly second grade. I knew enough about apples to know a pick-up when I saw one and this was a whole box of windfalls. Somebody had scrumped them from the long grass in an orchard. An illiterate scrawl told the rest. The giver was a husband of a patient who had just been discharged. He was a *bywoner*, a farm labourer, and this was all he could find to show his gratitude. Those apples were the sweetest I have ever tasted, when I managed to get them past the lump in my throat.

He clearly had a facility in expressing himself in words.

## Chris and Children

Chris's work with children was particularly pleasing to him, not only for the impact a successful operation might have on the child's future, but also because he had a special empathy with children who loved the attention he personally bestowed on them (Figure 6.iii).

Many people have written about Chris's delight in being in the company of children. He obviously had a great affection for them and enjoyed them, and would prefer to spend time with a child than with adults. Professor Louw wrote that when Chris was a guest in his home, Chris would spend more time with the Louw's children than with him and his wife. It was possibly because of this that surgery on children with congenital heart disease became such an important part of Chris's surgical practice in those days. Deirdre recorded that her father believed that every child 'had a right to every opportunity life could afford them' and, furthermore, he was willing to accept challenges and risks in order to help them.

The internationally known South African cardiologist and researcher, Lionel Opie, a GSH colleague, wrote:

> What remained with me was the manifest warmth which Barnard showed to his young patients, giving them all that famous smile, and all of them returning equally warm and human smiles, despite their varying degrees of disability. A man who can build up such close human contact with such simple young patients, many of them severely disabled, could only have gained their love by his devotion and care to them. This is a little-known aspect of his early career.

Nazih Zuhdi, with whom Chris was later to work in Oklahoma City (Chapter 24), was also struck by Chris's rapport with children.

> My last test of a man's presence is for him to be placed in the background of a field of children. If the children themselves come flocking to him to be talked to, held and loved, the man has reached a state of bliss, for his kindness, simplicity of soul, and blessedness are transcendent. At any place where they are, children surround Christiaan Barnard, and he talks to them at length in ways they understand, telling them fantastic stories, even acting them out, and the children are mesmerised.

To illustrate Chris's compassion for children, Deirdre Barnard related a story that touched her father deeply (which was actually told to her by Marius Barnard). An African boy of about ten was in hospital with severe heart failure brought on by rheumatic fever and, sadly, because he was so sick, an operation was unable to help him. It soon became clear that the boy was dying. Marius visited the child, who was in an oxygen tent, and asked the young boy whether there was anything in the world that he would like to have. What the boy asked for was a piece of bread. Chris could hardly bear to tell this story, it moved him so much. He was filled with pity for the boy. Deirdre suggested that, in many ways, human suffering was a personal cross for Chris to bear.

Chris became emotionally involved with the children he operated upon. One of my colleagues at GSH told me that, when much younger, his sister had been friendly with Deirdre Barnard, who had shown her Chris's album that contained photos of many of his young patients.

In one of his later newspaper columns, Chris wrote, 'The suffering of children in particular is the most heart-breaking of hospital problems. Their innocence and their total trust in nurses and doctors makes it even more poignant when the outcome offers little hope'.

In another column, he demonstrated the strength of his passion and his sense of responsibility about his own children, when he wrote the following words:

> No law would prevent me from upholding what I thought was best for my children. And if it were a case of preventing harm, whether from hunger or anything else, then throat-cutting—let alone drug-running— was not beyond imagination. Apart from such cold considerations, who can measure the anguish of a child deprived of its mother? Scripture lays down clearly that a millstone about the neck and a watery grave would be preferable to the punishment that awaits anyone who harms the child.

Whether Chris personally lived up to these high ideals is debatable. His subsequent self-centred lifestyle and divorces certainly harmed some of his children psychologically. Like many of us, he did not always abide by his firmly held ideals.

Nevertheless, there is no question that he felt a strong empathy with children, particularly sick children. This concern was not just on a personal level; he was concerned for children worldwide. In his book, *Good Life, Good Death*, he drew attention to the plight of millions of children in less-developed countries:

> Certainly the lives of a vast number of the world's children are sagas of quiet desperation. According to figures released by the World Health Organization, of the 125 million infants that will be born this year [1980], at least twelve million are unlikely to see their first birthday. Another twenty million may die before the age of five, and of those who survive, a percentage will be physical and mental cripples.

## Chris and Publicity

Even at this relatively early stage of his career, Chris realised the value of publicity. Bob Frater remembered that, after he (Frater) had carried out one rather innovative operation, he could not understand how the newspapers had obtained and reported the story.

There was this article in the newspaper on 'Cape Town cardiac surgeons once again perform innovative operation.' I hadn't said a word to anybody. I went to Chris, and said, 'Chris, how the hell did this happen? I didn't know anything about it.' He looked me straight in the eye, and said, 'I don't know anything about it either.' He always had a special way of looking at you when he told an outright lie; he had a funny way of staring at you, challenging you not to question his lies. He had obviously informed the newspaper because he was hungry for publicity—always hungry. It was for the good of the unit. It wasn't for him then, but he wanted Cape Town to be in the limelight.

… it was apparent that there was a very direct connection between what went on in our operating room and the Afrikaans press. It was, of course, nice for the paper to be able to write about good things coming out of South Africa, even for local consumption, rather than the alternative—endless political and racial conflict. The critical other component was the consuming hunger for recognition that was part of Chris's complex make-up. Given all that we were doing in cardiac surgery at that time, there is no doubt in my mind that had the heart transplant never been performed, Chris would have been recognised as one of the exceptional cardiac surgeons of his generation. He understood what he had to do to gain that recognition. He had a very clear idea of his own value. He would not lecture to the students without a large attendance.

One rather bizarre episode during this period (1960) involved some experimental work in which the head and neck of a dog was transplanted onto another dog. Similar work had been carried out in the USSR by Moscow experimental surgeon, Vladimir Demikhov, who had received some international publicity; thus, Chris duplicated it in the laboratory. He must have become intrigued by this surgical *tour de force*, even though it would have been of no direct value to patients either then or even today. Although of some physiological and scientific interest, it was clearly a controversial experiment. It brought Barnard and his co-researchers some local publicity, but also considerable criticism. Indeed, the press reports raised a storm of protest and criticism from animal welfare societies and animal lovers. Chris realised that he had gone too far and terminated the experiment. On this occasion, the publicity was less welcome to Chris than usual, though perhaps he believed that any publicity is better than none.

John Terblanche recollected that he and Chris had performed several successful auxiliary head grafts on dogs and published a paper in a local medical journal. They included a picture of one of their successful 'two-headed' dogs; it was this that was picked up by the local press. Terblanche believed that this was Chris's first experience of bad press publicity, but 'he went on to continue flirting with the press' whereas Terblanche had learned his lesson and subsequently avoided press publicity for medical advances.

Other members of the staff of UCT became disillusioned with Chris over this research. One colleague, physician Peter Jackson, went so far as to say he thought 'this sort of cruelty' to be 'criminal'. It appeared to him that UCT did not have an ethical committee to oversee such research at that time.

Professor Louw had a placard placed in the laboratory that read, 'Do not toy with the Delilah of the press', but it disappeared overnight. Chris was clearly upset and, according to Louw, 'would not speak to me for some time'.

Despite the South African government's claim that Nelson Mandela (who was not yet imprisoned on Robben Island) and the African National Congress (ANC) were backed by communists, Chris visited Demikhov in Moscow to learn more of his work, particularly on organ transplantation. He found Demikhov's facilities very inadequate, but was impressed by the Russian surgeon's vision. If Demikhov could be so innovative in Moscow, he asked himself why he could not do even better in Cape Town, where his facilities were so much better.

## Reasons for the Early Success of the Open Heart Surgery Program

Chris once told me:

> I was just an average surgeon, but our strengths were the fact that we looked after our patients and didn't mind how much time we spent at the hospital. That is where the results came from, not from the fact that we did the operation particularly well. [Denton] Cooley [the Houston heart surgeon] did a valve replacement in half an hour, but I took one and a half hours to do it. But my results were better because I looked after the patient personally. When I had a patient who was sick and about whom I was worried, I couldn't do anything else because that patient was with me the whole day. I couldn't leave the patient in the hands of other people.

Chris was famous for the personal attention he gave to his patients. He would theoretically hand over the patient in the intensive care unit to the surgical resident and nurses, but would continue to supervise every aspect of care. When he felt the patient had stabilised, he would walk or drive to his office in the medical school building a few hundred yards away, but as soon as he arrived there, he would call the registrar or nurse to inquire how his patient was doing. If he were in any way worried, he would be back at the bedside within minutes to personally supervise the patient's care.

In Louw's opinion, Chris's success was due to his tremendous drive and discipline. 'He believes that champions must have a "killer instinct" and should be constantly "hungry" to remain at the top. He therefore drove himself to the extreme at all times and did not spare his registrars and nursing staff at the hospital [or] his assistants in the laboratory.' However, from Chris's perspective, there was more to it than just his concern for his patients. He admitted to me once:

> You know, I've stood at patients' beds when they died, and I've been upset with everybody around me. I feel so upset, but I realise that what I'm really upset about is that, when I write up my series of operations, I have one more mortality. It wasn't really the death of the patient—it is the ego that is hurt. I should not have had a death with this particular type of operation—I'm too good for that. When I present my series of cases now, there will be one more death. But in the end, the patient benefits from it [this attitude of the surgeon]—that's why it's not all bad. You kill yourself for your records, but at the same time you kill yourself to save the patient.

Although there is certainly some truth in this explanation, which is typical of Chris's disconcerting honesty, his opinion would not be shared by many other surgeons. Personally, a patient's death always distressed and depressed me almost entirely for that simple reason: a patient whose life I was responsible for had died—it was as simple as that; the fact that it was detrimental to my surgical results was very much a secondary consideration.

Rene Favaloro, the great Argentinian heart surgeon, who was the major pioneer of surgery for coronary artery disease (and who tragically committed suicide in 2000), summed up his attitude to the death of a patient when he said, 'a surgeon's life means assuming responsibility for the risk that accompanies his decision to operate. The deaths associated with surgery are personal and the surgeon must endure their burden as long as he lives'. Personally, I would certainly agree with this sentiment—patients who die remain in one's memory for ever.

In *Good Life, Good Death*, Chris addressed his response to a patient's death:

At such times, when the patient eventually died, I felt let down and often blamed the other members of my team for not pulling their weight. I would lie awake at night and relive those moments of defeat, searching for ways and means by which to beat death. The next morning, I would get out of bed in a state of depression, unwilling to face the day because I had lost.

Every conscientious and committed surgeon will have experienced this state of depression. Picking oneself up 'off the floor' and facing the next challenge helps in the recovery. In a later newspaper column, Chris expanded on his view that we are motivated largely by self-interest.

If you ever want to know the taste of defeat, try spending the night hard at work and then go home as the sun is rising—knowing that it was all for nothing. I believe we are all totally selfish. There is no such thing as perfect altruism. Martyrs give their lives for promise of an afterlife, heroes die for glory, do-gooders do their consciences no end of good, and even a devoted mother playing with her baby has an ulterior motive.

Although many might not agree with this possibly 'jaundiced' opinion, there is no doubt some truth in it. However, Chris was not the hard-headed, calculating surgeon he would appear to be from his statements on his self-interest as a surgeon. He showed immense compassion to his patients. Dene Friedmann remembered the great care he gave to many patients when their deaths would not reflect on his personal reputation in any way. He would often go out of his way to help patients when the only thing driving him was his compassion.

In addition, he was renowned for being loyal to his close friends and doing all he could for them when sickness afflicted them. He took great pains to obtain a drug from the USA when Dene's father was dying of lung cancer, and he persisted in treating his friend, Fritz Brink, when all the other doctors felt there was no hope of sustaining life. In the event, Mr Brink recovered and lived for several more years.

## International Recognition

Due to the demands he made on his team and on himself, and despite his tantrums, the GSH heart surgery programme grew from strength to strength, particularly in the field of children's surgery for birth defects of the heart. The results were outstanding, ranking with the best in the world. In those relatively early days of heart surgery, all the surgeons involved required a certain ingenuity and originality. New technical and post-operative problems had to be overcome by trial and error. Geographically distanced from most of the other major centres in the USA and Europe (so he could not always learn from their experience), Chris was forced more than most to demonstrate his own ingenuity, which he did successfully on numerous occasions.

Among his innovations during this time was the development and testing of a new mechanical heart valve prosthesis (to replace a diseased natural heart valve), based to some extent on the studies he had carried out in Minneapolis. This mechanical artificial valve has been variously called the 'University of Cape Town (UCT) valve' or the 'Barnard-Goosen valve', after the surgeon and his technician, who together designed and manufactured it. Louwtjie Barnard helped out by sewing a new material, 'Dacron', around several hundreds of these mechanical valves to allow Chris to implant them easily into the patient. The stitches that held the valve in place were passed through the Dacron ring. Chris's work on this prosthetic heart valve soon received international recognition, and the University of Cape Town mitral, tricuspid, and aortic valve prostheses were used with success for many years after 1962.

Manny Villafana, the entrepreneur who later introduced the very successful St. Jude prosthetic heart valve, later commented that, although Chris's UCT prosthetic heart valve was 'crude by today's standards, at its time it was one of the leading heart valves'. In 1976, Chris and his colleagues helped in the clinical evaluation of the St. Jude heart valve, which had some significant advantages over most existing heart valves. Villafana was grateful that Chris 'took time from his busy schedule and at no charge monitored a worldwide meeting on the new valve'.

Chris also designed a new operation for the rare heart abnormality known as Ebstein's anomaly. This is an abnormality of one of the heart valves, the tricuspid valve. In his first successful operation to correct this abnormality, Chris removed the abnormal valve and inserted a UCT prosthetic valve. Remarkably, this patient—the first in the world to undergo this operation and using a relatively new and, by today's standards, primitive artificial valve—remained alive almost thirty years later. This is an example of Chris Barnard's uncanny success when he introduced innovations into heart surgery. He also devised a new operation for a complex heart condition in which the positions of the two ventricles are reversed (known as transposition of the great arteries) that afflicts a small number of babies at birth, though this was soon superseded by a better technique introduced by a Canadian surgeon.

In order to keep abreast of surgical advances elsewhere, Chris made visits to heart surgery centres abroad, visiting surgeons in several centres in the

US, Europe, Australasia, and India, all funded by GSH and the government of the Western Cape. On occasions, his trips abroad extended over several weeks, one for more than three months. Bob Frater commented on Chris's frequent travels.

> He sought out overseas engagements and, in fact, travelled a lot. The travel was paid for, in those days, by the provincial authorities [the local government]. There was a proviso that you had to repay the money by working, and you paid it back at a rate of one thirty-sixth of the amount owed per month. Chris had soon accumulated enough travel that he was in hock to the Province for years to come.

The quality of the work of the unit gave Barnard early international recognition within the medical profession. Contrary to what is popularly believed, he was already recognised and well-regarded in international cardiac surgical circles (though not in other less-specialised medical circles) some years before the first heart transplant, though to the public and press he may have remained 'an unknown surgeon from South Africa.'

Donald Ross, the leading London heart surgeon at that time, recollected:

> The first time I became aware of his potential was at a meeting of the British Cardiac Society. He had already started to shine. I can't remember which year it was. He spoke on the surgical treatment of tetralogy of Fallot, one of the commonest congenital heart defects, and he clearly had the best results in the world at that time, and probably the biggest experience. I think everyone at the meeting was impressed, whether they said so or not. I'm sure I was. He had clearly made his mark.

Marius Barnard published a report with his older brother on the results the unit had achieved 'with 100 consecutive cases [of Fallot's tetralogy] and no post-operative deaths.' According to Marius, when Chris presented the paper at a medical conference in London (probably the one Donald Ross referred to), 'not only were the results questioned by jealous British cardiac surgeons, but there were even attempts to discredit him.'

Chris's reputation was now good enough for him to receive an invitation from the Albert Einstein College of Medicine in New York City to relocate there to head a new programme in open heart surgery. The facilities and funds available to him would have been greater than those he had in Cape Town. After much agonising, he decided not to accept this offer. The main factors that influenced him in making his decision appeared to be the difficulty and effort of establishing a new program, concern about litigation against doctors that was increasing in the US (whereas he never took out any insurance against being sued in South Africa where litigation at that time was rare), and his hope that he could push his daughter to the pinnacle of success as a water skier, which he thought would be difficult in New York. Professors Schrire and Louw played a part in persuading him to stay. The position in New York was eventually offered to, and accepted by, Chris's colleague, Bob Frater. Frater remembered this period at GSH.

> I had a strange relationship with Chris. I was ambitious and anxious to do things. I got three referrals (of patients) from outside of South Africa. Chris was very upset with that. He went to the professor of surgery and asked him to pronounce that, in the future, referrals from outside must all be referred to the chief of the department [i.e. to Barnard himself]. That was an ominous sign that Chris didn't really want any success on the part of his colleagues. I was the only guy doing independent cardiac surgery besides him, you see.
>
> The time came, eventually, when I accepted an offer to go back to America. In fact, Chris had looked at the job and had been offered it himself. His excuse for declining was that he owed too much to the Province to be able to afford to leave Cape Town. But I suspect that he knew that it would be extraordinarily difficult to duplicate what he had in Cape Town anywhere else in the world. I believe he gave my name to the people that he had been negotiating with, and so I ultimately had to tell Chris that I had accepted the offer. He said, 'How could you do this to me? Don't you know that I have arthritis—look at my hands. I won't be operating in another six months, and then what shall I do if you leave?' Nevertheless, we parted amicably—and Chris operated for another eighteen years.

After only three years in Cape Town, in 1964, Frater returned to the US, where he had a very successful career in New York City.

Despite this growing international recognition, Chris felt he was underappreciated at home. At one point, he was bitterly disappointed that he had not been promoted to associate professor at UCT, initially blaming Professor Louw, but then, according to Louw, turning 'his wrath on the university authorities for not appreciating him, and never forgave them for what he considered unfair treatment'. Whether there was some reluctance on the part of the UCT authorities to promote him or whether Chris expected promotion too rapidly is uncertain.

## Family Life

Chris's return from the USA (in mid-1958) was not initially auspicious, with his wife remaining convinced that he had been having an affair in Minneapolis. She greeted him coldly, questioning why he had bothered to return. Perhaps, Chris thought to himself, he had made a dreadful mistake in not accepting Wangensteen's job offer and, we might add, remaining with his girlfriend in Minneapolis.

The first few days after his return, Louwtjie wrote 'were like a charade. He treated us as if we were an unwanted responsibility. Although he behaved towards me like a husband, he seemed to live in another world. We were not part of that other world. He looked disturbed at times. Chris had something on his mind—a woman?'

It could, of course, have been that as he had been charged with setting-up a new heart surgery unit—a truly major undertaking in those very early days—he was distracted from his family by his new responsibilities.

Relations between Chris and his wife improved, however, when, not long after his return from Minneapolis (just ten days before he carried out the first successful open heart operation in Cape Town) his father died from cancer at the age of eighty-three. Adam and his wife had retired to Knysna, a small town near his birthplace in a quiet pastoral region on the south coast of South Africa. Although Chris hurried there when called, he did not arrive before his father's death.

He was racked with guilt, realising that he had always put his own interests first, and had 'failed my father in many ways'. He admitted that, long before his father's death, he (Chris) 'had practically disappeared from his life'. All his father had asked of him was 'a little time, a few words. Yet even this I had not given—nor had our children'. His father had given him so much in life, 'yet I had given him little in return—too little ... Why had I not given him more time?' He realised that he gave all he could to his patients, but his family, including Louwtjie and the children, received only 'leftovers: leftover love, leftover days and leftover nights.' He had become, 'A leftover man and a leftover husband.'

His distress was so great that he locked himself in a bedroom and wept for his father, for himself, and for all those he had failed who wanted more from him than he felt he could ever give. Chris always regretted that his father had not lived to see his son carry out the first successful open heart operation in Africa. It is not uncommon for ambitious men (myself included) to devote too much time to their work and not enough to their family. Many subsequently feel guilt. However, if given a second chance, their ambition is so strong that I suspect many would make the same choice and would again relatively 'neglect' their families. Indeed, many have admitted this to me.

At his father's funeral, held in Knysna (about 200 miles from Beaufort West) Chris was profoundly moved to see the balcony filled with the coloured people to whom his father had ministered for so many years. They stared at him without smiling. 'The preacher would soon talk about my father but nothing he could say would ever equal this—the mute presence of these coloured people who had come 200 miles to see the burial of a white minister who had loved them as he had loved his own family.'

The coloured folk carried his father's coffin to the grave. 'They said nothing. Their faces were heavy with sorrow, but there was no sound. They bore him onward, as though he was a part of them.'

Chris's brother, Dodsley, living far to the north of the country, did not attend the funeral, claiming he had been away and had not received news of their father's death until after the funeral had taken place. This led to a rift between him and Chris that was never healed, with the two brothers hardly being in contact again until Dodsley died in 1975.

Adam Barnard's death was a great loss to the Barnard family, but it brought Chris and Louwtjie closer to one another. 'Our life became more tranquil and normal,' she wrote. 'Chris stretched out a hand which was all I required. In his need, I could help him. That brought us together again.' Chris described their relationship during this period as learning 'to preserve each other's personality.'

The small family—Chris, Louwtjie, and the two children—was much like any other white family in South Africa in those days. Deirdre remembers their lives as very 'ordinary'. Chris owned two cars, though one was described as 'a beat-up 1948 Ford', the other being a Triumph sports car. Although Chris and his wife did not attend church very often, Deirdre and André were raised in the Dutch Reformed Church and given the necessary religious education. On a Sunday, their mother dressed them in smart handmade clothes to attend Sunday school. Louwtjie not only helped by making their clothes but also supplemented the family income by working as a company nurse.

Deirdre remembered having wonderful family holidays, a favourite venue being Knysna, where her grandfather had died.

I must say one thing about my parents. During their time together they didn't have much money but even so, they managed to give us some wonderful holidays. It was simple stuff but it was the most amazing fun. We stayed at Hentie's Botel. It was a very 'family' kind of place with family entertainment in the evening, and part of the entertainment was to put on a concert.

My father liked to play the role of a doctor with a patient all covered up. He did it in silhouette. He stood behind a white sheet with a light shining down on him, so all the audience could see was the shadow play. He would ask for his 'instruments' and an assistant would pass him a huge spanner or a hammer, the most enormous tools, and all the while a narrator would be doing a funny voice-over. I suppose it was, in its way, grotesque—a parody of all that was to come—but I sat there, a small barefoot girl, clapping and laughing along with the rest while the enormous silhouette wielded his huge, unsuitable tools over his invisible patient. Grand Guignol, I suppose it was the kind of theatre that makes you laugh even as it makes you the slightest bit scared.

She also remembered how Chris loved being 'Father Christmas' (or Santa Claus, as he is better known in many parts of the world).

One Christmas when I was a child and we were down at Buffels Bay for the holidays, we decided to extend our wonderful Christmas to others. That year my father had been given a gift of a huge quantity of sweets (candy) from a grateful patient who must have owned a sweet factory somewhere. We decided we'd take the sweets, drive into the surrounding area where there are some very poor people staying in the bush, and give our sweets to their children so they could have something special for Christmas as well. No-one knows how to make moments of magic, except maybe my Dad and David Copperfield [referring to the great American magician]. These Christmases must have made a big impact on my father because when his third family came apart it was something he missed very much. His biggest wish was to go to their house and be Father Christmas again.

Years later, during Chris's third marriage to Karin, when he was already in his seventies, for the benefit of his two little children, Armin and Lara, Deirdre's husband, Kobus, was pressed into being 'Father Christmas', wearing the entire costume, boots, beard, and face mask. He was a big hit with the children, and Chris was very happy that they had enjoyed it so much. He could not stop talking about the look of wonder and surprise on the children's faces. Christmas with children meant a great deal to him.

## Deirdre and Water Skiing

It was during one of their vacations at Hentie's Botel in Knysna that Chris and Louwtjie became aware of their daughter's natural ability as a water skier. The hotel owner and several of the guests commented on her skills in this respect. Although at first not taking their comments very seriously, and initially knowing almost nothing about the sport, a year or so later, Chris took on the role of her coach with great enthusiasm and commitment.

Many writers have drawn attention to his determination to see Deirdre's success as a reflection of his own wish to excel. Although his own sporting achievements were very much local ones (in Beaufort West, for example), he had a natural aptitude for most sports though he had never had serious coaching or the opportunity to develop this aptitude. He threw himself into training Deirdre with relentless—at times, almost ruthless—determination, and she responded as only a natural athlete can: by steadily improving.

Chris described this period as having 'wonderful times with my family', with children who were 'delightful'. When he realised Deirdre's potential as a water skier, he devoted all of his spare time to training her, time that otherwise he would have devoted to his clinical or laboratory work. In March 1961, he had a boat made, which he christened the *Louwtjie*, and bought a 45-horsepower outboard engine to pull his daughter (then aged twelve) across the water. Later, when the demands of Deirdre's training increased, a gift from the family of a grateful patient enabled him to purchase a more powerful boat to which Chris gave a 'cardiological' name, the *Pacemaker*. Deirdre captured his heart.

> [I spent every] minute away from the hospital either on the road heading for the water with Deirdre by my side and the boat on the trailer, or actually out there doing tricks-slalom-ramp, tricks-slalom-ramp. Sometimes the waves were so high we could hardly get the boat into the water. Sometimes my arthritis pained me so much I could barely lift the sandbags needed to set the boat deeper and so create a larger wake for tricks. Deirdre was always willing, always laughing—and always a delight. By this time, I was wholly waterborne. When she flew across the water, I was with her.

At the age of twelve, Deirdre easily won all of the events at her local club and, in the regional (Western Province) championships she again won everything (Figure 6.iv). Quite remarkably, at the same age, she won the South African senior women's title, and was awarded her national (Springbok) colours, the youngest girl ever to be so honoured.

Based on this performance, Deirdre was selected to represent South Africa at the Junior European Championships in Spain (before South Africa had been banned from entering international sporting events), and Chris was appointed team manager. In her first foreign competition, she placed second, and so was selected for the world championships that were to take place in France. Not surprisingly for such a relative novice aged only thirteen, she was outclassed there. In 1964, she again won all three events in the South African championships and was selected for the European championships in Italy, placing third in tricks, second in slalom, and fifth in ramp. Chris found it amusing when people in Cape Town began to speak of him as 'Deirdre Barnard's father'. His drive and ambition for himself as well as for his daughter are reflected in his comment that 'somebody in the family, at least, was going to make it'.

To increase her prospects of success and facilitate their arduous training program, he and Louwtjie purchased a modest cottage as their home, called The Moorings, adjacent to a beautiful lake, Zeekoevlei (Hippopotamus Lake) 10 miles or so from GSH, which was ideal for the purpose. Due to his peripatetic life until that point, they had lived in no fewer than sixteen homes previously, but this cottage became their home for a number of years—probably the best years of Chris and Louwtjie's rather rocky marriage (Figure 6.v). The purchase was only possible because Louwtjie's father had loaned them money on the understanding that the sum would be deducted from her inheritance. After Chris's second marriage, his new wife's father paid for another, much grander house.

In her memoirs, Louwtjie later wrote:

> Our house was ideally situated near the water which made practicing no problem. Chris attacked Deirdre's training with the same enthusiasm with which he approached his own career. All of us were thrilled with her progress, and the interest Chris was showing in her. André [their son], although completely ignored by Chris most of the time, was never jealous of his sister's place in her father's heart. He, too, was grateful that the tension had left our lives to be replaced by this shared happiness. It was in this house that we spent some of our happiest married years. We were very happy here, and it was from the quiet surroundings of this lovely little home that Chris went out to perform the first human heart transplant.

Although living at Zeekoevlei was much less convenient for Chris, who now had a longer commute to GSH every day, and for his children, who had longer commutes to their respective schools, the house was, of course, much more convenient for Deirdre's training.

Chris dedicated many long hours encouraging Deirdre, offering advice, and helping her practice. In early mornings (usually before 6 a.m. and often before dawn), he would drive the launch that pulled her across the water of the lake. A second training session followed in the evenings. Perhaps more than anything, he tried to impart to her his own will to succeed, a quality that he had in abundance, which had been fortified by his mother's urging. Although the 'drive' to succeed came to some extent from Chris, Deirdre herself was equally motivated and pleased with her progress, and recognised that she also liked to be an 'achiever'.

When many years later I invited Nick Enslin, a friend of the Barnard family during this period, to write his recollections of Chris, he described an incident that he believed demonstrated two of Chris's very strong characteristics, namely determination and a refusal to admit defeat under any circumstances. By this time (1965), Chris had become the chairman of the national water ski committee for the year. Chris and Enslin were part of a team that was preparing the Zeekoevlei lake for the South African water ski championships that were to take place on the following day. A set of buoys attached to heavy cement bricks and a knotted measuring rope had to be lowered into the water at exactly the correct places. The national chairman of the South African water ski association had come from Johannesburg to ensure that the slalom course was set out correctly.

The weather was atrocious and, although they were in wet suits, they were all bitterly cold. The first attempt to lay the buoys accurately failed, as did the second. Enslin wrote:

> Harry, who was still manning the boat, had crawled under the bows for protection from the rain and was trying to light a cigarette with shaking hands. Van, young and strong as he was, was almost crying with wet misery, and I looked across at Chris, wondering whether he would decide to call it a day in view of the appalling conditions. But I should have known better! He was already returning to the beginning for yet another try. His teeth were chattering like castanets and his hands could hardly grip the ropes, but there was no sign of capitulation. I could only follow him, my vision of a comforting hot bath and hot toddy fading rapidly.
>
> Harry flatly refused to get back in the boat as he was chilled to the bone, and Van also decided that he was well on the way to pneumonia. They walked up to the house together, leaving Chris and myself to make the third and hopefully final attack on the course. By this time the curtain of rain sweeping across the darkening sky made visibility very poor, but he carried on with the job with incredible determination and a complete disregard for the acute physical discomfort he must have been suffering. I realised then that he never gave up, whatever he tackled, for he possessed that extra force that transcended mere physical strength— as future events in his life were to prove.

Chris's involvement in, and commitment to, water skiing was much greater than most coaches would anticipate. At times, he was appointed team manager for the South African national team and accompanied them to international championships abroad. On occasions, he also acted as a judge at competitions. These were major commitments of his precious time, already stretched by the demands of his hospital work.

Deirdre's training steadily became more intense. Chris refused all social engagements and any activity (apart from his work) that distracted him from driving her towards becoming world champion, which was his goal. At home, they would talk of nothing else. However, the pressure he put on her—in addition to her own undoubted wish to excel—at times began to strain their relationship. They would argue 'and she cried and we would not speak for days—even while training'. Her mother suggested that the lake was made up entirely of Deirdre's tears.

In Australia in 1965, when she would have been fifteen, Deirdre came second in slalom, second in jump, and fifth in tricks, which gave her a ranking of second in the world, a magnificent achievement of which she remains rightfully proud. In March 1966, she won the Victorian State Championships in Australia, jumping a distance greater than anyone before her, though it was not recognised as a world record because this was not a world-recognised competition.

Chris was clearly very proud of Deirdre's achievements. During my brief visit to GSH in 1965, Deirdre came to the hospital after a day at school for Chris to drive her home. He introduced her to me and told me of her sporting prowess. She came across as a cheerful, almost 'bubbly' schoolgirl, and it was difficult for me to believe that this young girl had achieved so much in her chosen sport. I remember being very impressed.

Chris bathed in the publicity Deirdre received in South Africa, but he realised even then that his young son, André, began to suffer from a sense of exclusion. Chris made some effort to support André by helping him train for soccer and, whenever possible, attending his games, where he would run along the touchline encouraging his son as much as possible. However, the highly talented Deirdre still absorbed most of his spare time.

Despite Deirdre's immense success, Chris began to despair that she would ever be world champion. He knew she had the natural ability, but feared she did not have the essential drive and discipline. He thought he could make up for any she lacked, and tried to transfer his drive to her, but came to realise that he was failing in this regard. He commented that 'champions were hungry people' and that you could not transfer that hunger to them. In his opinion, she did not have the 'killer instinct', the 'ruthlessness' that he felt was required.

[She was] too nice a girl ... She would be beaten and laugh about it ... She would cry if she saw an overloaded donkey or a coloured child alone in the street. If I shouted at her, she would cry, too. But if she lost, she would laugh it off ... This caused me to drive her even harder, trying to instil something of myself into her own personality. Inevitably, this caused bitter moments on the lake.

Chris could be very impatient, criticising Deirdre if she did not do well by telling her that she did not listen to him. There were times when, if he was upset with her performance in training, he would leave her in the middle of the lake, and drive his boat to the bank and tell her she had to swim back. Usually others went out in boats to pick her up.

The strain began to tell on Deirdre. On at least one occasion, her frustration (and perhaps even resentment) with the continual pressure he exerted, made her fight back. She was once driving the boat pulling her father around the lake, simply as he wanted some exercise and relaxation. Chris wanted to do just one circuit of the lake, but Deirdre took him round repeatedly until he was close to collapse. He wrote:

> I kept signalling her to return to the shore, but this only sent her back out into the middle of the lake. Finally, I let go of the line, and she left me there ... Everyone at the water ski club thought it very funny: The slave had turned on his master. I knew it was not at all like Deirdre, and I should have taken it as a warning.

## Thoughts Turn to Heart Transplantation

By the early 1960s, Barnard's surgical group, having by this time carried out approximately 1,000 open heart operations, had developed sufficient expertise for Chris to give active thought to the possibility of heart transplantation. A small but increasing volume of experimental work pertaining to this topic was being performed elsewhere, notably in California by Norman Shumway and his colleagues at Stanford University. The published results of his experimental studies, and those from a handful of other centres, as well as developments in the field of human kidney transplantation, were available to Chris, as they were to surgeons the world over.

At about this time, in March 1963—a little less than five years before the first heart transplant was performed—he had been invited to lecture to the students at the University of Pretoria on the past, present, and future of heart surgery. While thinking what he would say, it occurred to him that nothing less than a heart transplant would be required for the treatment of patients whose heart muscle was irretrievably damaged. He decided to carry out some heart transplants in dogs, and also to prepare his team for a programme of heart transplantation in patients. Indeed, he filmed one of his early dog transplants and showed it when he lectured in Pretoria.

Although he could not remember exactly when, American heart surgeon John Kirklin remembered having a long discussion with Chris in a bar at a medical congress in the US. 'He told me that he was thinking of starting to do heart transplants. Although his hands looked fine to me, he said that he was developing arthritis in them and he was anxious to accomplish something really useful while he could still operate.

I have already recounted my own experience with Chris during my visit to GSH in mid-1965 when he surprised me by telling me that one of his patients needed 'a new heart'. Although he did not mention this to me, by this time, he must have carried out his early experimental studies in dogs.

Preparation for the first heart transplant in a patient required animal experimentation (primarily to practice the operative technique) and learning how to deal with the rejection that would almost certainly develop and which, if not treated successfully, would destroy the heart graft. Chris began his preparation by performing the operation in dogs, though Marius claims that he (Marius) carried out most of these procedures. Practicing the operation in dogs was not particularly difficult for someone with Chris's surgical experience. To understand rejection and its prevention and treatment, Chris wisely decided to learn from the kidney transplant pioneers who had been treating patients for several years, though often not very successfully.

Therefore, his own planning for the first human-to-human heart transplant was careful and methodical. Suffice it to say, the first human heart transplant was no spur-of-the-moment, rush-of-blood-to-the-head event, as it subsequently appears to have been in several other centres worldwide.

Let us take a brief break in the story of Chris Barnard to ascertain what experimental progress had been made by others in the transplantation of the heart by the mid-1960s when Chris began to prepare for the world's first heart transplant.

# 7

# Prelude to the First Heart Transplant

As we have seen, the development of open heart surgery in the 1950s was one of the great advances in medicine in the twentieth century. Organ transplantation followed as an equally important development. The first successful heart transplant epitomised both of these great surgical advances, at least in the public eye, and therefore represents a defining moment in surgery in the twentieth century.

By the mid-1960s, surgery had developed so that it could deal with most of the conditions that afflicted the heart, even though surgery for coronary artery disease was only just beginning. The one condition that remained untreatable was when the heart muscle had been so damaged by multiple 'heart attacks' due to coronary artery disease or following a viral infection (or sometimes from an unknown cause) that it could no longer beat strongly enough to support the circulation of blood, resulting in what we know as 'heart failure'.

By this time, a patient with kidney failure could be kept alive by frequent use of the artificial kidney (dialysis machine). No such alternative as dialysis or a truly successful mechanical heart or ventricular assist device was yet available to patients with advanced heart failure. It seemed to a handful of surgeons that this condition could only be treated effectively by actually replacing the heart. These surgeons therefore began to take an interest in the possibilities offered by heart transplantation, despite the mixed results hitherto associated with kidney transplantation. To most surgeons and cardiologists at that time, however, this suggestion garnered little support or enthusiasm.

## First Experimental Attempts

Some of the earliest experimental work on heart transplantation was carried out in Moscow by the rather eccentric research surgeon, Vladimir

Demikhov, who had carried out the head transplants in dogs that had intrigued Chris. Since he was not popular with the Soviet hierarchy, I am told that he worked in rather poor conditions. A senior British colleague of mine who visited Demikhov in the 1960s told me the Russian's laboratory was a converted public lavatory—at least, that is what it looked like. Nevertheless, he carried out some ingenious transplant operations in dogs.

For example, he designed twenty-four different techniques for transplanting an auxiliary heart, sometimes with an attached lung, into the chest. He carried out the first replacement of the native dog heart with a donor heart (i.e. what is known as an orthotopic heart transplant) on 25 December 1951, without the use of the heart-lung machine, a technically very challenging—almost impossible—procedure (unless deep hypothermia was used). The fact that this experiment was carried out in his laboratory on Christmas Day maybe tells us something about this remarkable man, despite the reduced interest in Christian holidays in the Soviet Union at that time.

Among his many other ingenious investigations, he explored the cross-circulation technique (in which the blood circulation of a small dog was sustained by that of a large dog), a very similar technique to that used in patients by the Minneapolis group (Chapter 4), although they were almost certainly totally unaware of each other's studies.

Many years later, I had the good fortune to meet Professor Demikhov personally, when he was honoured by the International Society for Heart and Lung Transplantation. Unfortunately, his complete lack of English and my complete lack of Russian prevented direct communication, although we were able to have some discussion through his charming, bilingual daughter, who was herself a physician.

With the availability of the heart-lung machine, the technical aspects of the operation of heart transplantation were soon worked out. The operation proved relatively straightforward for a competent heart surgeon (Figure 7.i), and indeed the technique (later used by Barnard and others) had first been described in the experimental laboratory in dogs by Russell Brock and a junior colleague at Guy's Hospital in London in 1959. Just as with kidney transplantation, it was preventing rejection that was the major hurdle that needed to be surmounted; this proved difficult to achieve.

These early studies were followed by experimental work by Norman Shumway in California, James Hardy in Mississippi, and a handful of others. The first systematic studies were those of Shumway and his junior colleague, Richard Lower, at Stanford University, which they began in 1959. These men can be considered Barnard's chief competitors and rivals, all working towards performing the world's first heart transplant, and so a brief look at their backgrounds and personalities is warranted.

# Norman Shumway: 'Laid Back' Persistence

Sir Peter Morris, formerly professor of surgery at Oxford University, described Shumway as 'the quiet pioneer of cardiac transplantation'. By this, he implied that, although Shumway did not receive the immense publicity and public adulation that Barnard achieved, those of us in the medical profession acknowledged Shumway's major contributions to the development of heart transplantation over a long period of time.

Norman Shumway (Figure 7.ii) is recognised within the medical community as the 'father' of heart transplantation. Although James Hardy and Christiaan Barnard both performed this operation in patients before Shumway, it was largely through his experimental studies that the feasibility of the operation became accepted. His group perfected the operative technique and demonstrated that the immunosuppressive drugs available at the time could prolong heart graft survival and reverse an acute rejection episode. Furthermore, they demonstrated that a healthy heart 'autograft' (i.e. removed and replaced in the same animal so that rejection would not be a factor) would work well for years, indicating that division of the nerve supply to the heart did not prevent regular contractions and function.

Shumway died in 2006, aged eighty-three. I had known of him and his work since the mid-1960s, and heard him lecture on many occasions subsequently. I met him informally at meetings of the International Society for Heart and Lung Transplantation of which he was honorary lifetime President. Subsequently, through our common interest in heart transplantation, I came to know him as a friend.

Shumway was a little above medium height and tended to be rather on the thin side. He had a receding chin, which was particularly noticeable when he laughed or smiled because his upper teeth were prominent compared with his lower, with the receding chin disappearing into a wrinkled neck. Whenever I spoke with him, he was his usual casual, pleasant self. Every now and then, a flash of his humour would creep in.

Neither in appearance nor style did Shumway give you the impression of being a surgical 'heavyweight', yet he achieved an immense amount in his professional career. His explanation that success was to some extent due to the luck of having good young surgeons and researchers around him may well be true, but he clearly had the ability to attract these men and women and to allow them to fulfil themselves, rather like Wangensteen and Lillehei in Minneapolis.

In this respect, he (unknowingly) followed the tongue-in-cheek advice of Keith Reemtsma, the chairman of surgery at Columbia-Presbyterian Hospital in New York. Reemtsma advised appointing as many bright young surgeons to your department as you could, provide them with the facilities to carry out their studies, and then 'steal their results and slides and give talks around the world using their data'. Shumway did not exactly do this, but several of his *protégés* told me that he virtually never wrote an academic or scientific paper himself, relying on his very able junior colleagues to do this, and then just giving his approval of the final manuscript. This was in stark contrast to surgeon-scientists like kidney and liver transplant pioneer, Tom Starzl, who wrote many of his group's manuscripts personally, despite crediting a junior colleague with 'first authorship'. Remarkably, Starzl published more than 2,000 medical and scientific papers and chapters in his lifetime.

Shumway was a very 'laid back' character, always seemingly relaxed, unworried, and irreverently, even cynically, humorous. One did not get the impression of a person who was 'driven' as one does with some of the other surgeons whose achievements are discussed in this book, such as Barnard, Hume, Calne, and Starzl (Chapter 8). His relaxed, casual manner, however, disguised an immense determination to achieve his goals. If it did not, he would not have achieved the medical advances that he did. Additionally, like Barnard, Hume, Calne, and Starzl, he was no respecter of authority, having frequently gone his own way in opposition to those above him—possibly only in this way were they able to achieve the breakthroughs that they did. In Shumway's case, outward appearances were very deceptive.

Examples of his humour (often dark) abound. For example, 'The Aztecs and Incas were the first to perform heart transplantation—at least, the donor operation.' Referring to the need for organs for transplantation from deceased humans, he would say, 'Where there's death, there's hope.'

The most glaring example of his black humour was perhaps his comments when he gave a presentation at a meeting in Minneapolis in 1988 celebrating the pioneering heart surgery of Walt Lillehei. It was well-known to the audience that Lillehei had, late in his career, been in serious trouble with the Internal Revenue Service (IRS) about unpaid taxes (Chapter 5). His trial in St. Paul-Minneapolis had been a showcase trial for the IRS, went on for several weeks, and received widespread publicity. Most of Lillehei's colleagues believed that his problems had largely been the result of the disorganization of his personal affairs rather than from any criminal intent. Nevertheless, he had been heavily fined and compelled to do many hours of community service, and was perhaps fortunate to have avoided a prison sentence. The trial put the last nail in the coffin of his active surgical career. To some extent, therefore, the 1988 meeting had been arranged by Lillehei's admirers as a means of 'rehabilitating' his reputation, which had suffered as a result of his personal problems, not least of which was the trial.

In his presentation, Shumway referred to the fact that many patients had died in the early days of open heart surgery. Then, with Dr Lillehei and those who had come to honour him in the audience, Shumway added that Lillehei in many ways reminded him of Al Capone (the notorious Chicago gangster who was responsible for the deaths of many of his criminal competitors and some police, but who was finally imprisoned on a charge of tax evasion). Looking at Dr Lillehei, he said, 'Like Al Capone, you killed a lot of people [referring to the high death rate associated with the early attempts at open heart surgery], but the government could only get you on unpaid taxes.' Although a wonderful example of black humour, to equate Dr Lillehei with Al Capone was probably not the most tactful comparison to make, particularly on such an occasion—but that was Norman Shumway.

Several times I had broached the subject of an interview with him when writing my earlier book, *Open Heart*. On each occasion, he expressed interest in the book, but courteously and casually declined my invitation. I wondered why he was so reluctant to participate in this small project. It could have been humility or shyness, of course, though heart surgeons are not generally noted for a lack of ego or a wish to avoid the limelight. I considered my close association with Chris Barnard, with whom I had worked for several years, might be the problem. In the eyes of many Americans, including many of Shumway's supporters and *protégés*, Chris Barnard had 'jumped the gun' when he performed the first transplant in a patient. The implication was that, if Barnard had been a decent and honourable man, he would have left it to Shumway, who had done so much of the background experimental work.

There is no doubt that, in the mid-1960s, we all anticipated Shumway's group would be the first to perform this operation in a human (with the exception of the unusual operation already performed by Dr Hardy in 1964—see below). After all, there were very few other groups seriously interested in this field. I remember attending the first International Congress of the Transplantation Society in Paris in the summer of 1967 at which I heard Shumway announce that his group was ready to go ahead with a heart transplant in a patient. However, in medicine, as in most other fields of life, competition is rife. One has to be on one's toes since others are likely to beat one to the post. Such was the case with Chris Barnard who pipped the front-runner, Norman Shumway, to the post. Shumway performed his first heart transplant—the world's fourth—in a patient on 6 January 1968, more than a month after Barnard's first attempt, and even a few days after Barnard's second attempt.

In response to criticism in this respect, Chris pointed out that Shumway's group had published all of their experimental studies in surgical journals, presumably for the benefit of other physicians and surgeons. If Shumway and his colleagues had not wished others to use the information they had provided, then presumably the data would not have been published. Those, such as himself (Barnard), who built on the background provided by these studies, should therefore not be criticised.

Whether this rivalry was a factor in Shumway's early reluctance to discuss his career with me is uncertain. I suspect, however, that it was not the only factor since I know he was also reluctant to agree to interviews with several professional authors and journalists who were compiling books or articles on heart transplantation. Perhaps learning from Barnard's experience, Shumway was not keen on too much publicity. Eventually, however, he kindly agreed to speak with me.

Many years earlier, when I had interviewed Walt Lillehei for another book I was putting together, he had commented that he believed Barnard had the necessary 'courage' to take that first step, whereas he doubted that Shumway did. As Lillehei had had a hand in the training of both of these men, his opinion has to be considered seriously. Although there may be some truth in it, I find it an oversimplification of the situation. It may have been that Chris, isolated as he was at the southern tip of Africa, did not have the local pressures on him that might have made him unduly cautious in this respect. Shumway was arguably working in a more critical and adverse environment, particularly in regard to the medico-legal consequences of a new operation. Medico-legal insurance was not required in South Africa at the time and, to my knowledge, Chris was never sued by a patient.

In any case, the outcome was that Chris 'broke the tape' ahead of Shumway. Despite this fact, and despite Chris's remarkably good initial results and the further contributions he made to the field, Shumway is arguably considered the major pioneer in the field of heart transplantation.

Shumway's light-hearted manner and humour gave you the impression that he was not a great intellectual, and this may be so, but he was clearly very intelligent. When established as a heart surgeon, he was one of relatively few surgeons in his day who devoted much of his time to assisting (and teaching) his trainees in the operating room. He would encourage them by comments such as, 'Isn't this fun?' Nothing seemed very serious to him. In contrast to the atmosphere in Chris's operating room, Shumway's surgical procedures were carried out in a calm and relaxed environment. He was also a man who did not bow down to the establishment very easily, and I think this was one major aspect of the success of his career.

Norman Shumway was born in Kalamazoo, Michigan, on 9 February 1923, and was therefore just a few weeks younger than Chris Barnard, though he looked older. He had one older brother who died in infancy. His father was a retail merchant, had a bakery and creamery, and also ran a little lunchroom for students. I asked Dr Shumway whether he had been a good student at high school.

'Yes,' he replied. 'I was the so-called valedictorian; the rest of the class wasn't too bright'—a typical Shumway 'throwaway' remark. He liked all sports and was also on the debate team. Initially, he had no intention of following a career in medicine. 'I was very interested in law at that time and so, when I went to college at the University of Michigan, I was a pre-law student. After only about a year, pre-law students went into the [military] service; this was 1943. After being sent to engineering school, the military decided they might need more doctors,' and so Shumway ended up at medical school at Vanderbilt University in Nashville, Tennessee.

> The War was just about over. We had one year at Vanderbilt, and they mustered us out of the service. I had to decide whether to go back to Michigan and pursue law or stay in medicine. I was beginning to be very much enthralled by medicine, and I enjoyed it. At Vanderbilt, we had a very small class of only fifty or so. We had a great collegiality and we had good teachers. So I decided I would rather stay at Vanderbilt than go back to a big school like Ann Arbor.
>
> I never finished anything but medical school. (He was ranked twelfth in the class of fifty-two.) I have no bachelor's degree at all, just an MD— and, of course, one of those phony PhDs from Minnesota.

Shumway was referring to the research degree he obtained in Minneapolis under Lewis and Wangensteen, where he felt the research requirements were not stringent enough to warrant a doctorate. As we have seen, Chris also received a PhD in Minneapolis for some of his research studies.

'I graduated and moved to Minneapolis in 1949. I had an internship and one year of residency. It was just an unbelievable stroke of luck that I got to Minnesota. The atmosphere in Minneapolis was unbelievable; it was really electric. We used to say there that you had to invent an operation to get on the operating room schedule.' He was quickly influenced by John Lewis, (Lillehei's surgical colleague) whom he subsequently always referred to as 'the great John Lewis'. Lewis was 'probably the greatest influence I ever had.'

Shumway did not have a high regard for the diminutive Wangensteen's operative skills since he later wrote that 'Wangensteen personified that old observation of Somerset Maugham (the British novelist) that mediocre man is always at his best.' However, Shumway did acknowledge that Wangensteen was a great supporter of his trainees. Richard Simmons, a surgeon who was later on the faculty in Minneapolis, told me:

Norman Shumway was a legend in Minnesota. He had a contempt for Wangensteen, which was allowed if you did it in a witty way. [After a very major operation] he once said to Wangensteen, 'That's the first time I've seen the patient removed and the cancer staying.' He never finished the residency at Minnesota, and had trouble getting his boards [certification as a fully trained surgeon] because of this. He had to finagle that after he became world famous. He was a wonderful man—straight and witty and basically modest. He was a good teacher and inspired people. He surrounded himself with good people and was able to maintain their loyalty and enjoy their success. He was a heart surgeon from the start and wasn't very interested in other kinds of surgery.

Shumway continued the story of his life.

I then had to go back into the services because I had received so much money from the government—basically my entire education—so I really owed them a couple more years. That was during the Korean War, so we're talking 1951 to 1953. I decided I had had enough of the Army— what little I had had of it, actually—and so I decided to try Air Force this time. I went into the Air Force for two years. For most of that time I was a flight surgeon in Lake Charles, Louisiana. I had just gotten married.

Then I went back to Minneapolis to finish my residency. I didn't finish the general surgery residency because I knew that general surgery wasn't going anywhere. By that time, Lewis had done the first successful open heart operation using hypothermia in September 1952. Lillehei was still working mainly in the laboratory on the cross-circulation techniques with Herb Warden and Morley Cohen, and that work was coming along pretty well. It must have been in September or October 1953, at a meeting on cardiac surgery held in Minneapolis, that Gibbon reported his successful atrial septal defect closure using his heart-lung machine. Almost everybody who was doing anything in cardiac surgery at that time was on the program. It was a very exciting, stimulating program. Everybody who was there will remember it.

Shumway later reminisced on his days in Minneapolis.

Those days of high adventure for us fortunate enough to have been there set the style for our future travels in cardiac surgery. We never panicked. We always had fun. We kept going after early failures. We learned to persevere in the face of seemingly insurmountable obstacles both medical and political.

I left Minneapolis in late 1957 (when Chris Barnard was in the middle of his time there). I went to Santa Barbara in private practice. I was in practice for six weeks ... I was sort of disenchanted with academia at that time. I wanted to stay in Minnesota, but there were a lot of people at my level like Herb and Morley who were just slightly ahead of me. Wangensteen offered me a kind of half-ass job at St. Joseph's Hospital. So I sort of rebelled and left town, as it were, in the middle of the night. But obviously, in retrospect, I could see it was a great mistake.

He ended up in San Francisco. I asked him whether, when he joined Stanford Medical School, he was interested in transplantation.

Yes. The only way I could get on the faculty there and get any kind of a stipend was to take over the artificial kidney program. The nephrologist was only available at night, and so we would run all of our patients on the old Kolff artificial kidney machine through the night. In the daytime, I would work in the laboratory. We were hoping that we could get heart surgery started.

## Richard Lower

Richard Lower (Figure 7.iii), who was six years younger than Shumway, was to become Shumway's main collaborator in research into heart transplantation; he was the resident assigned to the Stanford surgical laboratory at that time. He had a less outgoing personality than Shumway and my impression is that he was less innovative than his senior colleague. However, Lower was described by Shumway as 'a bright man, and the kind of guy you knew eventually would become an excellent surgeon'.

Lower's initial intention was to go into rural general practice, and he was at Stanford just to get two years basic training in general surgery. I asked him why he had therefore arranged to be seconded to Shumway's laboratory, which did not seem to fit in with his career plan.

It was a diversion. First of all, Shumway is a very entertaining and interesting person, and so that was probably the main attraction. Everybody was attracted to his wit and his irreverence, and his very interesting ideas on how to do things. He had been, of course, superbly trained by John Lewis and Walt Lillehei in Minnesota so he really knew his way around, both in the lab and in the clinic. And research was nice on family life too because you didn't have night-call and that sort of thing. So I traded around with some other residents who were scheduled to go to the lab.

Thus, the duo who became known locally as 'Norm and Dick' was established.

It was during this period that Shumway made his first major contribution to open heart surgery—the concept that cooling just the heart would enable the surgeon to operate inside it in a quiescent, ideal state (although this approach had been introduced earlier by surgeons in Stockholm). While the heart-lung machine pumped oxygenated blood around the body, the blood supply to the heart itself was occluded and the heart was cooled to very low temperatures of about 4°C (by continuously bathing it with cold saline or packing ice slush around it) in order to protect it from the lack of oxygen. The concept was, of course, the same as Bigelow's for cooling the entire patient, but Shumway restricted the cooling to the heart; this was innovative research at the time. Lower explained:

> Shumway was at the time working on a very important concept which was that, if you cooled the heart, you could operate in a nice, dry operating field. The operative mortality of most open heart surgery was around 50 per cent at that time, but we operated on a bunch of dogs with no deaths. Shumway's approach to myocardial [heart] cooling probably saved the lives of many more patients than did transplants.

As Shumway was not allowed to carry out open heart surgery at the Stanford Medical Center, he began doing a couple of operations each week with the surgeons at the Children's Hospital in San Francisco, using this local heart-cooling technique.

When Stanford Medical School relocated from San Francisco to Palo Alto (only about an hour's drive away), the new chairman of surgery interviewed Shumway, who was, by this time, thirty-six years old. According to Lower, 'the chairman said he would like Shumway to do the heart surgery until he could get "a really big-name surgeon". I think that's the only time I ever saw Shumway really mad. But this was an opportunity for Shumway because none of the recognised cardiac surgeons moved from San Francisco to Palo Alto with Stanford, but, of course, there also weren't very many patients.' Shumway was therefore able to establish a heart surgery programme in the treatment of patients at Stanford.

Quite remarkably, Shumway's interest in heart transplantation began almost by chance. Shumway explained to me what happened in the research laboratory:

> We would stand there for an hour with a dog supported by the oxygenator [the heart-lung machine], the aorta clamped, and the heart being cooled [in iced saline]. We [he and Lower] were both getting bored

as the dickens, so I said to Dick, 'We can take the heart out and put it in cold saline', which we were using for cooling the heart, 'and then we can stitch it back in. It will give us something to do while we're standing here for this hour's time'. Of course, we were trying to improve our surgical skills.

We started to do that. The problem we had was that we had just silk sutures at that time and there was a lot of bleeding [around the stitches where the heart had been stitched back in] and other problems. Lower said, 'Why don't we get another dog's heart, leave more of the atrial tissue on it so, as we suture, we can semi-bolster the suture line?' [The technique of implanting a donor heart is easier than replacing the native heart.] So that's how we started to do heart transplants. We'd take the heart out of one animal, and put it into another animal. To our amazement, these animals began to live. They would be jumping around the laboratory for a while. Depending on the degree of tissue incompatibility, this might be anywhere from three or four days to almost three weeks, without any immunosuppression. So that was pretty interesting. It wasn't long before it became a project.

Their first true technical success was just before Christmas in 1959, and was reported in San Francisco radio and television programmes and in the local newspapers. A week later, when the recipient dog was still alive, the story made *The New York Times*. The dog was euthanised a day later. When they first presented their work at a surgical congress, however, there were only four attendees present in the lecture room: them, the moderator (chairman), and the slide projectionist. This is not uncommon when research that is 'ahead of its time' is presented. The medical profession can be largely apathetic until the work is clearly established in clinical practice. Many doctors are very cautious—even critical—of innovations, particularly major ones. In 1960, *Time* magazine included an article about Stanford's pioneering studies and, by 1963, Shumway was quoted in the *Palo Alto Times* as saying that he hoped they would be transplanting human hearts within a decade.

Shumway and Lower found that, when they decided to give immunosuppressive drug therapy to prevent rejection of the dog heart, there was a high incidence of infectious complications. Lower noted changes in the electrocardiogram (EKG or ECG) when rejection was occurring, and so, to avoid infection, they gave the immunosuppressive drugs only at the time that EKG abnormalities developed. 'That was the only way we were able to get any long-term survivors,' said Shumway. 'Until then, we were totally unprepared to believe that heart transplantation would be clinically possible.'

It is perhaps remarkable that the 'father of heart transplantation' began research in this field because he had nothing much else to do. Shumway and Lower began these studies in 1959 and continued them throughout the early 1960s. However, long before they felt ready to carry out a heart transplant in a patient, Dr James Hardy surprised everybody by transplanting a chimpanzee heart into a dying patient in Jackson, Mississippi. Hardy's group had begun their experimental work in heart transplantation even before Shumway, but had perhaps made less progress. Nevertheless, by 1964, they considered themselves ready to attempt the operation in a patient.

## James Hardy: Two Unsuccessful Firsts

James Hardy (Figure 7.iv) had the unique distinction of being the surgeon who performed the world's first lung transplant in 1963 and the first heart transplant in 1964. His attempt at heart transplantation in 1964 has largely been forgotten in the wake of the immense publicity that surrounded Barnard's transplant in 1967. Furthermore, Barnard can still claim that he performed the first human heart transplant in that year because Hardy's attempt utilised a chimpanzee heart.

What perhaps makes Hardy's attempts even more remarkable is that they were made from his base as chairman of the department of surgery at a relatively new medical school at the University of Mississippi, and not from one of the better known academic hospitals in the US, which one generally associated with major advances in surgery in the mid-twentieth century. Although neither of his attempts was particularly successful, he was clearly a remarkable man who had a clear vision of the future of surgery.

Both operations must be viewed as 'experimental' surgery in human patients, but so are nearly all pioneering advances in surgery. The change in attitude towards such experimental surgery that has occurred in the last fifty years can be illustrated by a look at the informed consent form that Hardy used at the time of his first heart transplant. The patient was semi-comatose and not in a position to sign the form himself, and so a member of his family signed on his behalf. The consent form consisted of only one paragraph, whereas today a small book would probably be necessary to meet legal requirements to cover such a major surgical innovation. Although the consent form indicated that no previous heart transplant had been performed in a human subject, it failed to mention that the 'donor' was going to be a chimpanzee, or any other animal, for that matter. I mention this not to be critical of Hardy and his team, but purely to indicate the great change in what is considered 'informed consent' in medico-legal requirements that has taken place since that time.

Hardy was a bespectacled man of average height with a full head of hair. I met with him on several occasions over a period of fifteen years or so and always found him to be a most courteous and genuinely friendly person. I liked him very much.

Hardy was born in Newala, Alabama, on 14 May 1918, and had a twin brother. His father was a fairly successful businessman who produced lime (calcium oxide) and sold it for construction and to farmers for water purification. His mother was a teacher of Latin and a good musician, and she clearly influenced her sons in the field of education and music. By the standards of the community, the family was financially fairly well-off.

After high school in a nearby town, Hardy and his twin attended the University of Alabama in Tuscaloosa, where they received a good grounding in science in the pre-med course. They went on together to the University of Pennsylvania to complete their medical education. Hardy graduated in medicine in 1942.

> Before the War [World War Two], I actually started out as a resident in medicine [rather than surgery] at the University Hospital in Philadelphia. But then I got called into the Army, where I spent three years with the ground forces in Europe. We were heading for the Panama Canal to take part in the invasion of Japan when the captain announced that the ship was turning back as the atomic bomb had been dropped. That was about the happiest thing I ever heard. I got out in 1946, by which time I had come to realise that I wanted to do something that was more curative than what was then available for the treatment of conditions such as arthritis, leukaemia and renal failure. I wanted to go into surgery.

After surgical training at the University of Pennsylvania and three years on the faculty of the University of Tennessee Medical School in Memphis, he was appointed head of the department of surgery at a new medical school in Jackson, Mississippi.

> By this time [1955], things were moving right along in heart surgery. Dr Gibbon had turned his pump over to John Kirklin, and Lillehei and Varco were using DeWall's bubble oxygenator, which was a major contribution to heart surgery. When I arrived in Mississippi, one of the staff who I recruited was Watts Webb. Once I got to know him, I realised that he was a real jewel, and he became full-time with us. He was a pure thoracic surgeon and didn't do any general surgery. He was a fine

technical surgeon and a fine person. In 1956, it was his idea for us to get involved with heart transplantation.

Watts Webb, who I contacted, estimated that he had spent a third of his time in the research laboratory. He remembered:

> When the heart-lung machine first came into being, we started thinking about trying to transplant a heart into the chest. Our first one was an autotransplant, where we removed the heart and put it back [into the same dog]. That was the first one in the world. As I look back on it, I am just absolutely amazed at what we were able to do with what little we had. Everything was so crude. You made your own pump-oxygenators [heart-lung machines]. You were sewing with needles and thread instead of the fine curved needles that we have today. Everything was so primitive, I am just amazed that we accomplished what we did.

Hardy also had a young surgeon with him from Turkey, and the two of them started investigating lung transplantation. By about 1962, they began to consider doing a transplant in a patient. Hardy proposed this to the university administration and they agreed. He had already been doing kidney transplants in patients for some time (including the first in Mississippi), and their results were 'as good as most places at that time'.

I expressed surprise to Dr Hardy that the range of surgery he had been doing at this time included both kidney transplants and open heart surgery.

> I was trained that way. Transplantation happened to come along as I was getting through the system. We started doing kidney transplants in Mississippi because there was no dialysis in the state. Things were fairly basic then. For example, when I went there, there was only one certified anaesthesiologist and one neurosurgeon in the whole state.

## The World's First Lung Transplant

Watts Webb remembered that the administration accepted the proposal to carry out a lung transplant quite well.

> In today's environment, I'm sure they wouldn't have. In those days, you didn't have the investigative committees and those sorts of things that you have today. You could move along pretty fast, both in the experimental animal work and in the human experimentation work.

Medico-legal wasn't that important and certainly we didn't have the regulatory bodies, either local or federal.

They began to look out for suitable patients for a lung transplant. In retrospect, it is perhaps surprising that Hardy and his colleagues felt confident enough to go ahead. Although they had performed several hundred heart or lung transplants in dogs by then, and knew they were technically feasible, Webb recollected that, because the immunosuppressive drug therapy available was so poor, their dogs with transplants rarely survived longer than a week or two. They believed, however, that 'we could give patients much better post-operative care [than they could offer to dogs].' They had no doubt that, in Webb's words, 'transplantation would proceed and become a very common achievement: lung, heart, kidney, etc.'

'We finally performed a lung transplant on 11 June 1963,' Hardy told me. 'The donor came from our own emergency room, having died from a myocardial infarct [heart attack] in the emergency room. The family gave permission for use of the lung for transplant. We removed the lung and cooled it immediately, but it was probably an hour or more before we could transplant it.'

For the record, the patient was fifty-eight years old, Mr John Russell. After the operation, which was technically successful, Webb remembered feeling 'very elated—no doubt about it. We had been able to do it technically, and obviously we had never done it before in a human. The strategy and tactics of being able to get the donor and recipient together worked out amazingly well for a first attempt.'

During the operation, one of Hardy's surgical residents had to leave the operating room to go to the emergency room to attend to a black civil rights activist, Medgar Evers, who had been shot and subsequently died. Mississippi was embroiled in a similar racial discrimination fight as South Africa. When Hardy emerged from the operating room, he found that the clamour outside was not about the world's first lung transplant, but about the tragic event that had just taken place. On the following morning, the lung transplant, which might have been considered to be headline news, was relegated to the bottom of the first page in the local newspaper. Hardy continued:

> The patient lived approximately three weeks. We used azathioprine and prednisone [the two immunosuppressive drugs available at that time], and had irradiated his mediastinum [the central part of his chest in which are situated several lymph nodes containing cells that might be involved in the rejection process], for whatever that was worth. He died from renal [kidney] failure, but the transplanted lung showed very little in the way of rejection.

I asked Dr Hardy what had been the professional and public reaction to the lung transplant.

> Pretty good, as a matter of fact. There wasn't a lot of criticism. In fact, there was much interest. It so happened that the American Medical Association was meeting in New York City at that time, and so the next day I took the patient's chest X-ray to the meeting. The reaction was good.
>
> The public reaction was very favourable and very excited about the fact that we had demonstrated that it could be done. The Mississippians were very pleased just to have a 'first' in that area. The professional reaction was also really quite good. There was some reluctance, of course, and reservations that immunosuppression was going to be a problem.
>
> But over the next few weeks, there were a lot of letters to the Annals of Internal Medicine [which used to be the 'Bible' of the internists] criticising lung transplantation. Now that today everybody is doing lung transplants, I have often wondered if these fellows ever searched their consciences about what they wrote in those early days. But the criticisms were mild when contrasted to those we received after the heart transplant. We didn't get an opportunity to do another lung transplant for a couple of years.

## The World's First Heart Transplant

I then asked Dr Hardy to tell me something of the build-up towards the first heart transplant.

> We were pretty well gratified with the way the lung transplant had gone. I had been joining Dr Webb in the laboratory more frequently. We went again to the dean of the medical school, and once again laid out the situation to him and his colleagues. They said, 'It's a big move, but we will back you. Go ahead, but be careful.' I talked to a lot of other people about it who were more or less in favour of it; at least, they didn't take to the hills. But then Watts Webb decided he would accept the chair of cardiothoracic surgery at Southwestern Medical School in Dallas, and so he finally left us in about November 1963. But my colleagues and I continued doing heart transplants every day in the dog lab. We saw a number of patients for whom heart transplantation had been suggested, but we either didn't accept them or they died before we could prepare for the transplant. We got the nurses trained in the operating room and made all the preparations.

By that time, people were beginning to consider brain death as a legal definition of death. But it still wasn't generally accepted, and I had made up my mind that that was one criticism [taking a beating heart from a brain-dead subject] we were going to avoid.

Chris Barnard was to make the same decision three years later.

How did Dr Hardy come to have a chimpanzee available for the heart transplant?

We found it extremely difficult to get people to donate kidneys here in Mississippi. Most people had never heard of a transplant anyway. Keith Reemtsma was in Tulane [in New Orleans], where they had done a number of chimpanzee kidney transplants [in patients]. There was no chronic dialysis then [long-term use of the artificial kidney machine]. I went to visit him. They had two patients in the hospital at that time, one of whom was a young female schoolteacher who had had a chimpanzee kidney transplant some seven months previously. She was doing surprisingly well, and there was a man there who was also doing pretty well. So I decided that, if they can do this at Tulane, we could give it a try. After all, we had nothing else to offer. We bought four large chimpanzees, and had them available for kidney transplants. We may have gotten them from the zoo, but I don't fully recall.

In 1963, Keith Reemtsma transplanted both kidneys from six chimpanzees into six patients with kidney failure, one of whom (the schoolteacher Hardy had met) lived for nine months. Due to this experience, Reemtsma is known to many as the 'father' of xenotransplantation—the transplantation of organs from one species to another [Appendix I].

I did not ask Dr Hardy for details of the heart transplant operation as I knew these well from reading his reports in the medical literature. The patient, sixty-eight-year-old Mr Boyd Rush, a deaf-mute, was by no means an ideal candidate for a heart transplant, even by today's relatively liberal criteria. The report of this historic operation (performed on 23 January 1964) in the *Journal of the American Medical Association* describes the patient as a relatively large man 'who was in a stuporous or semi-comatose condition [of uncertain cause] and who responded only to painful stimuli [suggesting a serious brain injury, which would absolutely exclude him from a transplant today]. He had a tracheostomy and was being mechanically ventilated [to pump oxygen into his lungs].' His left leg had recently been amputated for gangrene. In other words, he was far from being a stellar candidate for the operation.

Due to his comatose state, Mr Rush's sister signed the consent form for the operation. The choice of 'donor' obviated any need to consider whether the heart could be taken from a brain-dead donor, a problem faced by Chris three years later.

The chimpanzee heart was successfully implanted, but proved too small to support the circulation of the patient, who died on the operating table. Several years later, a microscopic examination of tissue from the chimp's heart, taken after the death of the patient, was carried out by my late colleague from the University of Cape Town, Alan Rose, an experienced heart transplant pathologist. The appearances of the heart muscle suggested to him that a very rapid rejection response to the 'foreign' organ may have played a role in the failure of the graft so quickly after transplantation.

I asked Dr Hardy to tell me about the professional and public reaction to the transplant.

There wasn't so much criticism locally, but there was nationally. Editorials were written in various journals, and remarks were made at meetings. It so happened that within a week or ten days of the transplant, the [international] Transplantation Society was meeting at the Waldorf Astoria Hotel in New York City, and they called me and asked me to join a hastily organised panel on heart transplantation. Norman Shumway was on the panel and one or two others. The other members of the panel made their presentations.

When I got up to talk, the chairman, Willem Kolff [the Dutch pioneer of the artificial kidney and the artificial heart], said, 'I want to ask Dr Hardy a question before he begins. Dr Hardy, do they keep the blacks in one cage and the chimpanzees in another in the Southern states?' [referring to the bitter integration and civil rights struggle then raging in the Southern states]. That obviously didn't help, you know. [I thought this was the understatement of the year by Dr Hardy.] Anyway, I gave my presentation, reporting exactly what we had done and, at the end of it, there was not one single hand raised in applause. Not one. Afterwards, Kolff came up to me, and said, 'You realise, of course, I was joking.'

I replied, 'I didn't think you were joking, and I don't think that the worldwide audience thought you were joking either.' It was a bad day.

In Shumway's opinion, Hardy was 'an unbelievable enthusiast, but there was absolutely no evidence to suggest the damn thing would succeed. I always thought Jim was a naïve, enthusiastic, wonderful guy. I just thought it was kind of foolish. If you'll pardon the expression, we called it a "foolHardy" procedure.'

Richard Lower also felt Hardy's attempt was 'ill-conceived; it wasn't going to work at that stage of our knowledge, so why do it?' Although both Shumway and Lower were probably correct in believing that success was unlikely, we must remember that Hardy was influenced by Reemtsma's modest success. Dr Hardy continued:

> I just hunkered down and let things pass, and they finally came back to the norm. As the years passed, things got better, but I decided we weren't going to do heart transplants of any sort until Shumway or someone else did something to take the heat off of us. It wasn't that I couldn't take the criticism, but we were living off National Institutes of Health [NIH] grants at the medical school and, at about this time, the NIH became terribly suspicious of any research whatsoever on people. I knew if we did anything else that was to one side of the straight-and-narrow, we might lose our grant support, and that we couldn't afford to do.
>
> Before the transplant, I had asked people their views on heart transplantation. Most had never thought of it or heard of it. I asked people in the church. I didn't say we were considering a heart transplant, but I asked what they would think of one. I asked women more than men. What would they think if their husband had one? Then I gave a lecture in New York to a group of outstanding medical students. After a discussion period, I asked these students whether they would have a kidney transplant. Yes, they would, if they had to. Would they have a liver transplant? Finally, I got to the heart, and I have to say frankly that none of them said they would consider a heart transplant. I knew it was going to cost us, but we underestimated the reaction, which was more than I anticipated. After the transplant, my life consisted of mainly going from the house to the hospital and back to the house. And so I didn't know much of the reaction except what was in the newspapers, but I'm sure it was intense.

Did he feel that most of the criticism was related to the fact that he had used a chimpanzee heart?

> No question about that—a good bit of it was. For example, it was characterised as a monkey heart, and at one meeting a well-known Boston surgeon said, 'Hardy, every time I look at you, I think of a monkey'. But most people don't have any realization that the genetic composition of the chimpanzee is about 98 per cent of that of a human being, and a baboon considerably less than that and, of course, a monkey off the scale. But as far as they were concerned, all lower primates are the same. I don't think Keith Reemtsma got similar criticism—at least, I didn't hear that much of it. In the first place, to many, the heart was almost the seat of the soul. Certain religious people felt that it just shouldn't have been

touched. It was loaded with difficult problems. I think that using the chimp was certainly part of it, but doing it at all was so far from what people could imagine and accept that it just took years for it to sink in.

Had the controversy affected his career in Mississippi?

'No, it didn't. Of course, I was already chairman, and subsequently I received every honour in Mississippi they could ever give me, and nationally too. So it really didn't. I was surprised. But I was tainted for a while.'

I asked whether he had received any reaction from Norman Shumway to the heart transplant.

'No. On this panel that I mentioned at the Waldorf, just days after we had done the transplant, Norman, who had done the best work in the laboratory, said some nice things. I don't know what he really thought. He probably thought I shouldn't have done it but, nonetheless, he wasn't openly critical.'

Interestingly, in his two autobiographies (*The World of Surgery, 1945– 1985* and *The Academic Surgeon*), Hardy noted, 'When I travelled to Europe, I found that our heart transplant was known everywhere, and instead of all the carping and criticism going on in the United States, many surgical scientists in Europe simply wanted to know why we had not gone right ahead with another one. The answer was that Dean Marston [the dean of the medical school] could protect me just so far; beyond that, the opposition might well force the loss of my academic post.'

However, the controversy over the chimpanzee heart transplant clearly did not hinder Hardy's contributions to medicine in Mississippi. It also did not prevent his rise in the establishment of American surgery. At one time or another, he became president of most of the major surgical societies in the US, including the American College of Surgeons, and many elsewhere.

Not every medical society, however, was prepared to recognise Hardy's efforts to push forward the frontiers of surgery. In the last few years of his life, I personally tried on several occasions to persuade the Board of Directors of the International Society for Heart and Lung Transplantation to recognise Hardy's vision and pioneering efforts. I had in mind at least a statement, possibly in the form of a scroll or plaque, recognising his early work. I am sure this would have given pleasure to him as he neared the end of his life. Sadly, my approaches were to no avail. Even though his efforts had not met with success, I believed that his vision for the future of both lung and heart transplantation deserved the Society's recognition. I was disappointed and, frankly, incredulous that the members of the Board could be so small-minded and mean-spirited. It seems that Marius Barnard agreed that Hardy deserved recognition for his vision. In his memoirs, he wrote:

Whenever I spoke about the first human heart transplant during my talks, I always gave Dr Hardy the recognition I believe he deserved for his courageous attempt to save his patient despite the known risks and the small chance of success. For this, he expressed his great appreciation. So, although we [i.e. the Cape Town team] were projected as brave people who took such bold steps in history, it was a myth: such an operation had already been done before, albeit with a non-human heart donor. If anybody was brave, it was Dr Hardy.

However, Hardy was not the only pioneer the Board of Directors was mealy-mouthed about. Despite my urging over several years, it was not until 2000—almost thirty-three years after his first heart transplant and little more than a year before his death—that its members belatedly agreed to acknowledge Chris Barnard's contributions by inviting him to speak at the Society's annual congress. Ironically, by then, Chris's poor health did not allow him to attend, and I gave the presentation on his behalf. Dr Shumway, who was in the audience, kindly came up to me afterwards and commented on the obvious affection and regard I had for Chris.

Despite Hardy's early vision and enthusiasm, after Chris's first human heart transplant, Hardy and his team played little part in the future development of heart (or lung) transplantation.

## Another Contender: Adrian Kantrowitz

There were very few other groups seriously exploring heart transplantation in the research laboratory in mid-1960s. The only other surgeon with pretensions to take the technique into the treatment of patients was Adrian Kantrowitz (Figure 7.v), who headed the heart surgery programme at a relatively little-known community hospital in Brooklyn, New York: Maimonides Hospital. Kantrowitz, four years older than Shumway and Barnard, was a big man (six feet two inches, weighing 250 pounds) with a big personality. This had enabled him to develop a loyal and enthusiastic team around him, but also generated considerable opposition from some of his colleagues.

Kantrowitz's Jewish parents had immigrated to the US from Eastern Europe and settled in New York City, with his father becoming a successful doctor. The young Adrian had graduated from the Long Island College of Medicine in 1943, became a battalion surgeon in Europe towards the end of the Second World War, and eventually became chair of cardiac surgery at Maimonides in 1955.

With a very substantial grant from the US National Institutes of Health (NIH), reputedly of $3 million dollars (a huge sum, even though at the time it was relatively easy to obtain grant funding), he was exploring heart transplants between puppies with encouraging results. He selected puppies as this allowed him to cool the recipient to low temperatures (using the techniques introduced by Bigelow and Lewis) and did not necessitate maintaining life during the operation with a heart-lung machine. He and his team achieved survival of weeks or even months in several of his puppies, which was a major accomplishment in those early days.

Indeed, by June 1966, Kantrowitz felt ready to go ahead and carry out a heart transplant in a baby with a complex heart defect. To try to obtain a suitable infant donor, he sent 500 telegrams to hospitals around the US informing them of his need, and his plea was successful. He progressed as far as taking the infant patient to the operating room for the operation. To avoid ethical and legal problems, he turned off the donor's ventilator to await cessation of heartbeat (as Chris would do eighteen months later), but the donor heart failed and was deemed inadequate for transplantation. The operation was therefore cancelled. A few days later, a second opportunity was also cancelled for the same reason. The baby in need of a heart transplant sadly died before another suitable infant donor could be identified. Dr Kantrowitz therefore came so close to being the first to transplant a human heart; such are the vicissitudes of fate.

Dr Kantrowitz is most remembered in cardiothoracic surgery circles for his development of a balloon pump that augments the output of a failing heart, which is still used frequently today. The balloon pump has saved very many lives by temporarily supporting the patient's circulation during a period when the heart is struggling. However, it can be used only as a temporary support until either the patient's heart recovers or a more permanent mechanical device, such as a left ventricular assist device is implanted, or a heart transplant is carried out. In the field of balloon pumps and the development of mechanical devices to augment or replace the heart, Kantrowitz was a major pioneer (aided by his wife and his brother, who was a physicist). As early as February 1966, he had implanted a device in a patient that supported the circulation, though without great success. He had also been early into the field of implanting pacemakers. However, as we shall see, his role in the development of heart transplantation was ultimately less significant.

## Chris Barnard: Preparations in Cape Town

While Shumway, in particular, Kantrowitz, and a few others were refining their experience of heart transplantation in the experimental laboratory, Chris was considering entering this new field of surgery.

In the early 1980s in Cape Town and again in Oklahoma City for a year in 1987, I worked on an almost daily basis with Chris; we frequently talked about the first heart transplant, but I specifically had a long (recorded) conversation with him on this topic when we were in Oklahoma City in September 1987. He began to give consideration to heart transplantation when preparing his lecture to the students at the University or Pretoria.

My reading of the medical literature, 'revealed that the surgical technique of [heart] replacement had been developed over many years by a number of research workers, beginning as far back as 1951. To illustrate my lecture in Pretoria, I actually filmed an orthotopic heart transplant in a dog, and showed this film during the lecture. Subsequently, with my colleagues—my brother, Marius, and Terry O'Donovan [later a surgeon in Louisiana in the USA]—I spent many months practicing this technique in dogs. We perfected the surgical technique in the laboratory. We never tried to get long-term survival. All we were interested in was perfecting the surgical technique.

Marius's memory was slightly different.

Our experiments involving dogs were actually surgical exercises that served only to help me become more proficient in performing cardiac surgery. On only one occasion while I was working there did Chris enter the laboratory to show us how the transplant should be performed ... Not only did we have no record of the numbers, but we did not perform more than twenty heart transplants on dogs, if that. I performed at least 90 per cent of these operations ... Our primary objective was to hone our surgical techniques and procedures ... The truth is that Chris performed no more than five dog transplants.

Nevertheless, five transplants may have been enough for a highly trained heart surgeon, like Chris, to learn how to do the operation.

However, John Terblanche's memory was that 'I assisted him [Chris] with heart transplants in dogs in the laboratory in 1964. It is quite untrue to have insinuated, as occurred in other parts of the world, that he did not have expertise in the area.'

Chris continued explaining to me how he had prepared for the first heart transplant. He organised a meeting every Friday lunchtime with people whose interest was in immunology.

We would have a little lecture, and I used to provide sandwiches and coffee. There was a guy who is now at the Mayo Clinic who was a very good immunologist. He lectured to us very often. He explained all about cellular immunity [the basis of rejection] and that sort of thing, which I didn't know very much about. I became a good immunologist from those meetings and by reading about it.

During these meetings Marius 'sensed no wild enthusiasm from any of the attendees other than Chris. He was fiercely determined to press on, and most of us reluctantly followed.' However, interestingly, he also remembered that 'not once ... was it ever mentioned that we should expedite our efforts because there was a race on between Norman Shumway, Adrian Kantrowitz and others to perform the first heart transplant. This only came later, and was the fabrication of desperate newspapers and other reporters.'

When Chris was ready from a surgical perspective to embark on heart transplantation clinically, he decided he would get some experience with immunosuppressive therapy and the management of patients who were immunosuppressed. 'I had been already planning to do the heart transplant for a year or two,' he told me. 'I arranged a job with Dave Hume. This must have been in 1966. I studied kidney transplantation under him in Richmond, Virginia, for three months. Then I visited Tom Starzl's centre [in Denver, Colorado] for two weeks to see the work they were doing. Hume taught me more than anybody else to make a successful transplant. I did exactly like he did.'

It is not surprising that Chris should select the groups of Hume and Starzl under which to study. In the mid-1960s, these were the busiest kidney transplant programs in the world, and so he would be exposed to the most experience. He had clearly done his 'homework' about the developing field of kidney transplantation. I presume he did not choose to visit Shumway's group at Stanford because his aim was to learn how you immunosuppressed patients with organ transplants rather than dogs.

Chris also arranged for his colleague, Dr Marthinus 'M. C.' Botha, to visit Professor Jean Dausset (a future Nobel laureate) in France and Professor Jon van Rood in the Netherlands to study methods of tissue typing. Ten years previously, M. C. Botha had spent time with these two well-known immunologists and so had some background knowledge. He also spent time with Paul Terasaki, another expert on tissue typing, in Los Angeles. When he returned to Cape Town, he set up a tissue typing laboratory at GSH, specifically for a future heart transplant program.

Like Marius Barnard, M. C. Botha sometimes found it difficult to interact amicably with Chris. He told Peter Hawthorne, 'We are both temperamental sometimes. In fact, Chris and I have had scraps in this office that you could hear right through the building.'

What was the state of the heart surgery programme at GSH in 1967? Marius Barnard had just returned to Cape Town (in April 1967) from Houston, Texas, where he had trained primarily as a vascular surgeon with Dr Michael DeBakey, who he disliked, and Dr Denton Cooley, who he admired. As there was no opening for a vascular surgeon at GSH, he had accepted a position that Chris had offered him in his department, but with some misgivings (on both sides) in view of their volatile relationship.

Marius started his career as a cardiac surgeon 'at the princely salary of R600 per month'. He described his first few months in Chris's department as 'utter hell'. He was expected to assist Chris in the operating room.

> Unfortunately, in the team context, this arrangement didn't work. I found his behaviour unacceptable and, however hard we tried, our efforts were never considered good enough. My resentment was obvious, especially in front of the rest of the staff. A few weeks of fighting-back became untenable to Chris, and I was subsequently banned from assisting him. In retrospect, I don't blame him.

Having just returned from Houston, where DeBakey and Cooley had at least eight operating rooms available to them every day, intensive care units (ICUs) with thirty beds, and anaesthetists and staff capable of performing sixteen to twenty operations per day, Marius found the unit in GSH inadequate. 'The government and the provincial council had no interest in us, our funding was pathetic and few people even knew of our existence'. Their heart-lung machines were old and outdated, the ICU had no ventilators (i.e. respirators—machines that pump oxygen into a patient's lung—which, if true, was quite amazing for that era), and the heart team was compelled instead to make use of an oxygen tent. However, it must be remembered that the cardiologists and surgeons at GSH were outstanding.

If Marius's recollections were correct, it was in this relatively ill-equipped environment that Chris was planning to carry out the world's first human-to-human heart transplant.

# 8

# Studying Kidney Transplantation with David Hume in Virginia

If Chris Barnard were to carry out a heart transplant, he was going to have to learn at least the fundamentals of the mechanism of rejection of a transplanted organ and how to prevent this. He did this by reading, learning from his medical colleagues in Cape Town, and visiting two leading kidney transplant centres in the USA for three months between August and October 1966. To put in perspective his own efforts to transplant a human heart, we need to know what was the state of progress in the transplantation of other organs, particularly the kidney, in 1967.

## Organ Transplantation: The Early Years

The history of organ and limb transplantation goes back centuries to the realm of myth and legend. The legend of St Cosmas and St Damian is one well-known and frequently cited example. From a scientific perspective, however, organ transplantation really began with the experimental studies of Alexis Carrel in the early twentieth century.

With his Chicago associate, Charles Guthrie, French surgeon Alexis Carrel spent several years developing surgical techniques of joining blood vessels together, an obvious prerequisite if an organ is to be transplanted. Despite the primitive nature of surgical needles and suture materials in those early days, they achieved considerable success in experimental animals. Indeed, because of these studies, Carrel, who was the driving force behind their work and more skilled than Guthrie at promoting himself, was awarded the Nobel Prize for Medicine in 1912 (much to Guthrie's disappointment).

After Carrel moved from Chicago to the Rockefeller Institute for Medical Research (now Rockefeller University) in New York, he gave a lecture in 1914 in which he said that the technical surgical problems of transplantation were solved, but until some method was developed to prevent the destruction of the foreign tissue by the recipient—what we now know as 'rejection'—organ transplantation was not clinically applicable.

Based on Carrel's studies, a now-forgotten Philadelphia surgeon named Levi Jay Hammond had the temerity to carry out a testicle transplant and also a kidney transplant (both on 13 November 1911). Both operations were reported in *The New York Times*, but the kidney transplant was never reported officially in the medical literature. Both operations were considered technical successes. The testicle was clearly dead within a month, but there appears to have been no report on what happened to the kidney. The field of organ transplantation then lay relatively quiescent for more than twenty years.

However, on 3 April 1933, Yuri Yurijevich Voronoy (known as Yu Yu Voronoy), a Ukrainian surgeon working in Kiev, carried out the first in a series of six kidney transplants in an effort to treat patients dying from acute kidney failure from mercury poisoning, usually ingested in an attempt to commit suicide. He sensibly considered the transplant more of a 'bridging' therapy until the patient's own kidneys recovered. He believed that using live human donors was unjustifiable, and so he took kidneys from the recently deceased.

Under local anaesthetic, he attached the donor kidney to the blood vessels of the groin of the patient, with the kidney sitting on the thigh. None of the grafts were particularly successful, with the first patient dying within two days. The early failure of these grafts was probably related to the fact that Voronoy did not understand the damage that could be caused to the kidney during the period when, after death of the donor and before completion of the surgery in the recipient, the kidney was not being supplied by blood. He mistakenly believed that kidneys might survive in the dead subject for some long time after death—hours or even days— which is clearly not the case. It was only some years later that the benefit of cooling the organ to protect it from the lack of oxygen and nutrients that would occur during this period was fully recognised. Although Voronoy did not fully understand the reasons for graft failure, he clearly understood the need for some form of immunosuppressive therapy after kidney transplantation. Efforts to transplant kidneys then ceased again for another ten years.


## Renewed Attempts at Kidney Transplantation

In 1947, a young surgical resident, Charles Hufnagel, at the Peter Bent Brigham Hospital in Boston (now merged into the Brigham and Women's

Hospital, and hereafter referred to as the 'Brigham') was asked by the hospital's visionary professor of medicine, George Thorn, to try to help a patient in kidney failure by carrying out a kidney transplant.

The patient Hufnagel was asked to help was in a very poor condition, having developed sudden kidney failure. Many years later, Hufnagel told me:

> They wouldn't let us take her [the patient] to the operating room, because they didn't want to have a death in the operating room. So we got the patient transferred to the third floor of the surgical ward and operated there with a couple of gooseneck lamps. We knew the kidney wouldn't survive very long and we didn't want to get into a lot of trouble, and so we connected the kidney to the blood vessels in the arm using Lucite tubes [so that no stitching was necessary]. We kept it warm, wrapped in saline.

The kidney was not even placed under the skin. It is debatable whether the kidney made any urine as witness accounts vary, but the patient's own kidneys soon began to recover and the graft was removed. Unfortunately, the patient died several months later from hepatitis derived from a blood transfusion.

When Hufnagel had completed his surgical training, and had accepted a position as a heart surgeon in Washington, DC, another surgical resident, David Hume, assumed responsibility for the transplant program, and it was to Hume that Chris Barnard later turned when he needed to learn how to prevent and treat rejection.

Before the Brigham group could advance their programme much further, however, another American group (in Chicago) carried out a kidney transplant. The surgeon who 'took the plunge' was Richard Lawler, who performed a kidney transplant from a deceased donor into a patient (Ruth Tucker) with renal failure in June 1950. Crucially, however, he left one native kidney in place, and so the extent that the grafted kidney supported life is uncertain. There was evidence that the graft was functioning for a couple of months, but not after ten months. Nevertheless, the patient survived for almost a further five years, presumably on her native kidney that must have recovered to some extent.

Perhaps because he was ostracised by some of the medical profession, Lawler never carried out another transplant operation. However, although the 'success' of his only case is doubtful, his experience stimulated surgeons in France and the USA, several of whom had been exploring transplantation in the laboratory, to enter the field.

## The 'Forgotten' French

It was the French who took up the challenge in what surgeon René Küss termed 'the historic and heroic era of transplantation'. Initially, teams at three different hospitals in Paris carried out kidney transplants in 1950.

Without the French surgeons' enthusiasm and drive, coupled with that of a couple of American surgeons, the field of transplantation may well have died—at least temporarily—after Lawler's transplant. Even among the transplant community, the work of the French groups has been largely forgotten, to the point that I refer to them as the 'forgotten French'. This is in part because much of their experience was published in French-language journals, not usually read, then or now, by the Anglo-American transplant community. Nevertheless, the reality is that one French surgeon, René Küss, and one French physician, Jean Hamburger, played major roles in getting organ transplantation underway.

The first of these, René Küss, was one of the great characters of the early days of transplantation. His young life reads like an adventure story and, if not quite as charismatic or flamboyant as Chris Barnard, he certainly was an exciting character throughout life. For example, he had a love of fast cars, and in his younger days, he was very much 'a man about town', dating, among many young ladies, a dancer from the famous Lido nightclub.

Although there were one or two living donors (probably the first ever to provide kidneys for transplants) the usual donors were criminals who had been guillotined, with the kidneys being removed immediately afterwards, usually on the prison floor and with lighting provided by a torch. Many deceased donor kidneys were removed 'in the morgue, the autopsy room, under very precarious conditions, and with no trained assistants,' Küss told me. The team responsible for organ collection 'often had to be present—like vultures—at the potential donor's death … a very traumatic situation which was sometimes exacerbated by the need to obtain the family's consent for organ donation'. The attitude of the families of potential donors is summed up by the comment of one man who was clearly torn between the loss of his daughter and his wish to help others. When asked to donate her kidneys, he replied 'Yes, doctor, I agree it will save someone else, but please only take one kidney'.

Perhaps Küss's most important contribution was that he developed the surgical technique whereby the donor kidney is transplanted into the abdomen of the patient. This technique is still used almost unchanged today.

Under these primitive conditions and with basically no or very inadequate immunosuppressive therapy, it is no surprise that the results were disappointing. In 1952, Küss wrote, 'In the present state of knowledge, the only rational basis for kidney replacement would be between monozygotic [identical] twins' where, of course, the transplanted kidney would not be rejected. He went on to predict that, because of its much larger population, the likelihood of identifying a patient with terminal kidney failure who had an identical twin would probably be in the USA. He proved correct, and the first transplant between identical twins was carried out two years later by Joseph Murray and his colleagues in Boston.

Küss's major competitor in Paris was Jean Hamburger. Despite living in the same city, the two did not get on well together and rarely communicated with each other. Both British transplant surgeon, Roy Calne, and Joe Murray of Boston told me that, when they visited Paris, Küss would ask them what Hamburger was doing in his hospital and Hamburger would inquire what Küss was doing in his. This total lack of collaboration limited their progress.

Hamburger was not a surgeon, but a physician who specialised in treating patients with kidney disease: a nephrologist. He played a leading role in establishing nephrology as a medical specialty; indeed, it is claimed that he gave the specialty its name. He also played a major role in developing kidney transplantation, in setting up intensive care units, and in pioneering scientific clinical research. As a skilled medical 'politician', he was able to obtain government funding to establish the first dialysis programme in France.

Hamburger made major contributions to the early development of kidney transplantation—on a par with those of Küss. As early as November 1947, Hamburger published experimental results from dogs and pigs, though the actual operations were carried out by his surgical colleagues. The grafted kidneys functioned for varying periods of time, but in all cases were eventually rejected. Rejection seemed more rapid when the donor and recipient dogs belonged to different breeds, suggesting that genetic factors influenced the outcome of the kidney transplant, exactly as it did in mouse skin grafting.

Reviewing all the known data at that time, Hamburger concluded that several barriers had to be overcome in order to achieve successful kidney transplantation in humans: 1. There needed to be efficient protective measures against the deleterious effects of a lack of blood and oxygen (ischemia) on the kidney during its transfer to the recipient—in other words, the kidney needed some 'protection' until it was reperfused with blood and oxygen after transplantation into the recipient. 2. Tissue compatibility groups should be found and applied in the same way that compatible blood group typing allowed successful blood transfusion. 3. The discovery of anti-rejection techniques or drugs was necessary.

Hamburger's conclusions are more or less a prediction of what was to occur in the following years, and illustrate his remarkable insight into the problems that needed to be overcome. These very same barriers had to be overcome when heart transplantation was introduced.

Over the next decade or more, his group investigated these problems. For example, Hamburger heard of the preliminary work of his compatriot, Jean Dausset, who was trying to identify tissue 'groups', similar to blood groups. Hamburger was the first to suggest to Dausset that 'tissue typing' of the white blood cells (the human lymphocyte antigen [HLA] system) might be important in selecting recipient-donor matches for kidney transplantation. Dausset took a long time to be convinced, but eventually a skin graft programme was set up, and it was rapidly shown that there was an association between skin graft survival and tissue antigens— genetic similarity between recipient and donor improved the results. As a result of these and other studies, Dausset was awarded the Nobel Prize for Medicine in 1980. In the mid-1960s, prior to the first heart transplant in Cape Town, Barnard's colleague, M. C. Botha, visited Dausset to learn his techniques.

While Küss and Hamburger were carrying out their first tentative (and competitive) efforts in France, the Boston group continued to explore kidney transplantation in the USA.

## Progress in Boston

George Thorn and his junior colleague, physician John Merrill, played a major role in establishing renal dialysis (using the artificial kidney) in the US, using a machine based on that of the Dutchman, Willem Kolff. In many respects, Merrill proved the American counterpart of Hamburger, becoming a pioneer in nephrology, dialysis, and kidney transplantation.

For a while, the only place in the United States able to dialyze somebody in renal failure was the Brigham. They were very selective in only dialyzing patients who they believed had a chance to recover function of their own kidneys—patients who had what we call 'acute' renal failure. After a month, if their own kidneys did not recover, the Brigham physicians would just allow them to die. However, the young surgeon, David Hume (Figure 8.i), got to know these patients very well and, rather than allow them to die, he wanted to give them a temporary kidney graft. If he could transplant a cadaver kidney, he reasoned, it would extend the period of time these people had for their own kidneys to recover. Like Lillehei, Barnard, and many other pioneering surgeons, Hume had the attitude of not quitting in the care of the patient.

Most scientists involved in the field did not believe kidney transplantation would be successful in patients because prolonged graft survival could not be achieved in experimental animals, but David Hume (and the French) demonstrated that patients with kidney failure did not reject a kidney graft as rapidly as a healthy dog or rat. That was how kidney transplantation was born in the US and France, and later elsewhere: out of human compassion for these patients. David Hume performed nine kidney transplants at the Brigham. He transplanted the kidney into the thigh, using a technique very similar to that of Voronoy. As the kidney was not expected to survive for long (perhaps only a few days) this approach was less stressful for the patient as it did not involve opening the abdomen (as in Küss's technique) and could be carried out under local anaesthesia. There were other potential advantages. For example, if the kidney was rejected (as would eventually be expected), it could much more easily be removed than if it were in the abdomen. It should be remembered that Hume left the patient's own kidneys in place, hoping that they might recover function.

Four of the nine transplanted kidneys developed measurable function and excreted urine for between about one and six months. Some of these patients, therefore, can at least be considered partial successes. However, Hume's conclusions were pessimistic. He echoed Küss's sentiments: 'At the present state of knowledge, renal … transplantation does not appear to be justified in the treatment of [patients with] renal disease.' A period of support while the patient's own kidneys recovered (from whatever insult they had suffered) was all that could be hoped for.

When Hume was called up into the US Navy in 1953 to complete his military commitment, responsibility for the kidney transplant research programme was passed to another junior member of the staff, Joseph Murray (Figure 8.ii).

In 1954, a patient with kidney failure was referred to the Brigham, and the very perceptive referring general practitioner drew attention to the fact that the patient had an identical twin. Now was the opportunity to test Küss's suggestion that transplantation would only be fully successful if carried out between identical twins. The twins underwent skin grafts and were fingerprinted in an effort to prove that they were indeed identical, which was found to be the case.

Murray carried out the transplant between Ronald (the donor) and Richard (the recipient) Herrick on 23 December 1954. The successful operation gained extraordinary media coverage (though nowhere near as much as Barnard's first heart transplant) and refocused the world's attention on the curative potential of kidney transplantation. In a romantic sequel, Richard Herrick (kidney recipient) married the nursing supervisor in the recovery room who had volunteered on that Christmas weekend to care for him. Sadly, he died in 1962, eight years after the transplant, from a recurrence of the original kidney disease that developed in the grafted kidney. His brother, the donor (who I later met), lived a normal life and died of heart disease at age seventy-nine. During the next few years, several further kidney transplants were carried out between identical twins in Boston.

Although this was an important step forward, and encouraged surgeons and patients that kidney transplantation might eventually have a place to play in the treatment of kidney disease, whether it was a major scientific achievement has been questioned. For organ transplantation to make an impact on clinical medicine, kidney grafts had to survive when transplanted between totally unrelated people. As a first step towards this goal, over the next few years, both the Boston and French teams carried out kidney transplants between non-identical twins and finally between unrelated donors and recipients. They frequently treated the patient with radiation in an attempt to suppress the rejection response. Only a handful of these attempts were truly successful. Indeed, in Boston, some members of the medical team began to be so stressed by the high mortality of their patients that, according to surgeon-author Nicholas Tilney, 'one senior medical resident in charge of the ward finally refused to involve himself any longer, telling John Merrill that he had officiated at enough murders.'

Rather like Lillehei, Murray attracted a series of gifted young men to work with him in his research laboratory, and it was one of these, Englishman Roy Calne, who did much to establish the efficacy of immunosuppressive drugs. Roy Calne (Figure 8.iii) is one of the two surgeons who I, and many others, consider to be the two greatest pioneers in the field of organ transplantation—the equivalents of Walt Lillehei in open heart surgery; the other is Tom Starzl (Figure 8.iv). I am very fortunate in having the privilege of knowing both of them well, in Roy's case, for more than forty-five years, having been a trainee of his in Cambridge in the UK in 1970–1971.

## Preventing Rejection: The Introduction of Immunosuppressive Therapy

As a medical student at Guy's Hospital in London (my own *alma mater*) in 1950, Roy Calne looked after a young man who slowly died from kidney failure. The patient's death impacted the young student who thereafter devoted much of his life to overcoming the barriers that prevented successful organ transplantation.

When Calne became a surgical registrar (resident) at the Royal Free Hospital in London (where, by the way, he contracted hepatitis after operating on a man with jaundice), he commuted between the hospital and the Royal College of Surgeons' research establishment several miles south of London where he carried out kidney transplants in dogs. Facilities at the research farm were primitive. For example, when operating on the dogs, the surgical light consisted of an 'Ovaltine' (a powdered drink) tin in which was an ordinary light bulb. Calne's wife, Patsy, provided major, unpaid help to him in these studies that were always carried out in the evenings (like Barnard's early research), often late into the night. Initially, he used radiation therapy to suppress the immune system, without much success.

He was then made aware of a recent publication by two Boston haematologists who had described an immunosuppressive effect in rabbits by treating them for two weeks with an anti-leukaemia drug, 6-mercaptopurine (6-MP). Roy decided to see if the drug could prolong kidney grafts in dogs, which it did. When he published his experimental results, he received a letter from one of Hume's team in Richmond, Virginia, saying that they also had quite good results with 6-MP.

Calne then obtained a scholarship to spend eighteen months in Boston working in the laboratory of Joseph Murray. On his way there, he stopped at the Burroughs-Wellcome Laboratories in Tuckahoe in New York, where 6-MP had been synthesised. The two research scientists who had provided 6-MP, George Hitchings and Trudy Elion, had subsequently synthesised a number of other drugs especially for the treatment of cancer (for which, in 1989, they shared the Nobel Prize). They gave Calne several analogues of 6-MP to investigate in renal transplantation, which he took with him to Boston.

One of the drugs, which became known as azathioprine, proved rather better than 6-MP or any of the others, and Calne demonstrated it prolonged kidney graft survival in dogs. Just as Calne was leaving to return to the UK, the Boston group began to use azathioprine in their patients undergoing kidney transplantation.

In 1961, Los Angeles transplant surgeon Willard Goodwin and Tom Starzl (then in Denver) independently demonstrated the efficacy of high-dose corticosteroid therapy in reversing kidney graft rejection. Starzl began treating his transplant patients with a combination of azathioprine and steroids, an improved regimen that remained the mainstay of treatment for almost twenty years.

This was Starzl's first contribution of many to the development of successful organ transplantation. Roy Calne explained to me that 'the observations that Starzl made were very important at that time because they gave some confidence to the field, which previously had been in almost complete despair. Some surgeons and scientists were leaving the field, but Starzl's series kept people working in it.'

After Calne's return to the UK, within about eighteen months, he was promoted to a senior position at the Westminster Hospital where his chief encouraged him to begin a kidney transplant program. They decided to concentrate on deceased donor kidneys, but the superintendent of the operating theatres would not permit dead bodies to be brought into her operating rooms, and so they had to remove the kidneys (behind curtains) in the open wards, which had changed little since the days of Florence Nightingale. In those days, wards of British hospitals were usually 'open' and the patient could only receive privacy if curtains were drawn around the bed. Calne had to remove the donor kidneys from the dead patient in the bed with only the curtains to shield his activities from the other patients.

He fully realised the disturbing effect this must have had on the other patients as they watched the surgeons go behind the curtains to operate on a corpse. Blood would sometimes trickle on the floor under the curtains. This outrage finally convinced the operating room staff that the donor operation would have to be done in the operating rooms, though there remained some resentment from the operating room staff. Calne described the results of kidney transplantation at the Westminster as 'markedly unsuccessful', but with the occasional longer-term 'success' that encouraged the team to continue.

Today, when a request to the donor family is largely acceptable and commonplace (and indeed legally mandated in some countries), we do not fully appreciate the difficulties of making this request in the early days, when organ transplantation was highly controversial and unacceptable to many.

In 1965, Roy Calne was offered the newly established chair of surgery at Cambridge University, where he soon initiated a kidney transplantation program. Perhaps with beginner's luck, his first patient lived for thirty-two years after the transplant and was 'a beacon of encouragement to us that transplantation could provide a wonderful cure when all went well.' He established a busy transplant service that soon expanded from kidney transplantation to include also liver transplantation, though this was not until about the same time as Barnard's initial heart transplants.

Several of the early transplant surgeons, including René Küss, told me that they considered the introduction of immunosuppressive drugs to represent the greatest advance in transplantation in their professional lifetimes.

# The First Hope of Real Success

By 1962, apart from the twin transplants, there had been only a handful of kidney transplants in the world over a period of four or five years that could be considered truly successful long-term.

In September 1963, a small meeting took place in Washington D. C. and was attended by more than twenty pioneer surgeons and physicians working in the field of transplantation. Several of the participants expressed doubts of the real value of kidney transplantation but, at the end of the meeting, Tom Starzl presented his results using azathioprine and cortisone, which encouraged the group significantly. Küss told me how impressed he was, and he decided to accompany Starzl back to Denver to see first-hand how he got such good results. He reminisced that 'in addition to his [Starzl's] operative virtuosity, we were able to appreciate the extraordinary vitality of his group and his already very promising results.' It was to Starzl's centre that Barnard also paid a visit while in the US in 1966.

Starzl also presented data on a new and quite different immunosuppressive agent, anti-lymphocyte serum (ALS). Chris Barnard was one of the first to use ALS to treat rejection of a heart graft in his second patient, Philip Blaiberg, in 1968.

The use of dialysis to improve the patient's condition before the transplant was a great advance. The surgeons also learned to transplant the kidney as soon as possible after removing it from the donor, and to keep it cold in ice to reduce injury from lack of oxygen. The demand for donor kidneys began to outgrow the supply. The physicians and surgeons were faced with increasingly difficult ethical questions.

When a patient was clearly undergoing severe rejection, one of the problems these early pioneers faced was whether to increase the immunosuppressive therapy (thus placing the patient's life in jeopardy from the possibility that the suppression of the patient's immune system would risk the development of a serious infection) or to sacrifice the graft and return the patient to dialysis. This, along with which patients should be offered long-term dialysis support (and which not) and which should be offered a kidney transplant (and which not), was one of the many ethical questions that the early transplanters had to answer. To the patients, of course, these were questions of life or death.

Chris Barnard and the other early heart transplant surgeons had to ask and answer many of the same questions. For example, in which patients should a heart transplant be attempted? In some respects, the ethical problems were different. For example, after a heart transplant, it would not be possible to allow the organ to reject because, in the absence of any life-support device like dialysis, the patient would obviously die. Once a heart transplant had been carried out, there was no backing out.

By 1967, the year of Barnard's first heart transplant, despite the efforts of Hume, Calne, Starzl, and others, the overall failure rate of kidney transplantation at most centers remained in the order of 50 to 60 per cent within the first post-transplant year. However, before Chris took his step into the surgical unknown of heart transplantation, Starzl had taken his own step to begin to establish liver transplantation, a much more difficult technical operative procedure. He had first attempted this in a handful of patients in 1963, but the results were so disappointing that he called a moratorium on this form of therapy. By 1967, however, he had carried out very many extra studies in the animal laboratory and felt justified in trying again. He performed seven liver transplants with all of the patients surviving the operation. On this occasion, these first few attempts were successful enough for him to persist with liver transplantation, which he (and, soon after, Roy Calne in Europe) went on to establish as a definitive form of therapy for patients with terminal liver failure, though it took them many years.

However, Starzl did not report his initial results of liver transplantation until April 1968, and so Chris did not have this minimal experience to encourage him when he entered the operating room on the night of 2–3 December 1967.

## David Hume

Since Chris chose David Hume as his major mentor in the field of kidney transplantation, let us take a further look at this surgeon.

I had the privilege of meeting David Hume on the occasion of his giving a lecture to the Harvard medical students and surgical staff of the Brigham Hospital in 1966. He had completed his surgical residency and been a junior faculty member at that hospital, and was, by 1966, chairman of the department of surgery at the Medical College of Virginia (MCV) in Richmond. He spoke on the then emerging field of kidney transplantation.

Not only was the subject greatly stimulating to a young man like me (and most of the others in the audience) but Hume's personality and charisma sparkled throughout. His enthusiasm for the subject and his energy and drive were immediately obvious, even to someone who had never set eyes on him previously. It was undoubtedly one of the most scintillating lectures I have ever heard. The Harvard medical students absolutely loved it, of course. Even today, some fifty years later, it remains one of the most vivid lectures I have been privileged to hear.

Those who remembered Hume from his residency and as a junior member of the faculty at the Brigham told me stories of his confidence and independence. For example, when he had been the chief surgical resident (i.e. the most senior of the surgical trainees, who had a good deal of independence in those days), he would sometimes present a patient with a complicated medical history to his seniors at the weekly 'Grand Rounds', and they would advise on management. Having listened to their erudite advice, it was by no means unknown for him to thank them, but then state that he would be following a different path of treatment—not perhaps the most tactful approach for a young trainee looking for a senior position, but that was Hume's nature. Some admired his independence of thought and deed, but obviously others were critical of what they perceived as his 'over-confidence' or even 'arrogance'.

Arnold Diethelm, later to head a very busy kidney transplant programme at the University of Alabama at Birmingham, was a research fellow and surgical resident at the Brigham in the mid-1960s. In his opinion, 'David Hume was the real starter of transplantation. He was very intelligent, very persistent, and very imaginative. He was an exciting person to be around.'

Richard Simmons, another pioneer in organ transplantation, was of the opinion that Hume was 'excessively competitive, but was probably the most important driving force in transplantation in those early days.'

From reminiscences of him by his chief associate in Richmond, H. M. (Hyung Mo) Lee, written after Hume's death, we learn:

He was a man of inexhaustible energy and optimism ... He had no concept of time. He frequently carried out midnight rounds on his patients, and this nocturnal activity extended into the research lab ... His intellectual curiosity was unlimited. He would not accept established rules or customs unchallenged, and he was arrogant against blind authority ... His compulsion to seek excellence influenced and inspired many of his students and colleagues ... He created a free and stimulating atmosphere for students, fellows, and associates.

With regard to energy and enthusiasm for his work, Chris clearly shared many characteristics with Hume. Chris himself recollected that, 'prodded by Dr Hume, we never slept and the drama never ceased'.

Maurice 'Taffy' Slapak, later to lead a kidney transplantation programme in the UK (and the founder of the Transplant Olympics) told me that his interest in organ transplantation was 'fired up' by working with Hume. He found that the approximate 50 per cent graft failure rate in those days, which usually resulted in the death of the patient, was not nearly 'as depressing at it might have been because David was an inspiring leader, and he was a guy who liked argument and liked discussion. I have never met anyone who was so open to new ideas. You could say anything you liked. His office was open to everybody, to all of us guys. He was highly innovative, very intelligent, very courageous, very kind—inordinately kind to his patients—a proper doctor.'

Many people I contacted for their comments on David Hume mentioned his undoubted 'charisma', that almost indefinable quality exemplified also by Chris Barnard. Joe Murray, who began his internship at the Brigham while Hume was still there, remembers Hume as 'a great guy, another enthusiast, very charismatic.'

When working with Murray in Boston for a year, Roy Calne visited David Hume in Virginia. He confirmed to me that 'Hume was a charismatic person with enormous energy and a relaxed approach. He had immense charm and a generous disposition. His role in transplantation was very important, and [if he had not died] he would certainly have continued to pioneer new areas of transplantation.'

Hume had become chairman of surgery at MCV at the age of thirty-nine in 1956. Some stories about him at that time provide insight into his complex character and personality.

G. Melville Williams, who was a kidney transplant surgeon in Richmond, recounts an interesting story about Hume's first few months at the MCV.

Hume was very good at some operations and not so good at others. This reflected his experience as a resident at the Brigham, where they did not do a lot of surgery, but what they did, they did very well. Hume's predecessor in Richmond had been a very good surgeon, and he recruited people who were also very good technically. These guys were kind of 'swashbuckling' people, and so the house staff and residents in Richmond were also technically good. Soon after Hume first arrived in Richmond, the surgical residents held a meeting, and said, 'We think this guy's pretty good, and is worth his salt. We ought to teach him how to operate.' So they called him for every single surgical emergency that came through the ER [emergency room]. They always encouraged him to do the operations. Hume was delighted and did not realise what was happening. He said, 'Oh boy, these guys really need me.'

When Peter Morris was in Richmond, he noted:

Desegregation was taking place, and there were some black surgical residents. There had been a hospital restaurant for black staff and one for white staff. After desegregation, the two were supposed to mix, but they didn't. The black residents continued to lunch at the former 'black' restaurant and vice versa. Hume heard about this and began to have lunch in the 'black' restaurant every day. Because of this, the white residents soon also started lunching in this restaurant. Hume did this for a couple of months till he was quite sure that the barriers had been broken down—and then he never had lunch again.

Mel Williams provided me with more information on Hume's unit at MCV in Richmond. After a surgical residency at the Massachusetts General Hospital and a year's research in Australia, Williams joined Hume at MCV.

I was very impressed with the transplant program—he was far ahead of what we were doing at Mass General. He had a whole special transplant unit, subsidised by the US National Institutes of Health [NIH]. He had a really crackerjack team. Hume was an extraordinarily charismatic man—brilliant—and a good person.

His major contribution in transplantation was possibly using kidneys from deceased donors. He showed that this was possible, that you could get good results [with about 50 per cent one-year survival at that time]. Second, he was largely responsible for defining that organ transplantation followed the rules of blood transfusion—he defined which ABO blood groups you could not cross. He also contributed to the fundamental technical principles of the surgery, for example, how you implanted the ureter into the bladder.

His major strength was his intellectual capacity. He was a very energetic and active person, and hated to sit down and put pen to paper. But when he did, it was just amazing. He would send H. M. Lee and me all over the place, digging up new data, examining charts in retrospect, and all that kind of stuff until he had a bunch of tables, figures, and data in front of him. With these and with a bunch of filing cards on which he had written down the relevant bibliography way before the days when a bibliography was easy [to obtain] with a computer—he would dictate an entire paper that subsequently needed maybe only four corrections. Whereas I would struggle to write and rewrite a manuscript, he just had this mind that was so clear about things that he could just do it. Once his secretary had finished typing it, he would show it to us and it was almost perfect.

## Hume and Heart Transplantation

In 1965, Hume determined that the Medical College of Virginia (MCV) should become involved in heart transplantation, with a view to taking it into the clinic in the treatment of patients. Having failed to persuade Shumway to leave Stanford (possibly because Shumway felt Hume would try to micromanage the heart transplant program, which in retrospect probably would not have been the case), Hume recruited Shumway's junior colleague, Richard Lower (aged thirty-six at the time), with the express aim of initiating a heart transplant program.

According to Frank Thomas, who was a surgical resident at the time in Richmond, 'David Hume had clearly pledged not only his willingness to let heart transplantation happen, but also his support for it. He was a very supportive person. I never could understand why Richard [Lower] didn't do a heart transplant sooner. People said there was reluctance on his part. My opinion is that he lacked courage in the sense that he was unwilling to do something that might involve a risk that was beyond the ordinary level of risk.'

I mentioned these comments to Dr Shumway, and asked why he thought Dr Lower had not pushed ahead, even before Barnard. He reputedly had several suitable patients, and so why not do it?

'I think he had the same problem we had: the declaration of death,' Dr Shumway replied. 'There was a question about the public and the professional acceptance of brain death.' In other words, would the surgeons be criticised (or even sued) for taking a beating heart from a subject who had lost all brain function? I asked Dr Lower the same question: had Hume been pushing him, and why hadn't he gone ahead with a heart transplant in a patient?

Before I left Stanford, everybody was thinking pretty soon we're going to do it. That's why Dave Hume got me to come to Richmond because he wanted to have the first. It was a race between me and Shumway. Hume used to push me quite hard every now and then when there was a suitable patient around. I think that's a fair statement, if not an understatement. He didn't have to push me very hard; we were definitely gearing up to do it.

As a matter of fact, a year or more before Barnard's case, one of my residents in Richmond and I obtained permission from several families to remove the heart for experimental purposes after the kidneys had been removed for transplantation. After the surgeons had removed the kidneys, which usually took about thirty minutes, the heart would be lying there in complete anoxic arrest [i.e. it had stopped beating because no blood or oxygen was circulating around the donor]. We would take it out, cool it quickly, and keep it cold until we could prime a pump and resuscitate it in the lab. [They would perfuse the isolated heart with warm human blood and it would start beating again.] The hearts functioned incredibly impressively; they would be beating hard. So we thought that maybe the heart could be used after it had arrested, which would circumvent this emotional problem about beating-heart cadavers [the ethical problem of removing the beating heart from a brain-dead donor].

In fact, on one occasion, we transplanted a human heart into a very large baboon. It actually beat for a while, but we couldn't get the baboon's chest closed [because the human heart was too large], and so we terminated the experiment. This was a little more than a year before Chris's first transplant. It was kind of 'hush-hush' because we didn't want to publicise the fact that we were resuscitating human hearts.

We were actually identifying patients at that time, as was Dr Shumway. A short time before Chris visited Richmond [which was in the third quarter of 1966], we had an almost perfect situation in terms of donor-recipient, except for ABO-incompatibility. [In such a situation, where the blood groups of the donor and recipient were incompatible, there would have been a high risk of immediate or very early hyperacute rejection.] That's where I think the story got out that Hume was pushing, and I said, 'No'.

Some years later (after Lower's death in 2008), I had the opportunity of speaking with Mel Williams, who knew Hume and Lower well; I asked him about this period of time.

Dick had done all the groundwork for the transplant. He had shown that if you did a transplant in a dog, the denervated heart functioned perfectly. He had one movie of a dog that he had transplanted a year previously, catching a Frisbee, and that's all you needed to show—that a transplanted heart did not need nerves. Up until that time, there was a lot of speculation that without nervous connections, the heart would not speed up when it needed to, or pump strongly when it needed to. Well, Dick showed that it did work. And his dog that was a long-term survivor was studied at the NIH [in Bethesda, Maryland], put on treadmills, to show that the denervated heart worked perfectly well.

After we would take kidneys out of a deceased donor [to transplant into patients with terminal kidney failure], he had permission to take the heart, and he would start it beating again on the bench. I'll never forget the day that he did this the first time. I think I had taken out the kidneys and had done a kidney transplant. I came back to my office, which, at that time, was across from the laboratory, and went across to see what the heart was doing. There, on a bench, with a little gooseneck lamp shining on it to warm it up, was a human heart [being perfused with human blood] beating outside the body. It was very spooky. But he showed that even after the heart had stopped in the donor and we had removed the kidneys, which would take half an hour, the heart would start up again outside the body and [could] function pretty darn well. He was then chided by Dr Hume, saying that's all well and good, but that doesn't really show that the heart can function and produce a blood pressure.

So we did what Dick Lower said would be a 'reverse Hardy' procedure. Jim Hardy had done a transplant with a chimpanzee heart in a human, and it functioned for a little bit and then quit. Well here we decided that Dick would resuscitate a human heart and transplant it into a baboon, and see if it worked. The first time we did it [which I believe was in May 1967], he got the heart started, but we couldn't close the chest because the heart was too big. I also remember transplanting a smaller heart—I think it was a child's heart—into a baboon. That baboon lived for five days with a human heart. I remember it so well because my job was to give him immunosuppression, and I would make slits in a banana peel, stick pills in it, and feed the baboon a banana with the pills in it. The baboon would eat the banana and spit the pills out. But this was just an anecdote. He [Lower] didn't think it was worth publishing, but it settled the issue that you could take a heart from a dead subject and make it work.

Chris Barnard was there when [some of] this was going on in Richmond. If we had a patient that Dick [Lower] could not resuscitate from the heart/lung machine [at the end of an open heart operation], and a cadaver donor [became available] at the same time, we had decided to do a heart transplant.

One day [in October 1966], soon after Chris Barnard had left Richmond, we had a deceased donor and I went into the operating room to see how Dick was doing with a [routine] heart operation. I said, 'Do you need a donor?' I had kidded him in the past, but this time he did need a donor. This time, we really had a donor. He sort of perked up and he said, 'Are you kidding, Williams?' I said, 'No, we've got a donor.' He said, 'I'm not having any luck here with this patient. I think we're about ready to let him go.' I said, 'Well, let's get serious here.' So we kept the patient on the heart/lung machine, and we met in Dave Hume's office.

We were all very much excited—ready to go, but there was a blood type mismatch. [The donor's ABO blood type was incompatible with that of the recipient.] Hume said, 'If we go ahead and do the transplant, we might learn something. And, of course, the recipient is going to die anyway, so what could be worse than that. New knowledge is worth taking a risk for.' He made the case that we ought to go ahead. I was kind of swayed by that argument, but I think Dick was less enthusiastic. He said, 'I think there's a lot of ballyhoo with all this heart transplant stuff, and I really think the first one should be done right.' And he won the argument. Hume supported the decision, and I don't think I've respected a man more in my life than I did Dick Lower at that time. He wanted to do it properly.

This story may provide an example of how Hume and Barnard might have had the courage—being prepared to take the relatively high risk of failure—that Lower (and possibly Shumway) lacked.

## Chris Barnard in Virginia

Chris Barnard was in Richmond for three months at about this time (August to October 1966), primarily to learn the rudiments of immunosuppressive therapy in patients with kidney transplants. While there, he was visited briefly by Marius, who was at that time still working in Houston. Despite Marius's long journey to see his brother, Chris did not make him feel welcome and did little to introduce Marius to what was taking place surgically or socially in Richmond.

Chris's temporary absence from Cape Town gave Deirdre, now in her mid-teens, her first experience of living without her father who had become such an important figure in her young life that Chris believed she almost looked upon him as her 'boyfriend'. Many years later, Chris recalled his experience there to me.

> During the time I was with Dave Hume, I was working in the laboratory. I was aware that they were doing cardiac transplants there, but I wasn't interested because I had already done what I wanted to do back home [i.e. he had practiced the surgical technique of heart transplantation in dogs]. One day I watched Richard Lower for a maximum of half an hour. He was busy doing a cardiac transplant in a dog. That's the only time I ever spent with Lower. If they say that Lower taught me, I must have been a bloody good scholar to learn everything that I needed to learn in half an hour.

It appears that Chris's memory might have been playing tricks on him because Dr Williams remembers:

> Dick [Lower] taught him how to do heart transplants in dogs, and he [Barnard] practiced a lot of those. As far as I know, he never got a dog

off the table [i.e. no dog survived the operation]. A dog aorta doesn't hold stitches well and technically it is difficult in the dog. It took Dick a while before he perfected it. Barnard was a careful surgeon, but he had a tremor. I wouldn't ever have considered him a brilliant surgeon at all, technically. But he was very intelligent, and delightful to talk to—full of stories, wisdom, and so forth—and enthusiastic and energetic.

I mentioned to Dr Williams that Chris had once told me that he only spent one afternoon in the dog lab with Lower during the time he was there. 'That's not correct,' he said.

Particularly in view of my own visit to Groote Schuur Hospital in 1965, I have no reason to doubt that Barnard had been contemplating heart transplantation for a year or two before his sabbatical in Richmond. Yet it does appear that he did take the opportunity of practicing the operation at the MCV. While there, he admitted to Carl Goosen (who had relocated to MCV after leaving GSH) that he was aiming to carry out a heart transplant in a patient in Cape Town. Goosen passed on this news to Lower, who, because he knew that Chris had little research experience in the field, did not believe him.

Although Chris played down the impact that watching Lower had on his aspirations, and claimed that he had long been planning heart transplantation, it may well have provided a major impetus. London heart surgeon Donald Ross remembered:

[Barnard] developed a habit of traveling back and forth from South Africa to the States to attend medical meetings and so on, and would always come through London, where I was working. He would always visit the National Heart Hospital, where I was at that time, and was particularly attracted to it, not necessarily because of me but because of the very pretty nurses we used to have. On one occasion, he came through on his way back from the States, where he had seen some experimental work involving heart transplantation, and said, 'Christ, Donny, I'm going to do that!' I thought nothing more of it until, soon after, his historic operation was announced on the radio … I know he got the idea there during that visit. As I say, I remember it dramatically. And I'm not taking sides on this issue whatsoever. But he had just seen Shumway or Lower's group transplanting hearts in animals, and he came back determined to do it himself.

With his by then extensive experience in open heart surgery, I do not believe Chris intended to make a sudden career switch to become a kidney transplant surgeon. The only sensible and logical reason for wanting to spend time seeing the work of Hume and Starzl must have been to gain first-hand experience of immunosuppressive therapy in patients with an organ transplant. I am convinced that his purpose was to use this experience to return to Cape Town to carry out a heart transplant. Therefore, he must have decided to embark on a programme of heart transplantation well before his visit to Richmond and his work in Lower's laboratory.

## Chris Barnard and Liver Failure

At MCV, Hume began to take an interest in liver transplantation. Dr Williams described:

> Some experiments that people might consider to be outlandish now. But they were interesting because we were searching for ways to sustain life in a patient who had liver failure—somewhat analogous to the dialysis machine for sustaining life in the patient with kidney failure. The notion was that maybe you could do this with exchange transfusions [i.e. passing the blood of the patient, which contained the toxins that the liver could not excrete, through the liver of a healthy 'donor' so that the donor's liver would get rid of the toxins in the blood]. We thought you could do this with a surrogate animal. There had been some reports of cross-circulation of blood between a child with severe hepatitis and her mother.
>
> It was actually Christiaan Barnard, who was visiting at the time, who said, 'Why don't you use a baboon? I bet you a baboon could live on human blood'.

With his liver specialist colleagues, Chris had already carried out this experiment in Cape Town.

> So we embarked upon these experiments. The first stage was to take a baboon and put it on the heart-lung machine, drain all its blood out—wash it out with salt water [normal saline]—and then infuse in human blood to see if the baboon could live and what the liver function was like. The baboon lived three or four days on human blood. We then connected the blood vessels between a baboon and a patient in liver failure. Many of the patients who had been very, very sick [in a coma] woke up. We kept the animal walled off from the patient. One of the patients actually recovered well enough to leave the hospital, but succumbed a few weeks later, but none of them had a permanent recovery.

# The Fateful 'Transplant Lung'

Dr Williams then told me a story that has great relevance to Chris's first heart transplant.

> Obviously we had problems with rejection and infection [in patients with kidney transplants], particularly virus infections in the lungs. We at first thought the shadowing on the chest X-ray was due to a cross-reaction between a rejecting kidney and the lung, causing pulmonary failure, and we called it 'transplant lung'. Actually, it was a viral infection of the lungs.

The fact that a pneumonia was misdiagnosed as an inflammatory reaction in the lungs to rejection in the kidney was a major error, but was part of the 'learning curve' in how to manage patients with kidney grafts, just as there is a similar learning curve for almost any innovation, whether it be in medicine, space travel, or any other endeavour. Chris was to see this same situation (shadowing in the lungs on chest X-ray) in his first heart transplant patient. Possibly through his misleading experience of 'transplant lung' in Richmond, where at the time of his visit they had not determined that it was the result of pneumonia, he treated it as an indicator of rejection of the heart, whereas in reality, it was an infection of the lungs. The outcome of the world's first human-to-human heart transplant might have been very different if Chris had not had the idea of 'transplant lung' at the back of his mind.

## Surgeons as Risk-Takers

Hume's enthusiasm for flying his personal plane began to worry his colleagues. Mel Williams told me:

> This bothered everybody because, if there was ever anybody who would challenge the clouds and the rain and the weather in an airplane, it would be Hume. Flying became his main interest for a while. He bought a little island in the Bahamas, and would fly there frequently. Everybody was nervous about it, but he loved it. He once tried very much to persuade me to fly to a meeting in New Orleans with him. I chose not to go with him, thank goodness, because when I got down there, he bragged about how he had 'outwitted the weather'.

Taffy Slapak had a similar experience. 'I got to Richmond one time, and it was snowing. I got off the plane and David was there to meet me, and said, "Ok, you've got to see my new airplane. Let's go right up now." I said, "Christ, Dr Hume, it's snowing." He said, "Yeah, but it's got all the controls, you know." I said, "I don't think so, thank you very much."'

It was this enthusiasm—or recklessness—for flying that caused Hume's untimely death. He was killed in 1973 (when aged only fifty-five). He had flown himself to Texas and from there to California, and was returning to Virginia when, in bad weather, he hit a mountain and was instantly killed. Dr Joe Murray explained to me the accident occurred because Hume 'was dogmatic—actually, that is what killed him—he wasn't going to turn back in the plane.'

This willingness, even enthusiasm, for taking risks may be a personality trait in innovative surgeons who pioneer a new field of surgery. In Hume, it also took the form of willingness to take risks in challenging the elements in his small plane. It can take many different forms, perhaps most commonly as the 'maverick' personality. Several surgeons whose names feature in this book—perhaps most of all, Walt Lillehei—were mavericks, all willing to 'buck the system' in one way or another.

Lillehei, for example, not only was willing to take risks in the operating room that other surgeons felt were prohibitive (the use of cross-circulation, for example), but he took risks in his personal life with his relatively heavy drinking and partying. Chris Barnard took personal risks with his womanising (jeopardising his marriages, for example), and there are several other surgeons, one or two featured in this book, who did similarly, but did not receive the publicity that Chris did, and so their activities remained unknown to all but a handful of close associates.

It is impossible to introduce a new surgical procedure without being prepared to accept the risk of failure. Of course, the patient carries by far most of the risk, but may have little choice if he or she wishes to remain alive, but the impact of failure, particularly if it involves the death of the patient, may hang heavily on the surgeon's shoulders for some time. When a patient died during or soon after the operation, Dwight Harken termed the pain that these pioneer surgeons experienced as 'the pain of the pioneer', and said it was 'the most heinous creation of Satan in his most diabolic mood.' Many surgeons are not prepared to accept the 'pain' of failure, preferring to pursue only surgical paths proven to be successful by their pioneer colleagues.

Chris Barnard and the few other truly innovative surgeons had the courage to risk the 'pain of the pioneer'.

# 9

# Life's Defining Moment:
# The First Human-to-Human
# Heart Transplant

*My moment of truth—the moment when the enormity of it all really hit me—was just after I had taken out Washkansky's heart. I looked down and saw this empty space ... the realization that there was a man lying in front of me without a heart but still alive was, I think, the most awe-inspiring moment of all.*

Christiaan Barnard

'On my return to Cape Town (from Richmond),' Chris told me, 'I decided I would do a kidney transplant first to get experience in the management of a patient who is immunosuppressed.'

He had begun to plan this before going to Richmond (in August 1966), but it was not until October 1967, a year after his return that he felt finally ready to proceed. This would not be the first kidney transplant in South Africa as a kidney transplant programme had been established in Johannesburg in the previous year, and had attracted considerable public interest. According to Marius:

> The first kidney transplant in South Africa had been performed in Johannesburg in 1966. Cape Town was lagging behind and still had to do its first kidney transplant. Chris decided that the cardiac team would go over the heads of the urologists and perform such a transplant. Although there was strong opposition from other departments, especially the Department of Urology, Chris went ahead.

The patient selected was a Mrs Edith Black, who, ironically, was white. The casualty department was alerted and, although six potential donors were referred to Chris's team, they were all in one way or another unacceptable or incompatible with the patient. The seventh potential donor was a coloured youth with severe, irreversible brain injury from an automobile accident, and the transplant went ahead on 8 October 1967.

Chris recollected, 'I remember the headlines [in the Cape Town newspapers] were "Mrs Black gets black kidney".' It is interesting that, for a kidney transplant (that presumably they believed would not receive the same publicity as a heart transplant), Chris's team was prepared to use an organ from a coloured or black donor and transplant it into a white recipient, which they were not prepared to do when the time came for the first heart transplant.

At the time Chris told me this, it had been twenty-one years since that transplant, and my understanding was that Mrs Black was still alive (although Marius records that she lived for fifteen years). In any case, as this was the only kidney transplant Chris ever performed, he would subsequently point out—with tongue-in-cheek—that he was the only surgeon in the world who could claim 100 per cent long-term success in patients with kidney transplants. Today, GSH has a thriving and innovative kidney transplant program

Shumway intermittently announced at medical conferences that his team was ready to go ahead with a heart transplant in a patient. 'The time has come,' he would say. Chris and Kantrowitz (and the few others with an interest) would get to hear these comments and knew that perhaps time was running out if they wished to be first in the field. My impression was, however, that, despite his competitive nature, Chris was not obsessed with being first and he did not think of it as a race. He just wanted to carry out a heart transplant because he thought this was the next step in the development of heart surgery.

## Selecting the First Patient for the Heart Transplant

According to Marius, 'after the kidney transplant there was no stopping Chris. All he could talk about was the heart transplant. Most well-educated people had never even heard about this procedure at the time, so to have to explain the procedure to simple, uneducated, God-fearing folk was an extremely difficult task.'

Chris explained:

I went to Professor Val Schrire, who was the [chief] cardiologist, and I said I thought we were ready now to do a heart transplant. I explained to him the work we had done in the laboratory—we had done about fifty or so heart transplants—and the preparations I had made to manage the immunosuppression. We laid down a list of indications and contraindications [in the selection of a suitable patient], which differed little from those still followed today. The patient would clearly have terminal heart disease for which no other surgical or medical therapy would be of value. We planned a whole protocol of studies to monitor rejection.

How would we diagnose rejection? Clearly, the patient would develop early signs of heart failure, which we could detect by careful and frequent clinical examination and by changes on the chest X-ray. We also knew that changes in the electrocardiogram would occur, as several previous research workers had documented these in dogs which had received heart transplants.

In November 1967, Norman Shumway was quoted in the *Journal of the American Medical Association* that his experimental experience had given him confidence that his team could move their programme into the clinic, and to the care of patients. Shumway's source of a suitable donor was slightly hampered by the fact that his Stanford hospital was not a major trauma centre. By this time, Adrian Kantrowitz had an infant baby, James Scudero, in Maimonides Hospital in New York City who was in urgent need of a heart transplant.

Chris recalled that Lower and Shumway had suggested that the first transplant should be carried out in a patient who could not be weaned off the heart-lung machine at the end of an open heart operation, but to Chris, this seemed unrealistic as it was extremely unlikely a suitable donor would become available at exactly that time. Instead, he felt the first recipient should be a patient with a heart condition that was irreversible and for which all other potential treatment had failed, and who was likely to die within the next few days or weeks.

Chris's first suggestion for a suitable potential recipient was a black African with a cardiomyopathy, a disease of unknown cause that afflicts the heart muscle of black Africans and leads to severe heart failure. There is no known cure and in 1967, there was very little effective treatment. These patients are often young with no other health problems—and thus would be ideal recipients and should do well after the transplant. Professor Schrire would not go along with this suggestion as he was adamant that they should not be perceived in any way to be 'experimenting' on black patients. In the light of the worldwide condemnation of the South African government's policy of apartheid at that time, Schrire was concerned that the transplantation of a heart from a non-white donor into a white recipient—or, indeed, the transplantation of a heart from any donor into a non-white patient—would be seized upon by the critics of that country.

In contrast, Schrire's opinion was that they should select a patient with a common heart disease about which they understood a great deal, such as patients with severe heart failure from coronary artery disease (related to atherosclerosis—thickening of the arteries until they become completely blocked, resulting in irreversible damage to the heart muscle). He knew that when medical therapy failed to control their heart failure, they would continue to deteriorate fairly rapidly until they died. He was confident that he could predict which patients would die within weeks unless a dramatic new therapy, such as heart transplantation, were offered. Schrire also felt it was very important that he knew the patient well as a person so that he could select a patient who would be able to cope with the demands that would be made on him by the operation and the long-term immunosuppressive therapy.

'In my surgical unit in Cape Town,' explained Chris, 'all patients, regardless of ethnic background, were treated equally, but Professor Schrire believed that selection of a non-white recipient or donor might be misinterpreted by the political critics of South Africa. I therefore agreed that both recipient and donor should be Caucasian [white] ... Two weeks before the actual transplant [on 22 November 1967], I got a very suitable donor, a young black man. I didn't take this black donor, even though I was very tempted to do so, but Professor Schrire said, "Please don't do it."' In fact, in the South African government's eyes, the potential donor was a 'coloured' man, rather than 'black'. Perhaps to ensure Chris did not go ahead, Schrire found some abnormalities on the potential donor's ECG (EKG) that suggested that the heart was not perfect, which was persuasive in convincing Chris to wait for a white donor.

Furthermore, Schrire said his team of cardiologists wanted to play no part in the treatment of rejection because they knew nothing about it. In any case, he and his cardiological colleagues had more work than they could handle; they saw 6,000 patients each year at Groote Schuur Hospital, of whom only a small percentage were candidates for surgery. Professor Schrire said he would look for a recipient.

During the last two weeks of October, Chris 'plagued' Schrire continually to find a suitable patient for the operation. Chris suffered such anxiety that his rheumatoid arthritis flared up and made him wonder whether he would be able to operate even if a suitable recipient and donor were identified.

'Eventually, he [Schrire] called me and introduced me to Louis Washkansky [Figure 9.i], who was a fifty-three-year-old diabetic [though there was some doubt about his correct age]. He was in severe heart failure, and was so sick that he had to remain in the hospital; he was terribly ill.'

Mr Washkansky's personal physician was Dr Barry Kaplan, who Chris described as 'a most human and sensitive physician.' Kaplan was fully aware that Mr Washkansky was dying and had been urging Schrire to think of some treatment that might help his patient. When Schrire mentioned to him that they were considering transplanting a heart into his patient, Kaplan admitted he had never heard of such an idea, but he agreed to discuss the approach with Mr Washkansky. When he explained the plan to Mr Washkansky and emphasised it was a 'gamble', his patient had no hesitation in accepting this opportunity. When asked if he wanted to think about it, Mr Washkansky replied, 'There's nothing to think about. I can't go on living like this. The way I am now is not living.'

When Chris reviewed the angiograms (X-ray movies) that had been made of Mr Washkansky's heart, the muscle hardly contracted at all, indicating the very advanced nature of his heart disease. Two of his three major coronary arteries were completely blocked. Mr Washkansky was far from an ideal recipient by today's criteria, being a diabetic and a smoker with peripheral vascular disease, meaning a poor blood supply to his legs (and therefore possibly also to his brain). His heart failure had resulted in his inability to excrete fluid through his kidneys, and the fluid had accumulated in his legs and feet, a condition known as oedema. Today, there are potent diuretic drugs that would have helped his kidneys clear the fluid, but in 1967, the fluid had required drainage by needles placed into the subcutaneous tissues of the lower legs—an old-fashioned method that was rarely used in the 1960s. Ominously, the puncture sites had become infected.

To Chris's surprise, when he first visited the patient, Mr Washkansky had no questions to ask him and, before Chris had left the room, he had returned to reading a Western novel. Chris wondered how he could read 'pulp fiction after being suddenly cast into the greatest drama of his life'.

When Mr Washkansky told his wife, Ann, that he was to get a new heart, she thought he was delirious and did not believe him. When he pointed out Dr Barnard to her, she was shocked as the surgeon looked to her like 'a young boy' (Figure 1.i). Mr Washkansky was ready to go ahead as soon as possible and, indeed, became impatient, particularly when he saw the surgical team leaving the hospital for the weekend, not realising that they would all be on call to come in immediately in the event a donor was identified.

## Selecting the First Donor

We next had to clarify the legal position relating to donation of hearts in South Africa. Here I consulted the Professor of Forensic Medicine, Professor Lionel Smith, who informed me that the legal authorities had wisely left the definition of death imprecise, and that, if a doctor so deemed, death of the brain was legally acceptable as evidence of death. He thought there was no problem because the law in South Africa at that time simply said that a patient was considered dead when he was declared dead by a physician. Therefore, because the law did not signify what sort of death you should declare, he was quite happy that we could use brain death as a criterion for declaring a patient dead.

In this respect, there was precedence in the experience of Guy Alexandre in Belgium, although I am not sure that Chris—or Shumway or Lower, for that matter—was aware of this. Guy Alexandre was a young kidney transplant surgeon who, as early as 1964, had taken the very bold step of transplanting kidneys from donors who were 'brain-dead'—their brains were totally damaged and had no chance of recovery, but their hearts were still beating. He had made enquiries from legal experts as to whether there was anything in Belgian law that addressed this point, and found there was nothing. He had therefore gone ahead and used brain-dead donors, when hearts were still beating at the time of donation, to perform the kidney transplants.

Nevertheless, when I discussed this topic with him, he admitted that initially he had been reluctant to publish the results of these transplants because he was uncertain—indeed, afraid—of the public response. Within a few years, following discussion undoubtedly stimulated by Barnard's first heart transplant, the use of brain-dead donor organs became the norm. In my opinion, Dr Alexandre has not received the recognition he should have done for taking this bold step, which greatly increased the number of donor organs that could be procured and, furthermore, improved the quality of those organs.

If the organs are to be utilised from a brain-dead donor, it is, of course, essential that the patient is determined to be truly brain-dead and that there is absolutely no prospect that any brain activity will recover. Neurologists and neurosurgeons had worked out how to determine this accurately just by a careful examination of the patient—whether a potential organ donor or not. There is no purpose in maintaining any truly brain-dead patient in an ICU on ventilator-support, etc., if there is absolutely no chance of any recovery of brain function. One of the important criteria for diagnosing brain death is that, if artificial respiration is discontinued or withheld, there will be no spontaneous respiratory movements (no spontaneous breathing). However, there are several other criteria, and so the diagnosis of brain death can readily be made by any neurologist or even a competent general physician. It is not necessary to carry out tests, such as the measurement of electrical brain activity (an electroencephalogram, or EEG), but these can be performed as confirmatory evidence if the neurologist wishes. Importantly, it is usually required that the neurologist examines the patient on two separate occasions—at least several minutes apart, or preferably longer—to confirm the diagnosis. Furthermore, another neurologist or other physician should separately and independently confirm the first one's conclusions.

The diagnosis of brain death made independently by two physicians on separate occasions leaves no doubt that the patient's brain will not recover. Later, Chris likened it to saying that 'when a man is hanged you can restart his heart, but you will never get him to live again.' Once the diagnosis has been made in a potential organ donor, artificial respiration can be resumed to keep the heart and other organs supplied with oxygen until the organs are recovered for transplantation.

In South Africa at that time, any person dying from unnatural causes, such as a traffic accident, by law had to undergo a *post-mortem* examination (autopsy). One or more organs could be removed legally for teaching or research purposes as long as the next of kin gave permission. Chris thought he could remove an organ, such as the heart or kidney, for therapeutic purposes (to treat another patient) rather than for teaching or research as long as the next of kin had given permission. If the patient had died from a known natural cause, like a brain tumour, then permission for both the *post-mortem* examination and for removal of the organ would be required from the family.

Chris and his colleagues decided that, to avoid any risk of them being accused of malpractice, such as 'robbing' dead bodies (like the historic 'body snatchers' who provided bodies for anatomical dissection and study in the nineteenth century by digging up the graves of the newly deceased), none of the doctors involved in the transplant should participate in the pronouncement of death of any potential donor. This diagnosis would be made by a quite separate team of experts in brain disease and injury—the neurologists or neurosurgeons. The transplant team would only become involved with the donor once the neurosurgeons had declared him or her dead. There would then be no conceivable argument that the donor was, or was not, in fact dead.

Nevertheless, Chris decided that 'to be quite sure that I did not run into legal problems in the first heart transplant operation, I decided I would wait for the heart to stop beating before I removed it.'

The donor needed to be young so that the operating team would probably find a normal, healthy heart. It had to be from a donor of the right size—approximately the weight of the recipient—and of a compatible blood group. If the red blood cell match was not good, it was already known from the kidney transplantation studies of Starzl's and Hume's groups that very rapid rejection (within minutes) might occur. Tissue typing, which involved matching the recipient and donor white blood cells, as opposed to the red blood cells in blood typing, was still in its infancy and so, although this would be carried out by Chris's colleague, Dr M. C. Botha, the operation would almost certainly go ahead whatever the outcome. Botha and Barnard did feel, however, that if the tissue (white cell) typing showed a great disparity between donor and recipient, suggesting there was a high risk of early rejection, they might decline to use the heart.

This would have been unlikely because so little was known about tissue typing in 1967 that few strong conclusions could be reached. In one later case, the heart transplant was already well advanced when Dr Botha advised them that the match was so poor that they should not carry out the transplant because of the likelihood of severe rejection. This patient became one of their longest survivors. This reflected the paucity of knowledge about tissue typing at that time. It was then a very inexact science.

Finally, the donor had to be free of any infectious disease so that this would not be transferred to the recipient.

## A Very Surprising Move

Having made detailed plans for the heart transplant program, Chris made a surprising move that might well have prevented him from carrying out the first human heart transplant—at least in 1967. When he was experiencing frustrations and resistance to the idea of heart transplantation by some colleagues in Cape Town, Barnard applied for a prestigious position at London's National Heart Hospital where his former classmate, Donald Ross, was the senior surgeon.

The circumstances were as follows. About three months before he performed the first heart transplant, at a meeting of the staff of the UCT Medical School, a colleague had accused him of being 'selfish and riding roughshod' over his colleagues. Chris admitted, that's just the way I am—I expect perfection from myself and from those around me. Often I'm brutally honest, as many theatre nurses and sisters will testify. I've never changed.' He left the meeting feeling deeply hurt and, when I sat down in my office, I started idly paging through the latest *British Medical Journal*. I saw an advertisement for a surgical post at the National Heart Hospital in London. I thought, to hell with these people in Cape Town, and applied for the job.

However, according to Chris, partly as a result of a postal strike, his application arrived in London much later than he anticipated. Years later, Donald Ross gave me a slightly different story of Chris's application. Ross told me that he thought Barnard's application was 'a joke'.

I don't think he was serious about it—not at all—although, subsequently, he says he was. After the job had been advertised and applications had closed, a telegram suddenly arrived from him out of the blue [applying for the position] on the morning of the appointment. My impression was that Chris sent the telegram thinking it would carry all before him. His application wasn't considered seriously because the closing date [for applications] had been about a month before, the short-list had been drawn up, and the appointments committee was set up. On the morning the appointment was to be made, this telegram arrived. It's very hard to accept that [a last-minute application], no matter what sort of job you're talking about.

I asked Mr Ross what would have happened if Barnard had applied in due time. 'He would have been seriously considered, yes.'

I asked whether he would have been appointed. 'I don't know. I suppose I would have been attracted to him being South African.'

I wondered whether Mr Ross would have looked on Barnard as too big a rival. 'I don't think so, not at that time. You can't tell. So few doctors work together amicably, but I think he would have been acceptable to me.' This I could believe because Ross had the surgical skills, experience, confidence, maturity, and reputation not to be worried or threatened by any local competition. However, the outcome was that Chris was not considered for the position.

'I was very upset that I didn't get the job,' he told me. 'I was well-qualified, had a lot of publications, and had done a lot of original [research] work.'

Chris subsequently realised that perhaps 'fate' was playing a role. He told me:

My life has been changed in the direction that it went by *not* getting jobs. Many years earlier I had applied for a bursary to go to England, and I didn't get that either. If I had got that bursary, I would have never gone to America, and I would never have been exposed to Lillehei [in Minnesota], and probably never would have become a cardiac surgeon.

Losing two jobs [the earlier bursary and the senior position at the National Heart Hospital] made me, first, become a cardiac surgeon and, second, probably do the first transplant.

Having progressed so far with his plans to perform a heart transplant in Cape Town, it is very unlikely that, as a new member of the staff, he could have made the same preparations in London very quickly. It might have been particularly difficult because, as Donald Ross found out later, he would have had to rely on other hospitals to provide a donor as there was no emergency room at the National Heart Hospital.

## The First Patient: Louis Washkansky

Louis Washkansky admitted being a 'gambling man' all his life, and perhaps this explains the nonchalant way he accepted Chris's offer of a 'new heart'. Perhaps the first patients who undergo a novel surgical procedure have to be as much risk-takers as their surgeons. Furthermore, perhaps he had a sense of destiny, as he had frequently told his wife to 'stick around, kid. I'll make you famous'.

In his book, *The Transplanted Heart,* Peter Hawthorne summarised Louis Washkansky's life. He was born on 12 April 1914, in Kaunus, the capital of Lithuania, but was taken to South Africa with his Jewish family when aged nine. He followed his father into the grocery business. He was hard-working with a talent for building strong personal relationships with his customers and suppliers. Perhaps illustrating his 'fighting' nature, he had been a competent amateur boxer in his younger days. As a young man, he was known for living life to the full; he drank and smoked, loved dancing, and enjoyed a good party. He and his wife had one adopted son.

A relative was quoted as saying, 'He's a man of no fear and no enemies, generous to a fault, extrovert but with a kindly and happy disposition. With Louis around, there's never a dull moment. He's a warm and wonderful person and if anyone deserves a new lease of life it is he.'

In 1940, the young Mr Washkansky had joined the South African Engineering Corps and served throughout most of the North African and Italian campaigns in the Second World War. When demobilised at the end of the war, he set up his own wholesale grocery business, but was later bought out by a bigger company, after which he became a partner in another wholesale company in Cape Town. For many years, he was also in the South African Police Reserve, until he had to resign through ill health. He had something of a 'black' sense of humour. For example, he and his wife lived almost opposite the Jewish cemetery and, when he became sick, he would say, 'well, at least I haven't far to go, just over the road.'

All that was required now was a suitable donor heart.

## The First Donor: Denise Darvall

In the afternoon of Saturday, 2 December, a potential donor was identified. Denise Darvall (Figure 9.ii) was a twenty-five-year-old woman who suffered a severe brain injury after being hit by a car as she (and her fifty-three-year-old mother, Mrs Myrtle Darvall, who was killed instantly) crossed a street close to the hospital.

Denise, her parents, and one of her two brothers were out for a Saturday afternoon drive on their way to a friend's home for tea, and had stopped their car to buy a caramel cake from Mr Joseph Coppenberg's Wrensch Town Bakery shop in Main Road, close to Cape Town's crowded, largely coloured, districts of Woodstock, Salt River, and Observatory. Denise and her mother, Myrtle, crossed the road to the shop. At about 3.45 p.m., Mrs Darvall and Denise left the shop to cross Main Road again when they were hit by a car.

It is ironic that Mr Washkansky's wife, Ann, and her sister-in-law drove past the site of the accident only minutes after it had occurred. Mrs Washkansky saw 'this enormous crowd' and she said, 'Oh my God, I think there's been an accident.'

It took only a few minutes for an ambulance to arrive, and the two women—one already dead and the other seriously injured—were taken quickly to the nearby GSH. Denise had sustained a broken leg and pelvis, and a fractured skull, and was taken into the hospital. The duty doctor came to the ambulance to certify the fifty-three-year-old Mrs Darvall dead, and she was taken to the mortuary.

Within hours, Denise, by this time in an ICU and on a ventilator, was certified brain-dead by Dr Peter Rose-Innes, a Groote Schuur Hospital neurosurgeon, and two other neurosurgeons. Only then was Denise's father, Mr Edward Darvall, asked by surgical resident, Siebert 'Bossie' Bosman, if he would consent to her organs being used for transplantation. He remembered how his daughter was always giving things to other people and so he quickly decided she would have said 'yes' if she had been asked. He decided it was better to donate her organs than to let them die with her and bury or burn them.

Denise and her mother were said to be as close as sisters, going everywhere and doing everything together. Peter Hawthorne described Denise as 'a quiet, hard-working young woman, who worked in a city bank. She was courteous and kind, dressed conservatively, and had never had a serious romance in her life. She spent most of her time at home. She was very good to the family.' A senior staff member of the bank where she had worked described her as a pleasant-natured, bright girl, who could turn her hand to any job required of her, and was likely to be promoted in the near future.

Mr Darvall, then aged sixty-six, had worked for one of the city's top-quality men's clothiers for almost thirty years. He had suffered ill health for many years. During the past year, he had had part of his stomach removed and had suffered a heart attack. His wife and his daughter were the main breadwinners of the family. Later, at the suggestion of Mr Darvall's personal physician, the Mayor of Cape Town was asked to be patron of a fund to help Mr Darvall and his two sons—the 'Darvall Memorial Fund'. The fund was to help in the care and education of the boys. Any excess money would be donated for research into heart disease. Mr Darvall received many expressions of sympathy and kindness from people all over the world. A final tribute to Denise came from her colleagues at the bank in January 1968.

There is one more player in this tragedy who is generally overlooked. He is the driver of the car that killed Denise and her mother. Friedrich (Frederick) Prins was a thirty-six-year-old Cape Town sales manager and police reservist. He had been speeding (and some reports said drinking) and was remanded by Cape Town Magistrate's Court on a charge of culpable homicide. He appeared several times in court and each time the case was remanded without any evidence being led. He was allowed bail of R50.

He later commented that 'I'm the only unpopular character in the whole drama of the heart transplant. Professor Barnard is now famous and I've become infamous.' The continued publicity about the heart transplant simply added to his emotional state. 'Each time I switch on the radio or open a newspaper I am reminded of the accident,' he said.

Louis Washkansky's wife, Ann, was very upset that the identity of the donor had been made public. She felt strongly enough, she said, that had she known that Denise Darvall would be identified, she might have influenced her husband not to consent to the operation.

Miss Darvall's blood group was found to be 'O'—the universal blood donor type, meaning that she could donate organs or blood to anybody without risk of the graft (or red blood cells) being destroyed by the presence in the recipient of antibodies against her blood group. Mr Washkansky's blood group was 'A', but he, like everybody else in the world, would not have any antibodies against an 'O' graft.

As preliminary 'histocompatibility' studies had indicated that the result of tissue typing, that is matching of white blood cells, between donor and recipient would not be bad, the surgical team decided to go ahead before the final result was known. It is important not to try to maintain a brain-dead subject in the ICU too long because the function of several organs, particularly the heart, begins to deteriorate. The team did not want this to happen.

The surgical team was therefore called in. Chris was at his home at Zeekoevlei, where he had been resting after spending the morning at the hospital. He telephoned Mrs Washkansky to inform her of the pending operation. She was shocked to learn that the donor was a woman as she had presumed that her husband would have to receive a man's heart.

## The Operation

On the night of 2–3 December 1967 (actually the entire operation took place in the early hours of 3 December), Chris performed the world's first human-to-human heart transplant in his patient, Louis Washkansky. Today, when heart transplantation has become a relatively routine and commonplace procedure, we may be inclined to underestimate Chris's immense confidence and courage in undertaking this first operation. By any standard, it was a monumental step to take. In the late 1980s, I asked Chris to reminisce about the first heart transplant:

> I want to tell you one thing. Before the operation, I thought, 'I'm not terribly religious, but I must pray today. I don't usually pray before an operation, but today I must pray.' I thought, 'What shall I say?' I couldn't say, 'Let me be a brilliant surgeon,' because I'm not a brilliant surgeon, so I said to God, 'Please help me to do this operation as well as I'm capable of doing it.' You know, it's no use to ask God to help you run the mile in under four minutes when you don't have the capability, because it's not within God's power. But it is possible for a higher force to help you do it as well as you can. Sometimes you don't do as well as you can, but I think I did it [the transplant] as well as I could.

I asked Chris if he still believed in God. 'That's a difficult question. If you push me, I have to say I believe in a higher power. Yes, I do.'

I inquired further. 'Did you believe in God more then than you do now?'

'No. It's always been the same. It was common for me to pray when I had a difficult task ahead and wanted confidence. Prayers give you confidence. Is somebody going to help me during this operation? Am I going to do it well? When you start off like that, you operate better.'

He later wrote that praying before an operation gave him the feeling that he was not 'alone'. With his father having been a church minister—and a man Chris greatly respected—I asked why he admitted to not being a very religious person.

> I don't know. It doesn't always follow that, if your father is religious, you become religious. You start thinking your own ideas. When I was a kid, I believed in God and heaven and all those things because of my father. But when you start thinking for yourself, you start doubting certain things. Religion is a belief, and there is no way that you can prove it or disprove it. You believe it or you don't believe it. I believed in praying because I believed that it assisted me to do better. My religion is how I treat people around me, how much I harm them, how much stress I cause the people around me.

Like most of us, it does not appear that Chris was always able to adhere to these 'religious' goals—particularly in the operating room, where he not infrequently caused stress to a number of people.

> It may be hard to believe, but at no time before the operation did it ever occur to me that I was planning to do something that would so capture the public's imagination. To me, it was just one more new operation in the long list of procedures made possible by the development of the heart-lung machine. Furthermore, at no time did I ever consider that I was involved in a race to perform the first transplant. There was no sense of urgency in our planning; everything was organised methodically without hurry.

However, although he had planned for this moment for years, as he was walking towards the surgeon's changing room before entering the operating room, he had the strange feeling that he hoped he would never get there—that something would prevent him from going ahead with the operation. He wrote in his autobiography:

> The farther I went, the worse it became. With each step the weight of doubt grew within me, until it seemed almost unbearable. I wanted to turn back, but there was no turning … I was not so sure that this was the right moment. Maybe it was too soon. Maybe we were not ready for this. It was not a new emotion. Doubt was my oldest enemy. I knew it well. Yet I had never expected it to come this way, to arrive so suddenly and with such force at this crucial time.

Questions entered his head. 'How can you go into such an undertaking if you don't have some idea of how long it'll work? Have you the right to decide on how long a man can live? You're going to cut out Washansky's heart. That's a decision on how long someone can live—if ever there was one.'

Chris overcame these doubts and fears, and continued into the changing room. Terry O'Donovan, a junior faculty member of Chris's team, remembered sitting in the surgeons' tea room (lounge) of the operating suite, waiting for the neurologists to declare the donor brain-dead and for the result of the tissue match. 'While we were waiting Chris picked up the telephone and phoned the Minister of the Interior and asked him not to divulge that he was about to do a heart transplant in a human. His words (in Afrikaans) at the time were, "*Moenie met my twis nie.*" [Don't argue with me.]'

The fact that Chris phoned a senior government Minister indicates that he did realise that he was about to do something that might be of national importance, belying his claim that he thought this bold operation would just be another small step in the progress of heart surgery. However, I believe him when he said that he did not expect it to capture the public's imagination as it undoubtedly did.

Amelia 'Pittie' Rautenbach remembered Chris walking in and out of the operating room, seeming nervous. He asked her twice if she was ready, but 'he knew just how to control himself. He had enormous self-control when it was necessary … He was an excellent captain, in control of the last detail.'

I asked Chris to recount the operation to me.

The operation was performed utilising two adjacent operating rooms. Drs Terry O'Donovan and Marius Barnard prepared the donor in one, and I prepared the recipient with the help of Drs Rodney Hewitson and François Hitchcock in the other. The anaesthetists [anaesthesiologists] were Drs Joseph 'Ozzie' Ozinsky and Cecil Moss [the latter had been a Springbok rugby football player and later became coach of the elite South African rugby team], and the operating room nurses were led by Ms. Peggy Jordaan and Ms. Amelia 'Pittie' Rautenbach.

Eventually, we had Mr Washkansky in one operating room and Denise Darvall in the next. I decided that I would not take out Denise's heart while it was beating, not even open the chest. I was scared that I would be criticised. Although we had discussed it with the forensic [legal] medicine people, and they said there would be no problem, I decided not to do that. When we had Mr Washkansky's chest open and we were ready to connect him to the heart-lung machine, I went to the donor and

I disconnected the respirator myself. The patient now no longer received oxygen. We waited. She didn't breathe.

O'Donovan remembered Chris being impatient, and also Dr Ozinsky, the anaesthetist, encouraging him to start taking the heart out before the electrocardiogram was at a complete standstill. O'Donovan recollected:

> I remember saying to Chris that I would not pick up that knife until the ECG was flat. He said, 'Well, okay then,' understanding that obviously everybody has moral codes which they adhere to and that he would accept my decision not to make the skin incision until the heart had actually stopped beating.

Before the operation, Marius had argued that they should take the heart in the best condition possible. 'Our responsibility was to the patient into whom we were going to transplant it—not this girl who, although her heart was beating, was dead.' However, Chris insisted that the heart must stop before they operated. If Marius had had his way, they would have gone ahead before it stopped. Subsequently, after the operation, he changed his mind because Chris had proved that the operation could be carried out successfully even if the heart was removed after circulatory death (after it had stopped beating). 'I know now that my brother's approach is the only way, because it is the only means of guaranteeing to everybody, the public and the profession, that there was no hanky-panky going on.'

They had to be prepared for sudden cardiac arrest, at which point they would need to open the chest as quickly as possible to attach the heart-lung machine so the heart—and the kidneys—could be provided with blood and oxygen. Dr Johan 'Guy' de Klerk, from the Karl Bremer Hospital in Cape Town, was standing by to remove the right kidney, which was to be rushed across the city to his hospital (where it was later implanted in the body of a ten-year-old coloured boy, Jonathan Van Wyk). Just as a black man's kidney was given to Mrs Edith Black, so a white woman's kidney was given to Jonathan van Wyk. The kidney transplant was carried out successfully, but it was later reported that it failed to function satisfactorily and had to be removed. Unfortunately, a second kidney transplant also failed so the patient had to be maintained by dialysis.

'After about five or six minutes,' explained Chris, 'her heart went into ventricular fibrillation. I then said to my colleagues to open the chest and remove the heart.'

The chest was opened quickly by splitting the sternum (breastbone) as for any open heart operation. The heart was a little blue and was not beating at all. Once the heart-lung machine was connected and oxygenated blood was circulating through the body again, the little blue heart almost immediately became beautifully pink, tense, and firm. Yet there was no recovery of the heartbeat. Desperately, Marius told himself that this was not a damaged heart. He reasoned that it was not beating because cold blood was being pumped through it by the machine. This was aimed to reduce its metabolism while it was transplanted. The blood in the machine had been cooled and, as it passed through the donor's body, it rapidly cooled the heart to a low temperature and would thus protect it from damage during transplantation, but the cold temperature would also prevent the heart from beating again. O'Donovan later wrote:

> Obviously, later on when the technique was more widely accepted by the world, it was then possible to remove a beating heart. At that early stage, however, one felt that one's moral obligation was not to remove a still-live heart from a patient, but to remove it only when it was 'dead' ... I seem to remember that it took us eleven minutes in this first case to get the donor heart attached to a heart-lung machine to keep it perfused with blood ... I did not feel too badly that the heart had suffered too much in that small period of time at probably normothermia [normal body temperature].

O'Donovan, who seems to have been very conscious of the legal—and ethical and moral—aspects of the operation, insisted that Chris remove the heart himself, in part I believe for medico-legal reasons (to place full responsibility on Chris) but in part because he felt Chris should himself ensure that the heart had been excised correctly and there would be no mistakes that might complicate its insertion into the recipient. He was perhaps fully aware that Chris would not hesitate to criticise any mistake his assistants might make.

O'Donovan recorded, 'I was adamant about his removing the heart for our first case because I felt that, given Chris's nature, he needed to have sufficient confidence that the donor heart had been correctly prepared by him. Similarly, he could then, with confidence, proceed to the recipient theatre and remove Mr Washkansky's badly damaged heart.'

The heart was removed from Denise Darvall's chest and carried into the adjacent recipient operating room at approximately 3 a.m. They removed the donor heart in such a way that the donor heart-lung machine would continue to perfuse it with cooled oxygenated blood, thus providing protection from injury. Even after they had carried the heart to the other operating room (in which Mr Washkansky's operation was taking place), they were able to perfuse the donor heart with cooled blood and oxygen from Mr Washkansky's heart-lung machine throughout most of the operation. Thus, the heart continued to be protected from injury.

This approach is almost never followed today when the donor heart is simply cooled to a very low temperature by perfusing it with a cold saline-like preservation solution, then excised, and covered in ice or cold saline (as Shumway had introduced, and as was carried out in kidney transplantation in most centres). However, the continuous perfusion of the donor heart with oxygenated blood in Mr Washkansky's case may have been important as they had allowed the heart to suffer an insult and possible injury while it stopped beating, which is much less commonly allowed today.

Many years later, Marius Barnard was interviewed by a journalist, Donald McRae, who was preparing a book, *Every Second Counts*, on what he perceived as the 'race' to perform the first heart transplant. Marius evidently told him that the donor heart had been removed while still beating, which was contrary to anything I had heard from any of the other participants in the operation and in contrast to anything that had been written previously. I was stunned to read this, particularly because, if true, it meant that Chris and all the many other members of the team had been lying for the previous forty years or so. I could not believe that they would all do this; it also seemed inconceivable that the 'truth', if that is what it was, would not have leaked out.

However, in his autobiography, *Defining Moments*, Marius states that he purposely gave Mr McRae misleading information on this specific point.

> I'd learnt, whenever I gave information that was meant to be treated as confidential, to insert a single untruth which I could correct once my permission had been duly given. If this was then ever published, I would be able to trace the source.' Marius goes on to confirm that 'we waited until the heart had stopped beating, period.

To provide an author or journalist with incorrect information is certainly strange, though we can perhaps understand Marius's concern about being quoted without full permission. However, his autobiography lays this controversy to rest. The heart had stopped beating in the donor's chest (but was then protected from any further injury by the heart-lung machine) before it was removed for the transplant.

Although Chris and two of his colleagues, Marius and Terry O'Donovan, had carried out a relatively large number of heart transplants in dogs, his two major assistants on the day of this first clinical operation, including his most senior assistant, Rodney Hewitson, had never seen a heart transplant in their lives before. Of course, nobody except Mississippi surgeon, James Hardy, and his colleagues had seen a heart transplant performed in a human, but Barnard's main assistants on this day had not even seen one in a dog or other experimental animal. This was confirmed personally to me by Rodney Hewitson, a highly skilful surgeon in his own right, who we have seen was for many years Chris's right-hand man in the operating room, where his steady temperament was a calming influence or at least as calming as it could be in the presence of Chris's outbursts. I found it quite remarkable that the team had not practiced the operation together.

Even more surprisingly, Rodney told me that, as he had not attended the weekly teaching conferences that Chris had organised and had not been involved with the dog experiments, he was not even aware that a heart transplant was planned that evening until he was called in. This seems difficult to believe, but Rodney Hewitson was a private person who was not a member of Chris's inner circle and may well have been largely unaware of what had been progressing within the department in this respect.

When Chris returned to the recipient operating room, he connected Mr Washkansky to the heart-lung machine. In the operating theatre were fourteen people—nurses, doctors, and technicians—and the open amphitheatre was filled with doctors watching the operation. Clearly, word of the event had passed around the hospital. Many of the day staff and members of Barnard's cardiothoracic unit had heard of the operation and slipped into the observation gallery to watch. The atmosphere was tense and quiet. The heart-lung technicians and nursing staff whispered to each other. Chris concentrated on transplanting the donor heart, speaking rarely.

Mr Washkansky's personal physician, Dr Kaplan, had been out late at a party and did not get home until 2.30 a.m. Just as he was getting to bed, the telephone rang. 'I was tremendously excited,' he remembered. 'I'd never felt like this before. You could feel the tension in the air and the excitement.'

There was one technical problem. The heart-lung machine had been connected to Mr Washkansky using a catheter inserted into his femoral artery in the groin. As this artery was narrowed by atherosclerosis (the same narrowing of the arteries as had occurred in his coronary arteries), the blood flow through the catheter was less than optimal. Chris had to insert a second catheter into the aorta in the chest, temporarily stop the heart-lung machine, disconnect it from the femoral artery catheter and connect it to the aortic catheter, a diversion that could not have been welcome and would have added to the stress of the operation. However, by mistake, Chris ordered the tube from the heart-lung machine to be clamped before the machine had been switched off. The pressure in the tubing therefore rose steeply and one of the connectors burst. Blood from the heart-lung machine swished on to the floor. The machine was rapidly switched off and the line reconnected. However, the tubing was now full of air, which, if pumped into the patient, could cause major brain injury (air embolism) and so had to be hurriedly removed before the machine could be switched on again and the operation continued. All in all, not a good start to the operation.

When Chris made the first cut into Mr Washkansky's heart, his hand was shaking because he was so tense. He found it difficult to control the tremor.

'Louis Washkansky's heart was then removed, and, for the first time in my life, I stared into an empty chest.' Although by this stage of his career, he had carried out hundreds, if not thousands, of heart operations, he had never before looked into a human chest and seen no heart. 'At that moment, the full impact of what I was attempting became abundantly clear to me. The donor heart was quickly sewn in place [Figure 7.i]—the practice in dogs had clearly been worthwhile. The surgery went very well, without any hitches.'

Over the previous few years, Mr Washkansky's heart had become dilated (swollen) when it failed to cope with the blood it was struggling to pump around his body. It was therefore much larger than a normal healthy heart. Denise Darvall's heart was much smaller than even a healthy man's heart, and so it looked tiny in the large space left by Mr Washkansky's heart. Chris looked at it and wondered whether it would cope. Surely it would be too small to support the circulation in such a relatively big man. This observation must have been very disturbing to him, but he could do nothing about it now.

Chris allowed the blood from the heart-lung machine to perfuse through the new heart. By warming the blood as it passed through the heart-lung machine, he also raised the patient's body temperature back to normal. This was the critical point. Would the new heart begin beating?

We then waited for the heart to beat once again, but for some minutes it refused to do so [although it was 'fibrillating', which means that the heart muscle fibres were active but not beating in a coordinated way]. Had the heart muscle been severely damaged when I had disconnected the donor's oxygen supply, I wondered. As the minutes ticked by and no heartbeat resumed, I became increasingly concerned. Would the operation end in failure with the patient dying on the operating table? I electrically shocked the heart, and at last it began to contract normally. It began beating, but only weakly, and would not take over the circulation.

Chris was not able to turn off the heart-lung machine since the patient's blood circulation was dependent on it; the heart was not beating strongly enough to maintain an adequate blood pressure in the patient. Without the support of the heart-lung machine, the patient's brain would not receive sufficient blood and oxygen.

'I was horrified,' he told me. 'You could see the heart was not doing well.'

He allowed more time for the donor heart to gain strength, continuing to keep the patient alive on the heart-lung machine. A second attempt to 'wean' the patient from the machine also failed, with the donor heart still not strong enough to support the patient's circulation.

'Steadily the beats became stronger and stronger. Naturally, I felt a great sense of relief. At the third attempt (to discontinue the heart-lung machine), the blood pressure kept rising.' The heart-lung machine, which had kept the patient alive during the operation, could now be switched off, and the chest closed. 'We were very happy.'

'Jesus, *did gaan werk*! [It's going to work!]' Chris exclaimed, using his native Afrikaans.

It was 6.15 a.m. Chris reached across the operating table and shook Rodney Hewitson's gloved hand. 'We made it, Rodney.'

'It's still a bit early,' replied the cautious Hewitson.

As is common for heart surgeons, when he was satisfied the heart was beating well and the patient would recover, Chris left his colleagues to close the patient's chest. From 'skin-to-skin', the operation took almost five hours. If any of the surgeons worldwide involved in developing heart transplantation believed themselves to be in a 'race', it was now clear that Chris had broken the tape first.

## The Immediate Post-Operative Period

Chris went out and sat with Marius and Francois Hitchcock in the surgeons' lounge in the operating room suite. They were all very tired. For some reason, Chris asked Marius to feel the pulse in his wrist. Due to the stress he had been under, his heart was beating at 140 beats per minute, approximately twice the normal rate.

They were joined by Dr 'Bossie' Bosman, one of the surgical registrars (residents), who would play a major role in Mr Washkansky's post-operative care. Chris cadged a cigarette from Bosman, and drank some tea.

Chris decided he should inform the hospital administrator that he had carried out a transplant. 'It was then [dawn on] the morning of the third [3 December 1967], a Sunday,' he told me.

I phoned Dr Jacobus Burger, who was the superintendent of the hospital, and said, 'We've done a heart transplant tonight.'

He said, 'Why the hell did you wake me to tell me that you've done a heart transplant? I know you've been doing them on dogs.'

Then I said, 'We didn't do it on a dog tonight. We did it on a human, a patient.'

So he said, 'How is the patient doing?

I said, 'Well.'

He said, 'Thanks for calling me.'

I phoned Jannie Louw, head of the department of surgery, and I told him also. He said, 'Why didn't you call me to tell me that you were going to do that?'

I said, 'I didn't think it was necessary.'

Chris must have realised that the operation he had just performed was special because he also telephoned Dr LAPA Munnik, an old friend from their student days and by this time a member of the Executive Committee in charge of Hospital and Health Affairs in the Cape Provincial Administration, a political position of some influence. Some years later, Dr Munnik remembered:

On the Sunday morning of 3 December 1967, at approximately 6 a.m., my telephone rang. It was Chris Barnard, who said, 'I have just transplanted a heart.'

'A human heart?' I asked.

'Yes.'

'Is the patient alive?'

'Yes, and he's doing well.'

After a few further words, I replaced the receiver and told my wife. I lay awake for a while and then decided to telephone the Administrator of the Cape Province—who is similar to a State Governor in the USA— the late Dr J. N. Malan. On the following day, he told me that he also lay awake for a while after receiving my news and then telephoned the Prime Minister of South Africa, the late Mr B. J. Vorster, who later became a good friend of Chris Barnard. The sudden importance of this unique operation is evident through the fact that the Prime Minister of the country was informed within about thirty minutes of Chris Barnard telephoning me.

It surprises me to some extent how quickly the politicians understood the importance of this operation and its potential impact on the world. Dr Munnik and his colleagues in government recognised almost immediately that it could put South Africa on the medical map. Due to the government's official apartheid policy, about the only good media coverage that South Africans obtained in the years preceding the first heart transplant was related to the activities of their gifted golfer, Gary Player, who, with Americans Arnold Palmer and Jack Nicklaus, was 'ruling the roost' of golf in those days. Dr Munnik and his colleagues soon realised that any publicity relating to the heart transplant would to some extent redress the balance between bad and good publicity. The operation was more important for South Africa than it might have been for most other countries because of its poor international reputation resulting from its apartheid policy.

Today, to those unaware of medicine in general, it might be like North Korea or Cuba taking such a dramatic medical step forward. It would just not be expected of North Korea, just as it was not anticipated from South Africa, except possibly by a very few surgeons who knew of Barnard's abilities and ambitions. Dr Munnik remembered, 'The operation took the world by storm.'

In contrast, I do not think Chris had any idea of the impact the operation would make on South Africa's standing in the world. I do not believe any surgeon would have expected the worldwide interest that followed. However, these government officers—at these various levels—realised almost immediately that the piece of news they had received might be of significant political importance.

Chris left the operating room suite to speak to Mrs Washkansky, who was waiting anxiously with three close relatives to hear news of the operation. She was naturally pleased to learn it had gone well. Chris then returned to the doctors' lounge to call Val Schrire, who he wanted to come to examine the patient to determine how the new heart was functioning. He also called Louwtjie who was very pleased to hear the good news.

The patient was transferred to what Marius referred to as 'our rather inadequate isolation transplant unit, a two-bed ward that we had had to adapt by thorough cleaning to ensure that it remained sterile.' The room, ward C2, was clearly not sterile, but it was as clean as it possibly could be. 'To this end, strict rules had been applied to prevent the doctors and nurses from bringing infections into the unit.'

Catheters in Mr Washkansky's veins allowed blood and drugs to drip in and measure the venous blood pressure, a breathing (endotracheal) tube remained in his windpipe to ensure there was no obstruction to his airway and through which oxygen could be supplied, a stomach tube decompressed the stomach, two rubber drains in the chest allowed any blood or fluid that accumulated around the heart to drain into bottles, and a urinary catheter drained urine from the bladder.

Chris continued. 'The immunosuppressive drug regimen I prescribed for Mr Washkansky was exactly that which I had learned from David Hume in Virginia, and which I had used successfully on Mrs Black, the kidney transplant patient.' However, to help prevent rejection, Chris decided to give some radiation therapy to the heart, which was not part of David Hume's immunosuppressive regimen. It is doubtful if it added much to the regimen, and in later patients it was omitted. (It has rarely been used in the past fifty years.)

> Having seen Mr Washkansky settled comfortably in the small intensive care unit, I left the hospital … It was summer, so it was already daylight. There was not one photographer, not one television camera, not one newspaperman in front of that hospital. We hadn't announced it; we didn't tell anybody that we were going to do it.

He walked out of the hospital and spent a few minutes in the fresh air of the quiet Sunday morning, looking at the distant Hottentots Holland Mountains, savouring the moment that all surgeons feel after a successful operation. He felt very tired, not only because he had been working all night, but because of the emotional stress he had been under.

> I got in my motor car to drive home and I turned on the radio, and there was a news bulletin. Amongst the items, they said that a group of doctors at Groote Schuur Hospital in Cape Town had done a human-to-human heart transplant. That was all they said—nothing else. I don't know how they got that information. We didn't let the news out.

In his autobiography, Marius Barnard states that he had no doubt that Chris had provided this information to the press himself, but there is no evidence for this and the press has many different ways of obtaining 'inside' information.

After the kidney transplant, Chris had called in to see his good friends, Captain Bert Friedmann and his wife, Dolly (the parents of Dene Friedmann, one of the heart-lung machine technicians) and he thought he would do so again. Dene had already arrived and told her parents, but Chris updated them with news of Mr Washkansky's condition. He then drove home. Louwtjie came out excitedly to meet him. She had already phoned Deirdre and left a message for André, who was in school in Pretoria.

# The Media Onslaught Begins

Before the heart transplant, when Chris had told Dene Friedmann's parents of the planned operation, they had asked him whether it would make world news. 'Probably there will be a ripple in the medical world,' he had replied—how wrong could he be.

I got home and sat down to breakfast. A friend of mine phoned me. He said, 'Chris, I heard that news bulletin and they didn't mention your name. If they don't mention your name, I'm going to write a letter to the newspaper to tell them that you did the first heart transplant.' Of course, it was only an hour later when phone calls came from all over the world. I remember Australia was early to phone, and the United States. Sweden was early to phone, and England. Then, of course, the whole world just burst ... I was soon inundated with telephone calls, literally from around the world, seeking further information.

When the phone rang the first time, Chris thought it would be André or the hospital, but it was from London. The first question the journalist asked was 'Was it a white heart—that is, from a white person?' A New York television network asked if Washkansky was Jewish and what the religion of the donor had been. Chris said he did not know, but was certain that different religious faiths would not complicate the rejection problem. These questions illustrated the world's interest in race, colour, and religion, particularly in regard to South Africa at that time, and confirmed Professor Schrire's good judgement in recommending they avoid any controversy that might have resulted from transplanting a heart between donor and recipient of different ethnic groups.

Exhausted as he was, Chris found it impossible to get any rest or sleep as the calls kept coming in. Every time his phone rang, he thought it would be Coert Venter, the surgical trainee managing Mr Washkansky's post-operative recovery, but it was always another journalist or television station. A veritable 'avalanche of phone calls from around the world' came in. After about forty minutes, Chris called Venter to check on his patient's progress.

Chris told me many times that he and his colleagues were stunned by the interest the transplant engendered. He genuinely believed the transplant would be recognised as a small step in the development of heart surgery, but he had absolutely no concept of the public response. I can believe this because no photographs were taken of the operation or of the surgical team in the operating room. Surely if they had believed this was going to be a major historic advance in medicine, somebody would have suggested the occasion should be captured photographically or even recorded on film.

> There were no photographers at the first transplant, not because we wanted to keep them away, but because we honestly didn't think it was a big deal. If you look at the development of cardiac surgery, you will see that, after they introduced the heart-lung machine, the advances depended upon the introduction of new surgical techniques— closing holes with plastic patches, reconstructing valves, putting in artificial valves. All those were just surgical techniques. We considered transplantation to be the introduction of a new surgical technique, not something special.

Furthermore, when he left the operating room, Chris discarded his surgical gloves in the trash can as usual, only to learn a few days later that a newspaper was offering to purchase them for US$25,000. If he had realised what a big deal the operation would be seen as, he might have saved the 'historic' gloves. When the monetary offer was made, he clearly regretted that he had not kept them.

So great was the interest that the entire team was called back into the hospital that afternoon to be photographed (Figure 9.iii). Terry O'Donovan was tasked with gathering everybody together for the photograph. Everybody was, of course, tired. Pittie Rautenbach remembered:

> That same afternoon, we went back to the hospital to have pictures taken. The photographers wanted to take a picture of Professor Chris alone. 'Oh no,' he said, 'you must first take a photo of the whole group. I did not do this operation alone. Afterwards you can take all the pictures you like of me but my team comes first.' After that we were always referred to as Professor Barnard's Heart Team. We all felt very special.

Marius Barnard had not driven straight home, but had gone to church, and he did not attend the photograph because he gave priority to an event in which one of his children was participating. When he later saw the photograph, he commented that he had never previously seen some of the people in the group. 'The first photograph published of the heart transplant team duly appeared that morning in the *Cape Times*. I was amazed to see faces of 'members of the team' that I had never seen before, and have not seen since. The team had more than doubled. My face was not in the photograph, my preference having been to attend my children's carol service.' Although there may have been one or two interlopers, I think Marius's statement is a little exaggerated.

So great was the media attention that, in order to get some well-deserved sleep, Chris and Louwtjie stayed at Captain Friedmann's home the night after the first heart transplant because the telephone and the reporters had invaded their Zeekoevlei house and they could not get a wink of sleep. With great foresight, Bossie Bosman visited Mr Darval at his home and arranged for him and his sons to be collected and taken to a relative's home to avoid the press onslaught.

South African Prime Minister, Mr B. J. Vorster, sent telegrams of congratulations to Professor Barnard ('hearty congratulations to you and helpers on world achievement') and to the hospital administrator, Dr Burger ('congratulations on wonderful achievement.')

'On Monday morning [i.e. the following day],' Chris told me, 'I got a cable from Denton Cooley [the leading American heart surgeon under whom Marius Barnard had trained in Houston, Texas]. He was the first surgeon to congratulate me. He said, "I heard the news. Congratulations on your first transplant. I will be reporting on my first hundred soon."'

Cooley had a great sense of humour and this comment referred to the fact that he was famous for the very large number of heart operations he performed every day. Indeed, within the next few months, he did, in fact, carry out more heart transplants than any other surgeon in the world—but with relatively disappointing results—one of the first indications that, although most competent heart surgeons could perform the operation, very few centres had the expertise or experience to manage the immunosuppressive therapy that was required to prevent rejection.

'The same day,' continued Chris, 'an obstetrician came to me, and said, "Chris, I'll tell you something. You will never look back again." I said, "But why?" He said, "Because you have transplanted a heart."'

Pittie Rautenbach recollected that 'the next day we were back at the hospital again where Professor Barnard was interviewed by world television. He was just great—so relaxed it seemed as if he had been on TV and in front of cameras all his life.'

A brief meeting was arranged between Ann Washkansky and Edward Darvall during which she thanked him for his magnanimous gift and he wished her and her husband every happiness for the future. The meeting, of course, was highlighted in the media.

It may perhaps be difficult for some to appreciate what is meant by 'media attention'. Journalists and photographers flew in from all over the world and swarmed over Groote Schuur Hospital. For example, two days after the transplant, a chartered Boeing arrived at Cape Town airport full of television and press staff from the USA. Radio and television services worldwide provided bulletins and updates on Mr Washkansky's progress throughout the day. On the front page of several local newspapers, a photo showed Louis Washkansky with a nurse, Sister 'Georgie-Girl' Hall, who was one of the senior nurses caring for him, and was transmitted around the world within twenty-four hours (Figure 9.iv). Indeed, the whole world watched the patient's progress.

The first heart transplant generated more public interest and media coverage than almost any other event I can remember—more than events of global interest involving popes, presidents, or prime ministers, or royal events such as the wedding of Prince Charles and his bride, Diana, in 1981. The media attention must have been exceedingly distracting to Chris and his colleagues, taking their attention away from their major responsibility of caring for the patient. Their every decision was scrutinised by pundits and non-pundits around the globe. Barnard's youthful good looks, his articulacy, and his candid and honest responses to questions were surely a journalist's dream. These characteristics of his—as well as the dramatic nature of the operation—did much to heighten and maintain public interest. Within days, Barnard found himself on the covers of *Life*, *Newsweek*, and *Time* magazines (Figure 1.ii). There is no doubt he enjoyed being the focus of attention.

South Africans were justifiably proud of the heart team's achievement. The *Cape Times* wrote of the pride of every South African:

At the world reaction to the medical miracle carried out so unassumingly … on Sunday … South Africans can only repeat their original 'well done!' a thousand times. The needy rural beginnings of some of the team [referring to the Beaufort West childhood of the Barnard brothers] add a warming contrast to the crown they wear … The benefit of an event like this to the country's standing in the world is incalculable … It reminds anyone who had forgotten that we are in the Big League, not only as producers of gold, diamonds and rugby forwards … The Cape Town operation was heart surgery's 'first man in space'.

In their efforts to obtain information, some of the members of the press and media went to extreme lengths and became a nuisance to the medical team and the hospital authorities, disregarding all security measures. Journalists infiltrated everywhere, pretending to be doctors or orderlies, and even climbing trees outside the hospital window. One or two even inveigled their way into Mr Washkansky's isolation room to try to obtain a television interview. Dr Burger telephoned Dr Munnik to ask for help and advice. He was advised 'to call the police to clear all unauthorised people from the premises.' This corrected much of the chaos.

'Outside the ward we were under constant barrage from the news media,' remembered Chris. 'Special correspondents and television teams had flown in from around the world. It was impossible not to be civil to these men and women. It was also flattering to be the centre of such attention.'

Outside of Chris's office in the medical school, a crowd of correspondents and photographers waited for him almost continuously. Work for him became almost impossible; the telephone rang with calls from magazines, newspapers, and other doctors. His secretary found it impossible to protect him. He accepted an invitation to the United States to appear on *Face the Nation*—a nationwide news panel show. Yet it was equally impossible to accept all invitations or to satisfy all the demands of the press.

In an effort to answer the press's questions, on the Monday (the first post-transplant day), Chris and members of his team held the first press conference in the medical school, but the questions and requests to appear before television cameras were never-ending. Chris admitted that they lacked experience in handling the media, and the press soon began to take up too much of their time. The hospital received an offer of US$1 million for a photograph of the donor heart being placed into the chest of Mr Washkansky on the operating table, but, of course, no photographs had been taken.

Marius also realised that they 'were totally unprepared for this eventuality and had to handle it without, of course, having any previous experience. We received no assistance from the hospital or the provincial administrators. I was fortunately able to continue with our routine surgery and patient care, but Chris took to this new celebrity status like a duck to water'.

Marius was subsequently told by a visiting French doctor:

He had expected the hospital situation to have been similar to those conditions in which Dr Albert Schweitzer had operated in West Africa. He had expected to see mud huts in Cape Town with goats, sheep and cows grazing around Groote Schuur Hospital, but had been greatly impressed when he witnessed this hospital for himself and the world-class standards that were being upheld, despite our rather outdated equipment.

Indeed, by 1967, GSH had approximately 1,000 beds for inpatients, employed a staff of almost 3,000, and cared for 1,500 outpatients every day. To give some idea of the workload of the hospital, when I was on the staff in the early 1980s, the emergency department would see 700 patients with stab wounds of the chest each year, of which approximately

10 per cent involved the heart. In my entire surgical training over several years in the UK, I can recollect seeing only two patients with stab wounds of the chest.

Dr Munnik realised that Chris Barnard was in the centre of the turmoil that ensued. 'Most people would have crumbled under the pressure, publicity, praise and personal attacks that were showered on him,' wrote Dr Munnik.

> Chris Barnard had put South Africa and its medical standards on the world map. Some overseas medical men were overwhelmed, others resented his achievement because they were not first ... Invitations and congratulations, and even criticism, were streaming in from all over the world, and it was clear that Chris needed assistance in dealing with this avalanche of mail. I appointed a special secretary/public relations officer, a Mr Stofberg, to handle all public relations matters relating to the transplants.

The public relations officer tried to direct attention away from Chris and his team, though not entirely successfully.

Dr Munnik also recollected:

> All invitations for Professor Barnard and other members of the team to speak abroad were considered and, after discussions with Chris, placed in order of importance. Early on we decided that the Provincial Administration would bear the costs of all overseas visits by Professor Barnard or members of the hospital staff and that there would be no sponsorships by medical, surgical, or pharmaceutical companies. Universities in the countries being visited could contribute to the travel expenses if Chris were invited to lecture at their institutions.

## Mr Washkansky's Progress

Chris remembered:

> Mr Washkansky's immediate recovery was excellent. For the first time in medical history, we were able to observe the effect that a healthy transplanted heart had in a patient who, until that time, was in severe heart failure. Heart transplantation had never been done in animals that had heart failure. The fluid which had accumulated in his body was rapidly lost through the kidneys [over the next few days], and his swollen legs shrank almost before our eyes. Mr Washkansky 'poured' buckets of

urine. His oedema [the swelling of his body from the collection of fluid that resulted from heart failure] just disappeared. You could immediately see that he was doing very well. This was the beauty of it—to realise that this operation had a great future.

Although Dr Hardy's patient had heart failure, the chimpanzee heart unfortunately failed so quickly that there was no opportunity to see its effect on the patient's heart failure.

Chris later wrote, 'the immediate effect of our treatment was to give Washkansky a remarkable state of well-being that lasted five days—five glorious days of new life for a man who had been dying.' The transplant had had an almost immediate effect on his sense of wellbeing. Mr Washkansky is later reported to have said, 'I woke up and it was all different and I wondered why it was different. Then I realised that I was breathing. I could breathe again. I was not gasping for air. I could breathe because my heart had been fixed up.' His family could immediately see the change in him. He had been transformed from a dying man to one with a new life.

'And it was the first time that anyone had used a brain-dead donor,' said Chris. In the experimental animal laboratory and in Hardy's only clinical case, the 'donor' had been anesthetised and the heart had been excised from a living animal, whereas Denise Darvall was brain-dead. In addition, her heart had been allowed to stop beating, increasing the risk it might not function satisfactorily.

Once he was able to speak, Louis Washkansky told the nurses, 'Look at me—I'm the new Frankenstein. How about that?

Chris decided that he and his main medical colleagues should meet twice daily—morning and evening—to examine the patient and review his progress. They met each morning at ten o'clock (Figure 9.v). Each specialist, including surgeon, cardiologist, and infectious disease expert, examined the patient and reviewed the nursing charts and laboratory results.

It seems some minor jealousies between members of the team arose quite quickly, which is often the case when publicity is involved. Marius noted that Dr M. C. Botha, who had very little involvement in the care of the patient 'before, during, or after the transplant,' would sit next to Chris at most media conferences.

On Wednesday, 6 December, Mrs Darvall and her daughter, Denise, were cremated at Maitland Crematorium in Cape Town. Among the large crowd of mourners were Drs Marius Barnard and Terry O'Donovan.

For several days, Mr Washkansky made excellent progress, and spirits were high throughout the team and, indeed, throughout the millions of the worldwide public who were following his recovery.

On Thursday, 7 December, the fourth day after the transplant, a unit from the South African Broadcasting Corporation was allowed a half-minute interview with Mr Washkansky, who spoke into a sterilised microphone in his room. After that, Mrs Washkansky was allowed in to see him. It is perhaps a reflection of the way in which the hospital became caught up in the media onslaught that the patient's wife did not see him personally until after the first media interview. On the Friday, Mr Washkansky, gave his first bedside radio interview. He described Professor Barnard as 'the man with the golden hands'. When he heard this, Chris said 'I looked at my [arthritic] hands on the [steering] wheel of the car and thought: the man with the swollen hands.'

Marius, who had absolutely no sympathy with the government's apartheid policy and no love for its members, wrote:

Within a few days, we received visits from Dr Carel de Wet, the minister of health, and Dr L. A. P. A. Munnik ... They arrived in our ward with photographers accompanying them. These were image-polishing exercises more than anything else: the government realised that the transplant could be used as a means of trying to improve its deservedly poor international image. In many respects these efforts succeeded. Poor Chris, who was always ready to please, would be increasingly drawn into this distasteful plan ... There is no doubt, though, that the direction of publicity towards some and not others was a cause of great tension. Professor Schrire wanted nothing to do with it, and his disenchantment with Chris's behaviour very soon resulted in a cooling-down of his relationship with Chris.

Later, Dr Munnik reported that he 'personally witnessed two transplants and invited Dr Carel de Wet to attend one with me. What an experience it was to see the maestro and his team at work! Most of us who knew Chris Barnard were immensely proud of what he and his team had achieved, not only for mankind but for our country'.

After the first week, Mr Washkansky began to feel tired and less well. In retrospect, it is clear that his recovery was impaired by allowing him to have too many visitors and interviews. He was seen by visiting surgeons, politicians, as well as by his wife and family. He was photographed by the German *Stern* magazine, interviewed by the British Broadcasting Corporation (BBC), and televised by the Columbia Broadcasting System (CBS). Perhaps too late, Chris decided to allow no more interviews until Mr Washkansky felt better.

After approximately twelve days, Mr Washkansky's condition began to deteriorate, and he developed radiographic infiltrates in the lungs (shadows on chest X-rays). The surgical team was uncertain whether these were associated with heart failure from rejection (which would have been associated with fluid collecting in the lungs), or possibly with 'transplant lung', or with infection (pneumonia). The technique of endomyocardial biopsy, by which a small piece of heart muscle is taken to be examined under the microscope to determine whether rejection is occurring, was not introduced until some years later [Chapter 21]. They were influenced by the fact that Bossie Bosman reported some reduction in the voltage of the ECG, which Shumway's group had documented to be a feature of rejection (though some years later, my own observations led me to have grave reservations about this conclusion). Mistakenly, Barnard's team initially elected to treat for rejection, intensifying the immunosuppressive therapy. This was a critical mistake as the patient had pneumonia. The increased immunosuppressive drugs weakened his resistance to infection further, thus worsening the pneumonia.

This might seem a serious error of judgment by the team—and indeed it was—but one must remember that this was the first such operation in the world, and there was no previous experience to call on. Furthermore, we must also remember that, as described earlier, the kidney transplant team at the Medical College of Virginia, headed by David Hume, had reported a complication following kidney transplantation in which they attributed shadowing in the lungs on chest X-ray to result from an immunological response that they called 'transplant lung' (Chapter 8). Chris had been in Richmond when this complication had first been described and erroneously identified. This almost certainly influenced the thinking of Barnard's team at Groote Schuur Hospital.

'Transplant lung' was later disproved, and today, any shadowing in the lung on a chest X-ray always makes the medical team think first of pneumonia, although heart failure from rejection remains a possibility. Today, if rejection is occurring, an endomyocardial biopsy will confirm the clinical diagnosis.

A clue that something serious may have been wrong was that Dr Arderne Forder (in my personal experience, an outstandingly good infectious disease expert) had cultured potentially dangerous bacteria (*Klebsiella*) from Mr Washkansky's nose and leg from the sites where the fluid had been drained before the operation, suggesting that he could also have an infection in his lungs. Furthermore, the patient had by now developed a high temperature, much more likely to be related to an infection than rejection.

By Saturday, 16 December, the thirteenth day, the chest X-ray appearances became worse, with shadowing in both lungs. The threat of infection now seemed more likely, and so antibiotic therapy was initiated. Soon, Mr Washkansky began coughing up sputum, and it was now fully obvious that he had pneumonia. The press got wind of this complication and began calling Chris at any hour and from everywhere in the world (Figure 9.vi). He had to leave the phone off the hook to get some unbroken sleep.

In his immunosuppressed state, Mr Washkansky's condition deteriorated quite quickly. He struggled to breath, lost his appetite, and developed diarrhoea (possibly a side-effect of the antibiotics). Despite increased antibiotic treatment, he deteriorated hour by hour, suffering more and more as he entered the night. Chris reported that his patient developed pain in his chest, which spread to his arms and legs, 'so that he refused to be moved, preferring to lie in his own faeces rather than suffer the agony of movement.'

On Tuesday, 19 December, he had an episode when he became mentally confused and incapable of coherent speech. Coert Ventner quickly discovered this was because the patient had too low a blood sugar, and corrected it by giving him glucose. Despite all of their efforts, it became necessary to put their patient back on artificial respiration, which meant that with an endotracheal tube in his throat, he could no longer speak to those around him.

Throughout this entire period, the transplanted heart had been working perfectly, with no sign of it failing. However, Mr Washkansky continued to deteriorate. Grasping at a last possible straw, Chris suggested to Schrire that they support the patient on the heart-lung machine (which would provide oxygen directly into the blood) while they searched for a second donor heart, but Schrire wisely advised against this desperate approach that was in any case illogical as the new heart was working well and was not the cause of the problem.

'You have done your best, Chris,' Schrire said. 'Let your patient go.'

As a surgeon who has cared for patients in this situation (desperately ill with no improvement despite every effort), I can imagine the mental and emotional anguish that Chris and his colleagues felt at that time. Deep down he realised that the patient was doomed despite all the efforts being made to keep him alive. It is an agonising state for the surgeons and nursing team as well, of course, for the patient's family and friends.

Mr Washkansky's family was informed of his critical state. Shortly after 5 a.m. on Thursday, 21 December, there was a rapid deterioration.

In *One Life*, Chris wrote eloquently, but perhaps rather melodramatically, about his patient's death. It is said that many patients die at dawn, probably when the body's metabolic activity is at its lowest. Chris wrote:

This was to be his (Mr Washkansky's) last dawn and the last one for that incredible heart—two deaths at dawn. Living, they were together. Dying, they became two. It was this division that ended it all, taking with it one life and something of myself. For my life was also under this dawn. From birth, it had built toward one moment in an operating theatre when a blue heart turned red with life, and a man was reborn. At that moment, two lives had been fused into one. My life had found its meaning there, nowhere else, and now the dying of this one life was my death, too.

Although perhaps overly emotional (the writing almost certainly influenced by Chris's professional co-author, Bill Pepper), I fully understand Chris's feelings at that time. When a patient dies, it is as if a little part of the surgeon has died with him. It is an incredibly painful experience.

Sadly, with the world hanging on every word from Chris and his exhausted team, Mr Washkansky died in the early hours of the eighteenth day (21 December 1967). Ironically, Denise Darvall's heart was the last organ to fail in Mr Washkansky's body. One can imagine the anguish the patient's family experienced and the disappointment that the surgical and medical team felt.

Chris walked to his office in the medical school; it was shortly after 7.30 a.m. The corridor that had been filled with noisy and bustling journalists for the past several days was now empty. A copy of *Time* magazine, with Chris's picture on the cover (Figure 1.ii), was on his secretary's desk. His own desk was covered in mail, telegrams, and invitations to speak at universities and medical congresses from all over the world. Among them was a letter from CBS informing him that arrangements had been made for him to appear in the near future on their nationwide news show, *Face the Nation*, to which he had agreed when Mr Washkansky was doing well.

## Autopsy

An autopsy (*post-mortem* examination of the patient's body) was carried out immediately by the professor of pathology, Professor James Thomson. He could find no features of rejection of the heart, and confirmed that death had resulted from pneumonia. By inspecting the suture lines, he ascertained that Chris had performed the operation faultlessly.

Too distraught and depressed to remain in the room, Chris walked through into the nearby animal laboratory. There, alone and mentally drained by the stresses and strains of the previous several days, he wept at the outcome of his efforts. He was both exhausted and depressed. He walked out of the building and stood gazing at the Hottentots Holland mountains in the distance (the same mountains he had stared at after the exhilaration of completing Mr Washkansky's operation only eighteen days previously) before returning to his office.

He later recorded his feelings when staring at the mountains alone:

Deep sorrow. A great sadness overwhelmed me and it was impossible to speak to my colleagues in the morgue—for fear that I would start crying. I have always been easily moved emotionally and I laugh or cry quite spontaneously. The events of the past eighteen days had sapped my strength completely.

[Mr Washkansky had become] a friend rather than a patient. We had talked a lot, laughed at each other's jokes, got to know each other as people each with his own problems. And we had both known before the transplant that we were facing a number of unknown factors. I felt his death strongly. It was a personal loss as well as a professional defeat. In the days immediately after, it became a driving concern to examine all aspects of the operation. To look for the cause, the possible fault, the thing we might not have foreseen.

Perhaps Marius summed up this initial experience aptly when he said to Chris, 'Well, we climbed Everest. Next time we'll know how to get down.'

When the world heard the news, some people, just strangers in the street, cried. To many people in Cape Town, it was as though a close friend had died. Louis Washkansky's name had become a household word. When people had met in the street, they would ask each other, 'How's Washy?'

Cape Town City Council members stood in silence as a sign of respect. The Administrator of the Cape, Dr J. N. Malan, sent a telegram to Mrs Washkansky:

After the brave and historic fight put up by your husband, his passing has come as a great personal shock to every citizen of the Republic. With you and your family we mourn the loss of a man who, in his last weeks of life, was called upon to make a great contribution to medical science.

Another telegram from the Administrator to Chris said, 'We rest in the knowledge that what was humanly possible you and your medical team have done. May this setback be an incentive to proceed with your untiring struggle in the interests of humanity.'

The death of Louis Washkansky was a great shock to Mr Edward Darvall. 'I feel empty now that Mr Washkansky is dead,' he told a reporter. 'After the operation, there seemed to be at least a part of my daughter still alive in Mr Washkansky. Now I have nothing more to look forward to.'

The Belgian daily paper, *Le Soir*, suggested that funds be raised throughout the world for a monument commemorating Louis Washkansky. The London *Daily Mail*, in an editorial headed *Heart of the Matter* said, 'The past eighteen days has seen a succession of big news stories ... but one above all has appealed to the deepest emotions of men and women everywhere. It is that of Louis Washkansky.'

The funeral of Louis Washkansky was held at the Pinelands Jewish Cemetery in Cape Town on Friday, 22 December. Among the 300 or more mourners were Drs Marius Barnard and M. C. Botha—both fighting back tears—and many other members of the staff of Groote Schuur Hospital. Mrs Washkansky generously asked people not to send any floral tributes, but to donate money to the Darvall Memorial Fund or the Groote Schuur Hospital Heart Clinic. She was secretly disappointed that Chris had not attended the funeral personally (an opinion with which I personally agree). Her subsequent relations with Chris and with GSH were never completely amicable as she felt the surgeon and hospital received most of the glory and rewards, and her late husband less than he was entitled to.

## Report in the *South African Medical Journal*

Despite the pressures of attending to the patient and responding to the immense media attention, the hospital team rapidly wrote several articles on aspects of this first transplant attempt. These were printed in a special edition of the *South African Medical Journal*, which was published before the end of December, thus enabling the report of the operation to be referenced in 1967. No other heart transplant, except an unsuccessful case by US heart surgeon Dr Adrian Kantrowitz (see below), was carried out in 1967. This must surely rank as one of the most rapidly published medical reports of all time.

Terry O'Donovan was initially asked to put these articles together. He recollected:

> Because I was acting as 'editor' for this special edition, I asked Marius Barnard to prepare an article on the experimental work that we had done on heart transplantation. I felt that this would give him at least one article, and I did not want to take on too much myself as I was going to edit this entire edition. For my part I wrote down all the events that had occurred around the first transplant. As it got closer to the publication date, and the word was out that this operation was really an earth-shattering event, everybody wanted to get in on the act. Originally Chris was not particularly interested in making notes about the first transplant,

but he then took over the notes that I had already made, embellished them, and wrote that section himself. It was then decided that Dr Burger, the hospital superintendent would be the editor of this special edition and so, in fact, I ended up not really being represented in it at all. This was disappointing to me as I was really responsible for putting the whole thing together.

Among the papers published in this issue was that by Marius Barnard on the experimental work they had carried out in Cape Town, and by Val Schrire on the preoperative assessment of the patient, but the major contribution was 'an interim report of a successful operation' by Chris himself. It is interesting that he should include the word 'successful' in the title of his paper. Although the surgical procedure was certainly successful, and the importance of this should never be minimised, the outcome for the patient was clearly unsuccessful. It is not at all unknown for surgeons to claim that 'the operation was a success, but the patient died.'

Richard Lower was critical of the fact that the report on the actual operation was authored solely by Chris Barnard. 'How many surgical papers have you ever seen written with one author?' he asked me. 'Chris's paper on the first heart transplant is a classic—one author! It's as if he did it by himself in his basement. It was pathetic.'

In Chris's defence, he was not an author on any of the other papers in the special issue, for example, on selection of the recipient. Furthermore, it is noteworthy that he took pains to acknowledge the research of others, stating that progress had been made through the work of many 'brilliant men and, in particular, through the invaluable contributions of Shumway and his associates'. He cited five references to the work of Shumway's group as well as eleven to the prior contributions of others that had made heart transplantation possible. No one can accuse Chris of not acknowledging the contributions of his predecessors in the field of heart transplant research.

Author Chris Logan reported that the GSH transplant team also cut a long-playing record in which they described their roles in the operation. I never heard any of the members of the team mention this, and do not know if any record is in existence.

## Local Recognition

The University of Cape Town was quick to recognise Chris's major contribution to heart surgery by conferring an honorary degree of Doctor of Science on him only a few days after the operation; I believe this made him the first member of the university staff to receive an honorary degree from the university (Figure 9.vii). Until then, he had been an associate professor, not a full professor. He recollected the events of 14 December 1967:

> After the transplant, the University gave me an honorary doctor's degree (Doctor of Science honoris causa) and they made me an associate professor of surgical science. My salary stayed the same. Later, they made me an ad hoc professor. That's just an appointment. It's an honour. It's not a chair [i.e. it was not a formal and established professorship]. You don't get paid, and you don't fall under university rules. I was never a full professor in my life. I was upset that they never created a chair for me.

Professor Jannie Louw recalled:

> In 1961, the University of Cape Town [had] promoted him to principal specialist and head of cardiothoracic surgery, in recognition of his outstanding contributions to surgical research and cardiac surgery, and, in 1962, he was granted the ad hoc associate professorship which he had wanted so badly when he arrived back from the USA in 1958. In 1967, he was elected a Fellow of the University of Cape Town. These honours did not satisfy him because he felt that he should have been offered a full professorship, but no such chair existed on the establishment, and so his attitude towards the university did not improve. In July 1968, the university awarded him a personal full chair, but even this did not change his attitude because, he said, 'I am now a professor of nothing.' Chris is an ambitious man, but he could also be stubborn and even vindictive.

To outsiders, it does seem incredible that Barnard's immense contributions to the reputation of the University of Cape Town were never recognised in this way. I believe that for the rest of his life he remained quietly disappointed—if not slightly bitter—about what he saw as a slight to his importance to the university. I cannot believe that, with the Province's and indeed the country's enthusiasm for the first transplant, it would not have been possible to obtain sufficient funding to create an endowed chair to fulfil Chris's wish. Ironically, some years later, after his retirement, the university created an endowed chair—the Chris Barnard Chair in Cardiac Surgery—to which subsequent heads of the department have been appointed.

Cape Town itself played its role in honouring their native son. Chris received the Freedom of the City of Cape Town. At that time, only two other people had been honoured in this way.

Ever critical of his brother, Marius pointed out that Chris's team was not invited to any of these awards ceremonies. 'While he basked in the glory, we were bending over the patient in the operating theatre.'

The South African government's enthusiasm for the transplant provided the prospect of increased funding for medical research, particularly into heart disease and organ transplantation. Within days, it was announced that a National South African Heart Foundation was to be formed by doctors throughout the country. The objects of the foundation would be the furtherance of cardiac research and to seek private and public support for this purpose. The Administrator of the Cape Province announced the establishment of a research fund to be known as the 'Chris Barnard Fund' also for research in heart disease and organ transplantation. The Prime Minister, Mr B. J. Vorster, promised even more government funding for medical research; more funding did become available, at least until the mid-1980s when international sanctions on South Africa began to cut into the government's budget.

Dr Hannah-Reeve Sanders, then a junior administrator at GSH and later the first woman appointed Chief Medical Director and Head of GSH, wrote:

> The immediate effect of the heart transplant on the hospital system was the incredible pace at which bureaucratic red tape was suddenly cut, in no small measure due to the euphoria that accompanied the whole episode. It was not only cardiac surgery that benefited but, because of the rather closely knit hospital society, virtually every unit or department was involved. To his credit, Chris Barnard really shared his hour of glory with everyone in the Groote Schuur Hospital.

The South African Chamber of Mines, representing the mining houses in Johannesburg, particularly those involved with gold mining, donated R1 million (one million rands, at that time equivalent to more than US$1 million) to the Chris Barnard Fund and the University of Cape Town to construct a building dedicated to research in heart disease and organ transplantation. I had the pleasure of working in this well-designed building for seven years in the 1980s.

For Marius, the transplant had another welcome result. He was promoted to the rank of Senior Lecturer and Senior Surgeon, and his monthly salary was increased from R600 to R900.

The impact of the first heart transplant was therefore immense, affecting members of the surgical team, the hospital and university, South Africa as a nation, and the world of medicine. Chris was to ride on this wave of interest for many years.

# 10

# The Heart Transplant Heard Around the World

There is no doubt of the importance of the heart in literature and the arts. Marius Barnard reminded us that the Bible refers to the heart 743 times, whereas the kidney, the next most frequently mentioned organ, is cited only thirty times, and the liver a mere thirteen. The heart is viewed entirely differently from most other organs, and it was partly for this reason that the first human heart transplant gained so much publicity and interest. In his 1968 book, *Heart Transplant*, South African journalist, Marais Malan pointed out:

> The heart has been, from time immemorial, the symbol of life. It is associated with a lot of religious mysticism and over the centuries has been endowed with properties it does not possess and actions of which it is incapable. Few anatomical structures have inspired so much sentimentality and so many metaphors and expressions. The heart may be tender or hard, light or heavy, it breaks easily and can burn with indignation or envy [or from a common digestive ailment].

To many people, the heart was not merely a pump, but the seat of emotion and even of the soul.

There was also the drama associated with heart surgery, in particular, the question of the risks the patient and surgeon undertook. In those early days, whereas a surgeon who transplanted a kidney put the patient at risk from death within the next few days or weeks (unless he or she could be supported by dialysis), a surgeon who transplanted a heart that did not function immediately was effectively condemning the patient to instant death.

Due to the special place of the heart in world culture and the emotive nature of the surgery, the media and the lay public response to the first heart transplant was overwhelming: generally of admiration, but with some criticism. The achievement was greeted by a tidal wave of emotion: a mixture of awe and unease. The media attention resulted in the first human-to-human heart transplant being certainly better known by the public than the first operation carried out painlessly under general anaesthesia at the Massachusetts General Hospital in Boston in 1846, although this latter operation had much greater significance to the future of surgery. However, what was the response of those who were also working towards introducing heart transplantation as a means of treating their patients—surgeons such as Kantrowitz, Hardy, Shumway, and Lower, for instance?

Adrian Kantrowitz was told of the Cape Town operation by his teenage daughter who heard the news on the radio on that fateful Sunday morning. He later admitted that he was disappointed that he had not been first, and surprised that it was Barnard who had taken this first step and not Shumway or Lower, whom he believed to be his major competitors.

What was James Hardy's reaction when Barnard did his first transplant three years after his own attempt?

I'll tell you exactly when I heard it. It was at a Christmas party for my department, which we had each year. I came up the stairs at the club where we were holding it, and the resident who had most recently been transplanting hearts with me in the dog lab said, 'Dr Hardy, I just heard on the radio that somebody in South Africa has transplanted a heart. Dr Hardy, we should have done that years ago.' He had ruined my night—I'll tell you that. I felt like shooting myself. I wouldn't have minded it that much if it had been Norman Shumway who had done it—in fact, we were waiting for that to happen—or even [C. Rollins] Hanlon's group, which was very active in St. Louis, a very good group. But I just thought, doggone, we sat around and the NIH kept the pressure on, and somebody in South Africa has done it. We should have done it in this country, and we, the St. Louis group, or Shumway should have done it.

I asked Dr Hardy whether he felt any bitterness towards Barnard.

Oh, no. Of course not. It didn't really have anything to do with South Africa. If the man on the moon had done it, I'd have felt the same way. We had been waiting for someone to take the heat off of us because I wasn't going to risk our grant structure to do one more transplant until somebody else had done one. We had every intention of going right on, but we had to have somebody to take the heat off of us. We should have done it. We should have gone on and done it, and not procrastinated, and said the heck with NIH. But I think that, in the situation in which I found myself after the first heart transplant, I made the right decision. I regret that I had to make that decision. I would like to have gone on and done a transplant that worked.

It is of interest that Dr Hardy remembers exactly where he was when he heard this news. In my own life, there are very few occasions when I remember very clearly where I was and what I was doing at the time I heard news of events that were of global interest. Three that remain embedded in my memory are: first, the assassination of President John F. Kennedy; second, the announcement of the first heart transplant; and third, watching the television as the first man stepped on the moon. I think many others who were alive in those days (all in the great 1960s) remember those occasions clearly. Larry Stephenson, later to become a leading heart surgeon himself, had similar recollections.

> Although there were many important national and international events which occurred during my eight years of college and medical school, there are only three that I remember so vividly they seem as if they happened yesterday—the assassination of President John F. Kennedy, the astronauts landing on the moon, and the heart transplant performed in South Africa on 3 December 1967. In retrospect, the latter event was to have a profound influence on my life.

That was because it was a major factor in his desire to follow a career as a heart surgeon.

I know others in whom hearing the dramatic news of the first heart transplant changed the course of their lives forever. My former colleague in Cape Town and Oklahoma City, Dimitri Novitzky, who was a medical student when he heard the announcement, decided on a career in heart surgery at that moment, and eventually became a major contributor to progress in heart transplantation. Our former trainee in Cape Town, Eduardo Becerra, told me that it was this news bulletin (that he heard at the age of eleven) that determined him to work towards becoming a heart surgeon, which he ultimately did. In fact, some years later, he carried out the first heart transplant in a public hospital in his homeland, Chile. American cardiac surgeon, Bill Frist, later to become a US Senator, attributed his determination to become a heart surgeon to the day when, as a teenager, he had heard of Barnard's first heart transplant operation.

When Watts Webb, Hardy's former colleague, heard news of Barnard's transplant, 'I could only applaud him because that was great.' Webb was not disappointed that the operation had not been performed in the US.

After Barnard's heart transplant, Hardy recollected:

The attitude of our national governmental institutions changed overnight. All the transplant teams in the United States, plus outstanding heart surgeons who had not been interested in transplantation, were called by the National Institutes of Health to a meeting at O'Hare Airport in Chicago on 28 December, barely three weeks after the heart transplant in Cape Town, to plan for the future. Barnard (who was in the USA at that time for the CBS television program) addressed the meeting. He reviewed the details of his case.

What a dramatic change in the attitude of the leadership of the NIH.

Among the attendees were Shumway, Lower, and Kantrowitz. According to author Chris Logan, it appears that Barnard was not formally invited to this meeting, but the CBS television team persuaded Kantrowitz to invite him as a guest. Many of the surgeons in the room resented Barnard's presence, feeling that it 'rubbed salt in their wounds'.

'Once again,' continued Dr Hardy, 'I was besieged by reporters and telephone calls asking for a review of our 1964 heart transplant. This time there was none of the adversarial hostility that had characterised such interviews in 1964.' He later wrote, 'Thus, Dr Barnard's universally acclaimed operative success was immediately enlarged enormously by a second major contribution, namely, the unleashing and liberation of heart transplant groups throughout the world.'

In his book, *Every Second Counts*, author Donald McRae reported that Shumway's group was devastated by the news that Sunday morning, and felt they had been upstaged by an 'opportunist'. The small group sat forlornly in the hospital cafeteria in relative silence. For once, Shumway was not cracking jokes. When he was later interviewed by the press, he hid his disappointment and, to his great credit, was laudatory in his comments on the Cape Town success. Many years later, I asked him how he viewed Barnard's pioneering operation.

In Minneapolis [when they both trained there under Lillehei, Varco, and Lewis], he [Barnard] was smart enough to know that the future of surgery lay in cardiac work—and so he was a smart guy. Later on, he got interested in kidney transplants. He went to Dave Hume's place and there, of course, he encountered Lower [who had moved there in 1965]. Lower was continuing the same great lab work he was doing with us.

There, of course, Barnard saw immediately that kidney transplants were interesting, but heart transplants, my goodness! Lower told me once that the heart-lung pump technician who had previously worked with Barnard, but who had relocated to Richmond [Carl Goosen], said, 'You know, he's going to go back home and do a heart transplant.' Lower thought, 'No, no he wouldn't do that.' Then, of course, he did. So he is a clever guy and could see what was an opportunity.

Lower confirmed this story to me. At the time, not knowing of Chris's preparation over the previous two years, he told the technician that Barnard 'had no real background in this, so why would he do it?' Lower added to me, 'So, big surprise! I'm sure I felt a little disappointment maybe. I thought it was going to be fun whether we [in Richmond] or Stanford did the first one. And it wouldn't have mattered.'

It seems that neither Shumway nor Lower wanted to expose their disappointment publicly; instead, they acted with grace and dignity. Lower continued:

Of course, I think the biggest surprise was what happened regarding the publicity. The media just went crazy after the Cape Town event. That certainly surprised me. I was kind of relieved not to be in that. That may be superseded any disappointment. I'm sure there was some disappointment, but I would not have been happy with dealing with that kind of situation.

Melville Williams told me about Hume and Lower:

[They] were surprised, but I think they had to give him [Barnard] credit for it. He had done enough ground work and felt that he was entitled to do a transplant. They didn't think, 'Oh gosh, the guy is blowing himself up,' and so on. I think later, when he went around the world and dated movie stars and all that kind of stuff, they didn't think much of him. Early on, though, I think that they did respect him. I don't think they were sad or disappointed. Dick was not all that much out for his own glory. I think Hume was disappointed more than Lower was.

I asked Shumway whether he resented Barnard's intrusion into the field.

No, I don't, because we were having a heck of a time trying to get our people to come around to accept brain death as a diagnosis and confirmation of death. Had it not been for his December 1967, case, I don't think our people would have ever submitted to acceptance of brain death. What it did was open the door to brain death. Our neurosurgeons would go by a brain-dead patient, disconnect the ventilator, and then come back twenty minutes later when the heart had stopped and say, 'Well, now he's dead.' That sort of mentality was broken by Barnard's case. If Barnard made any contribution, it was in this aspect of it. Within a year of Barnard's case, a Harvard Medical School committee [Ad Hoc Committee to Examine the Definition of Brain Death] came out with the criteria of brain death. That's the contribution I see from Chris that really helped all of us.

These comments by Shumway much later give the impression that he thought Barnard had taken the beating heart from a brain-dead donor, which, as we have discussed above, was not the case. Although Denise Darvall was, indeed, brain-dead, her heart was allowed to stop beating, and so she fulfilled all of the traditional criteria of death. For many years, there was a widely held misconception that one reason why the first heart transplant was carried out in South Africa was that the brain death laws were permissive in that country compared with those in Europe and North America. In fact, there were no laws relating to brain death in South Africa at that time, as elsewhere. The situation was no different in South Africa than anywhere else in the world, including the USA.

Any surgeon with the confidence and courage to do so could have done what Chris did—namely, allow the donor heart to stop beating so that there was no legal doubt that death had occurred. In such a situation, the arguments about brain death were irrelevant. Shumway or Lower could have done this, but they did not, and I believe it was Chris's courage that differentiated him from his 'competitors'.

Chris's former mentor, Walt Lillehei, clearly agreed. When I met with him, he told me:

Getting back to Norman Shumway, who was also one of my graduate students—I was very close to him—being very candid, Shumway might have waited a couple of years or more before performing the first transplant in man. He was ready to go on to the transplant, he had said—I think publicly—a month or so before Chris did his famous operation. I don't know whether Chris was even aware of that because he was in South Africa. But both Shumway and Kantrowitz, who was also poised to do a heart transplant, were very troubled with the problem of brain death in the donor. I know from talking to Shumway in earlier years, he couldn't really conceive that the public would accept taking the heart out of the donor while it was still beating. I must say it's hard for me to imagine it at that time too. I think as open-minded, or maybe even radical, as I was in those days, I might have hesitated. As it turned out, as you well know, brain death proved to be a very acceptable criterion when it got defined. But it took a great deal of courage from Barnard.

To carry out a heart transplant was a courageous step, but to do so with a heart that you had allowed to stop beating for lack of oxygen—to 'die'—was immensely courageous. This was particularly so because in the transplants that Chris and his colleagues had carried out in dogs, he does not seem to have tested whether the heart would recover after such an insult. This would have been a very sensible (and relatively easy) investigation to have carried out before embarking on a clinical program, and it is surprising he did not do this.

In the couple of years after the first heart transplant, while I was working towards a PhD research degree in London, I actually did some of the very experiments Chris should have performed. I found that the majority of hearts recovered relatively poorly if allowed to 'die' first, and so Chris was very brave to go ahead with his transplant under such circumstances. However, in his first case, the period of time during which the isolated heart was perfused with oxygenated blood from the heart-lung machine during the operation almost certainly enabled better recovery to take place. This idea of his—to 'resuscitate' the donor heart by supplying it with oxygenated blood as soon as possible and to continue that supply throughout the operation—was a brilliant move, and probably made all the difference between success and failure, and between life and death for Mr Washkansky.

However, Shumway was correct in that this first transplant certainly drew attention to the topic of organ donation after brain death. Any reasonable physician or surgeon would realise that it was not in the potential recipient's best interest to receive a heart that had stopped beating before it had been removed from the donor. This would have certainly been detrimental to the heart, and would reduce the probability of the operation being successful. Removing the heart while it was still beating would be much preferable.

Furthermore, to allow the heart to stop beating—and thus no longer supply blood and oxygen to any of the other vital organs, such as the kidneys—was detrimental to all organs, and reduced the chances of immediate good function of kidney and liver grafts, for example.

The eminent New Zealand heart surgeon, Sir Brian Barratt-Boyes, agreed with Lillehei's opinion. He felt that the hesitation of the US groups to begin clinical heart transplantation was 'a reflection of American ethics and restraints at that time. They were ready to do it, but they were scared to do it. It took someone in a place like South Africa—or New Zealand—

where you didn't have those restrictions, to jump in and do it first. As soon as they showed it could be done, away it went. Chris Barnard deserves full credit for that.'

I asked Shumway whether he had felt disappointment that somebody else had jumped in ahead of him.

> No, not really. I'll tell you one thing, we were really surprised. As soon as I heard about Chris's first case, I wrote him. First, I congratulated him, of course, on doing the first case, and then I sent him further information which I think and hope was useful. Since I knew he didn't know anything about the diagnosis of rejection because he had never had an animal live long enough, I sent him a fairly detailed account of how to diagnose rejection from the EKG, which had to be done at least once a day, and I recommended augmented immunosuppression when there was a threat to the heart.

As someone who has been involved in surgical research for more than fifty years, I cannot believe that Shumway, Lower, or even Hume were not very disappointed to have the 'prize' of being the first to carry out a human heart transplant snatched from them. Shumway and Lower, in particular, had put an immense effort into developing this field of surgery and to not be able to take this advance into the clinical realm before anybody else must have been deeply disappointing for them. I suspect that the many years that had passed had made them forget the psychological pain of hearing the news of Barnard's operation.

Surgeons (and, indeed, physicians and scientists) are highly competitive people and, although their major aim may be to advance medical science, they usually anticipate recognition and some reward for their efforts. The man or woman who is first in any field generally receives more recognition than those who follow. For example, how many of us remember the name of the second man to 'discover' America, the astronaut who led the second expedition to the moon, or the second man to run a mile in under four minutes?

Although the public reaction to the first heart transplant was generally one of awe and admiration, there were, of course, many critics of the procedure. Some of those in the field of health service administration were clearly concerned at the potential costs of such operations if they became commonplace. Many others felt it was 'against God's will' to transplant a heart, 'the seat of the soul'. Surely, the surgeons were 'playing at being God' to take such a step, forgetting that transplantation of a kidney, which had been taking place for several years, was equally life-saving and audacious.

Chris commented that 'laymen, theologians and politicians all of a sudden knew far more about the definition of death than the doctors.' Many journalists, and some doctors and other 'doomsday' people around the world, of course, concluded that the world was not yet ready for heart transplants. As we shall see later, several critics of apartheid (both within South Africa and elsewhere) took the opportunity to use the transplant to condemn South Africa in general.

In his later book, *South Africa: Sharp Dissection*, Chris recollected that 'when hearts were first transplanted, a storm of indignation based on moral and ethical issues broke loose. This is because, as so often happens, issues are created by people who seek publicity through exploitation.'

In his autobiography, Chris gave one such example of how people could use the transplant programme for their own aims.

The moral aspects of heart transplantation were actually investigated by a Congressional Committee of the United States Congress and I was invited to give evidence. It soon became clear to me that the chairman of this committee was raising issues aimed primarily at achieving political publicity and thus promoting his own political career. For example, he asked me whether I thought that the man in the street should have some say on how heart transplantations were done, when they were to be performed and which donors were to be used. When I told him that I totally disagreed as the doctor was the man with the training, expertise and responsibility and these matters should accordingly be left in his hands, he asked who paid for these operations. I explained in South Africa the provincial government paid and, on hearing that, he looked very pleased with himself and said: 'In other words, the taxpayer pays.'

'Yes,' I replied, 'the taxpayers pay for it.'

'Well then,' he enjoined, 'if they pay for these operations, don't you think they should have some say in the matter?'

'No,' I replied emphatically.

'Why not?'

I replied by asking a question: 'Tell me,' I asked, referring to the Vietnam War that was then raging, 'is it not the taxpayers who foot the bill for the Vietnam War?'

He readily agreed with me. 'If they pay for it,' I said, 'don't you think they have the right to tell the generals when to attack and when to withdraw, and what weapons to use?'

There was a roar of laughter from the press gallery and the chairman of the committee, looking rather sheepish, mumbled something to this effect: 'Well, I think they would like to'.

# 11

# The Controversy over Hamilton Naki

Many years after the first heart transplant, and even after Chris's death (in 2001), a news item appeared, first in the UK daily newspaper, *The Guardian* (25 April 2003), then repeated in several other media outlets worldwide. This article claimed that a black laboratory assistant at the University of Cape Town, Hamilton Naki (a member of the Xhosa ethnic group, as was Nelson Mandela) had played a leading role in the performance of the first heart transplant. Although he had no medical degree, or any formal educational qualifications for that matter, the news item claimed that Mr Naki had been a key member of the surgical team, and implied that his contributions had been hushed up because of the apartheid policy in South Africa in 1967. It would have been embarrassing for the South African government to have to admit that a black African had played such a significant role.

This revelation came as a huge surprise to me. Having spent seven years in the department of cardiac surgery at the University of Cape Town in the 1980s and knowing many of the participants in the first heart transplant personally, it seemed inconceivable to me that I would not have heard rumors of Mr Naki's contribution earlier if the story were true. Although fully aware of the excellent contribution of the staff members of the experimental laboratories in the departments of surgery and cardiac surgery at the university medical school, with whom I had worked personally throughout my time there, I could not remember ever hearing about Hamilton Naki. I thought it was strange that, if he had played such an important role in the first transplant, I had never heard his name mentioned.

My own research at UCT had personally benefited immensely from the important contributions of men and women with no medical or other qualifications, just experience, such as Frederick Snyders (who acted as anaesthetist and oversaw the administration of the immunosuppressive drugs to the animals in our studies), Ferdinand Barends (a naturally gifted and excellent surgeon), Prescott Madlingozi (who ran the heart-lung machine in the laboratory faultlessly), John Roussouw (animal care), and Joanna Kloppers (operating room nurse), and I had heard the names of several of their predecessors as laboratory technicians, such as Victor Pick, but I had not heard of Hamilton Naki.

It would have been very surprising (and probably illegal) if a medically unqualified laboratory technician (of any ethnic background) had participated in a patient's operation at Groote Schuur Hospital in 1967. However, Mr Naki may possibly have been the equivalent of Vivian Thomas, the African-American laboratory technician who indubitably helped develop the Blalock-Taussig shunt operation carried out at the Johns Hopkins Hospital in the US in the 1940s (Chapter 4). Mr Thomas was definitely present (and was photographed) at the first clinical performance of this operation on a blue baby by Alfred Blalock in 1944, although his role was confined to providing advice to the surgeon, but not actual 'hands-on' participation.

Mr Naki's personal story is a remarkable one. As a young man, he migrated to Cape Town from the rural Eastern Cape looking for work. After considerable difficulty in being granted a work permit, he was employed by UCT as a gardener, but later obtained a position caring for the animals in one of the laboratory facilities. By assisting the surgeons in carrying out their experiments, he steadily learned surgical techniques until he was skilled enough to teach medical students and trainee surgeons in the animal laboratory. When recounted by the press, this story, of course, had all the elements to capture the public's attention and, indeed, it is a remarkable and inspiring one.

Subsequently, so much did the rumour of Mr Naki's participation in the first heart transplant grow that several of my former colleagues at GSH and UCT clarified the situation by contributing letters and articles to the press and to medical journals. They drew attention to his valuable work in the experimental laboratory, but emphasised that he had played no role whatsoever in any aspects of the clinical heart transplant program. Marius Barnard also wrote definitively on this topic in his autobiography, and Deirdre Barnard also commented on Mr Naki in her memoirs.

Deirdre Barnard later wrote:

> The reality is that, in those days, animals were used for research and there were people who took care of them. There were two assistants in the animal laboratory. Both of them were black men. One was called Hamilton Naki and the other Frederick Snyders [who was officially

'coloured' under the apartheid rules] … I want to tell this story simply because references to Hamilton were a part of the day-to-day talk in my early life and because my father so much admired him … My father was angry and frustrated that children should be born into this world imperfect, with heart defects … you should also know how great his frustration was that so many people of potential ability in this country were fettered because of their race.

Hamilton was an incredibly neat and dapper dresser and an extremely dignified and upright man. His tie was always straight and beautifully knotted and his shoes gleamed. This pride in his appearance reflected his perfectionist attitude to his work. 'Everything he did, he did well,' said my father. Hamilton is retired now, but during his forty-two-year professional life he helped to train a generation of young doctors [who were taught the rudiments of surgical techniques in the animal laboratory].

Marius Barnard, who we must remember played a leading role in the animal research that preceded the first heart transplant (performing the majority of the transplants in the laboratory) and who was present at the operations on Denise Darvall and Louis Washkansky, had a rather different view of Mr Naki. In his autobiography, he wrote:

Also present [in the animal laboratory] was the now well-known and highly controversial Hamilton Naki. He was our reluctant anaesthetist—we all understood he had other interests around the medical school and hospital. Hamilton could administer the basic anaesthetic and intubate animals, but he was lazy and his concentration and dedication poor.

If it [his participation in the first transplant] were true, we would never have been able to hide it from the press: they would have had the story out the next day. I find it interesting that Naki kept it a secret until after Chris's death. What I cannot understand is why this blatant lie is still being perpetuated by certain elements in the media. It is very sad that Naki allowed himself to be used by unscrupulous reporters and others to spread this misinformation around the world, but it is also exasperating that he never once repudiated this misinformation.

My medical associates and I have, for many years now, tried to rebut the articles that reflect such false allegations. We even wrote to The Guardian stating the facts of the matter but, until today, this newspaper has ignored us and our letter has never been published. I cannot understand why, because this would finally dispel this myth and, after all, the press prides itself on only reporting the truth. So why this gross exception?

These comments are perhaps particularly important coming from someone renowned for his anti-apartheid beliefs and activities. Marius Barnard certainly cannot be accused of any racial prejudice or racially motivated criticism.

It appears that the role of Mr Naki was 'hyped' by the media and, although he should receive full credit for his important contributions in the laboratory and in the training of medical students and surgical residents in surgical technique, he was not present and played no role in the first clinical heart transplant at Groote Schuur Hospital or, indeed, any of the subsequent transplants.

When he retired from the university (in 1991), he was given a present as a token of appreciation for his many years of work. Much to his dismay—and to his wife's disgust—this gift consisted of a water jug, perhaps not a gift worthy of his lifetime contribution. However, it seems that the University of Cape Town and Groote Schuur Hospital were not in the habit of giving generously to its staff on retirement. Chris Barnard's retirement gift was a hospital necktie with a laundry instruction attached that declared it to be washable.

In later life, Hamilton Naki finally received recognition for his contributions to the work of the university (but not for any contribution he made to the first heart transplant) when he was honoured by the provincial government of the Eastern Cape, where he was born. In addition, in 2002, the South African government awarded him the new Order of Mapungubwe, and in 2003, the University of Cape Town gave him an honorary degree (a 'hybrid' Master of Science in Medicine degree) (Figure 11.i).

This was reminiscent of the Johns Hopkins Hospital's belated recognition of Vivian Thomas. Although the innovative Vivian Thomas certainly deserved the honour of an honorary degree, whether Hamilton Naki deserved it any more than several other skilled research technicians who worked in the laboratories of the University of Cape Town medical school—men like Victor Pick, Frederick Snyders, Ferdinand Barends, and Prescott Madlingozi, for example—I am not so sure.

At the time of Mr Naki's death (29 May 2005), several respectable newspapers published obituaries that repeated the claims made originally in *The Guardian*. They later had to retract these claims.

# 12

# The First Survivor:
# Barnard's Second Heart Transplant

## Adrian Kantrowitz and the World's Second Heart Transplant

Before Mr Washkansky's death, the world's second human heart transplant had been carried out at Maimonides Hospital in Brooklyn by surgeon Adrian Kantrowitz on 6 December 1967, just three days after the operation on Mr Washkansky. The patient was a three-week-old baby, Jamie Scudero, with a severe developmental abnormality of the heart.

Dr Kantrowitz had explored heart transplantation in puppies, obviously with a view to carrying out heart transplants in babies with congenital heart defects. He had obtained very encouraging results, with one puppy surviving for more than two hundred days, an excellent result in those early days. To be able to organise and perform a clinical heart transplant within three days of Chris's first effort indicates that Kantrowitz was fully prepared for such a procedure. He certainly had been planning to go ahead even if Chris had not taken that first courageous step.

Dr Kantrowitz cooled the baby to a very low body temperature, much lower than the temperatures used by Drs Bigelow and Lewis in the early days of hypothermia. He was then able to carry out the heart transplant without the need for the continuous support of the heart-lung machine (as the brain would not be damaged by the absence of oxygen at such a low temperature) thus facilitating the technical procedure in such a small patient. Although the surgical procedure seemed to be successful, the baby survived only a few hours, when the heart stopped beating. The cause of the sudden failure of the heart remained uncertain.

Subsequently (on 8 January 1968), Dr Kantrowitz performed one more heart transplant, this time in an adult, which was also unsuccessful. He then withdrew from the field and never attempted heart transplantation again. I later asked Dr Shumway what contribution Adrian Kantrowitz had made to the development of heart transplantation; he was dismissive of his role. Personally, I do not think this gives sufficient credit to Kantrowitz for his excellent experimental studies, although I agree he did not contribute a significant advance to the establishment of clinical heart transplantation.

## Barnard's Second Patient: Philip Blaiberg

Before Mr Washkansky's death, Val Schrire had identified a second patient for a heart transplant in Cape Town, Dr Philip Blaiberg (Figure 12.i), a local dental surgeon who had been forced to retire because of his ill-health. Chris had visited him in the hospital and Dr Blaiberg, who knew he was dying, had readily accepted the offer of a heart transplant. He enthusiastically clutched at this last straw to keep himself alive. As soon as Mr Washkansky died, Chris visited Dr Blaiberg again.

> I immediately broke the news to him. I said, 'Dr Blaiberg, you probably heard that Mr Washkansky died [in fact, he had not heard this] and I just want to tell you that if you don't want to go ahead with the operation, then I understand.' He said to me, 'No, I want to go ahead with it because, the way I am, it is not worthwhile living. I'd like you to do the operation. I have no alternative.'

He declared that, if he could not regain his health, he would rather be dead, and asked how soon the operation could be carried out. Chris told him he had to go overseas for about ten days, but would carry out the operation as soon as possible on his return. Dr Blaiberg stressed that he wanted his operation to be successful, not only for himself but for Barnard and his team. Chris replied by saying that the most helpful thing Dr Blaiberg could do was to 'stay alive until I get back.'

Chris's spirits had begun to be raised at the autopsy on Mr Washkansky, when he saw the perfect technical result of his operation. The suture lines were perfect: there were no surgical errors. 'At that moment,' he wrote in his autobiography, 'I began to build again. I had not failed. I had succeeded. The first attempt, with all its pain and sorrow, had been made for the second. To now turn back would be to deny the first—to turn away from Louis Washkansky's dream.'

Philip Blaiberg was fifty-eight at the time of the transplant. He had been born in Uniondale, a town not unlike Beaufort West, and brought up in Oudtshoorn, a town in the centre of the ostrich-farming industry in the Karoo. Like Mr Washkansky, he was Jewish and his home language was Afrikaans. After local high school, he attended the University of the Witwatersrand in Johannesburg and then transferred to London to study dentistry at the Royal Dental Hospital. He combined a good academic record with playing rugby for the dental school team, his strong build making him an above-average player. He returned to Cape Town to set up in practice, but soon volunteered as a dentist in the South African Medical Corp, serving in Abyssinia (now Ethiopia) and Italy in the Second World War.

It would appear that he had a similar personality to Mr Washkansky as, throughout life, his ability to relate to others made him a popular person who enjoyed life to the full. He was an equally good 'solid citizen' as his predecessor as a candidate for heart transplantation.

After many years in practice in Cape Town, he suffered a series of heart attacks that forced him to take early retirement. Again like Mr Washkansky, Dr Blaiberg's heart failure was related to severe coronary artery disease, for which he had received all of the treatment that it was then possible for Professor Schrire to offer.

Philip Blaiberg underwent heart transplantation on 2 January 1968— the world's third heart transplant. He was to live for a remarkable nineteen months. Dr Blaiberg wrote a short book about his experiences, *Looking At My Heart,* published in 1968, the title being based on the fact that he was the first human in history to actually inspect his own heart and, indeed, hold it in his own hands.

A patient's view of his doctor is always of interest, and Dr Blaiberg's view of Barnard is particularly important. In *Looking At My Heart,* Dr Blaiberg described his first meeting with his surgeon.

> The day after my admission to Ward D1, I was lying in bed with eyes closed, feeling drowsy and thoroughly miserable, when I sensed someone at the head of my bed. I opened my eyes and saw a man. He was tall, young, good-looking with features that reminded me a lot of General Smuts in his later years (Second World War soldier and former prime minister of South Africa). His hands were beautiful; the hands of the born surgeon.

I do not think even Chris would have agreed with this. His hands were already slightly swollen from rheumatoid arthritis, and he was not one of the few surgeons 'born' to the profession. Like most of us, he had to learn his trade the hard way over years of experience. Dr Blaiberg continued:

> Though our conversation was brief and he stayed only a few minutes, I was immediately impressed with the stature of the man and his air

of buoyant optimism. He inspired me with the greatest confidence, an invaluable asset in the relations between a surgeon and his patient.

I felt somewhat better. Here was a man to whom I would willingly entrust my life. I came to know him well in the weeks and months that followed. He is a vital, determined, somewhat mercurial personality, utterly dedicated to his profession.

Geniuses are not like ordinary people. You have to forgive them their tantrums, irritability, ill temper and dogmatism. Some of those who have come in close touch with Barnard and experienced these facets of his character know he can be as charming as he is sometimes grim, as lovable as he is occasionally offhand, as wryly humourous as he can be impatient, as willing to listen as to be dogmatic. They know no one with greater grit and resolution, willing to do more for his patients, rich or poor, well-born or humble, white or non-white, he strives for them, suffers with them, devotes himself entirely to them. That is how I found him. I am proud to have been called the 'most famous' patient of one who has gained international renown and is now an outstanding heart surgeon of our time.

In the copy of his book that Philip Blaiberg gave to Professor Barnard, the author wrote, 'To Prof Chris Barnard, the boldest surgeon in history, from his most grateful and admiring patient.' These comments are dated 3 March 1969, some fourteen months after Dr Blaiberg underwent heart transplantation.

Philip Blaiberg had to wait and stay alive for at least two weeks for Chris to return from the USA before his heart transplant could be carried out. As a surgeon myself, who for many years had responsibility for caring for patients waiting for (or recovering from) heart transplants, I am struck by Chris's willingness to take leave of absence to appear on American television when his second patient was waiting, seemingly, from all the evidence available to us, at death's door, for a donor organ to become available.

Although Professor Schrire had promised Chris to keep Dr Blaiberg alive until his return—and indeed encouraged Chris to accept his invitation to appear on American television as he said Chris owed it to the people of the United States—with Chris out of the country, his team would have undoubtedly declined any donated organ that presented, and Dr Blaiberg might possibly not have survived until Chris's return.

It may have been Chris's intention to cut short his visit to the US and return hurriedly to Cape Town if a suitable donor became available, but flying back would have conservatively taken him at least twenty-four hours (unless a military plane was made available) and in my experience, many donor hearts failed within that period of time. He certainly could not have guaranteed getting back in time.

Many surgeons would not have been comfortable with leaving the country under such circumstances. I am sure there was great pressure on Chris to accept the invitation to appear on CBS in America, possibly from members of the South African government for whom the publicity for their country would be welcome, but he was certainly taking a risk. If Dr Blaiberg had died while Chris was abroad, particularly if a suitable donor heart had been declined because he was not in Cape Town, this would not have reflected well on Chris or his team. However, I believe this is just an example of Chris's ability to take risks that others might not. It was an important part of his character.

Fortunately, Professor Schrire was as good as his word, and did keep Dr Blaiberg alive until Chris's return. Remarkably, within a couple of hours of Chris's plane landing back in Cape Town, a suitable donor became available.

## The Donor, Clive Haupt

New Year's Day is a public holiday in South Africa. It being the height of summer there, Clive Haupt, a twenty-four-year-old coloured man of Salt River, Cape Town (the suburb where Denise Darvall had been killed in an automobile accident) went to the beach for a picnic with his wife and other relatives. Mr Haupt had married his wife, Dorothy, only three months before. He was a garment worker in a factory in Parow, near Cape Town, and one of a large family of thirteen. He had to provide a large contribution to the family budget since his father had died from a stroke (haemorrhage into the brain) in 1965. His mother took a job as a cleaner to earn extra money.

While on the beach, Clive Haupt, like his father before him, suffered a massive brain haemorrhage and was rushed to hospital. It was soon realised that he had sustained irreversible injury to his entire brain and would not recover; he was brain-dead. His wife and mother generously agreed to donate his heart and kidneys (which were to be transplanted into two patients elsewhere in Cape Town), and his brain-dead body was transferred to GSH.

Of interest is that the diagnosis of brain death was confirmed by GSH physician, Dr Raymond 'Bill' Hoffenberg. Mr Haupt was, in fact, the last patient Dr Hoffenberg would examine in South Africa as he had been banned from the country because of his opposition to apartheid. On the following day, Dr Hoffenburg left South Africa for the UK, where he had a very distinguished career, eventually being elected to the presidency of the Royal College of Physicians of London.

It is also of interest to note that Chris attended Mr Haupt's funeral personally, perhaps aware of the criticism directed towards him when he was not present at Mr Washkansky's funeral. As an illustration of Chris's by now godlike stature in South Africa, he was mobbed, with many of the mourners clearly intent on touching him.

Dr Blaiberg would, therefore, receive a heart from a coloured man. After the operation, this of course led to many comments and articles in the world's press in regard to the apartheid policy. Mr Haupt would not have been allowed into many venues which Dr Blaiberg, with his 'coloured' heart, was able to access. The ridiculousness of the policy was laid bare. Nevertheless, the operation was criticised by some of the diehard supporters of apartheid.

The surgical, anaesthetic, and nursing team that was called in was almost identical to that which had carried out the first transplant.

## The Operation and Post-Transplant Care

The operation (on 2 January 1968) did not begin well, with Chris (possibly because of tiredness after his flight back from the USA) making several mistakes that could have been disastrous. He began to regret he had taken the American trip. However, because of his experience and the help of his colleagues, he was able to recover from these errors. Furthermore, he was suffering from a flare-up of rheumatoid arthritis, which he again blamed on the stresses of his American trip. He found operating to be more than usually painful. However, after a shaky start, the operation went well and the donor heart began to beat strongly in the patient's chest.

In this operation, Barnard made one relatively minor modification to the surgical technique, which made the operation less likely to damage the conducting system (the nerves) in the heart, and which became the norm for the multitude of surgeons who followed. The exact nature of the modification is relatively unimportant, but it is interesting to note that, with far less experience of heart transplantation in experimental animals than several other surgeons, including Shumway, Lower, Hardy, and Kantrowitz, it should be the innovative Barnard who introduced this technical modification.

A member of the medical staff of the hospital—a haematologist, who Chris named as Dr Mibashan—surreptitiously took some photographs of the operation from the observation dome, which Chris reports the haematologist intended to try to sell to the media. He had done so without the permission of Dr Blaiberg or his family, the hospital, or Chris. He was exposed, and my understanding is that he was forced to resign from the faculty. It is strange that some people will risk their reputation and job just to 'make a quick buck', if that was truly his intention; if his intention was to record the operation for posterity, I presume he would have gained consent from those involved in it.

In preparation for this second heart transplant, the hospital authorities had transformed three rooms into an air-conditioned transplant suite, a greatly improved isolation facility in which the patient could be nursed after the operation with the hope that this clean environment would reduce the risk of infection. The hospital bacteriologist, Dr Arderne Forder, had been asked to draw up a report on Mr Washkansky's management and to make recommendations on how in future cases infections could be avoided. The rooms in the new suite had never been used before to nurse post-operative patients, and therefore would likely not be contaminated by previous patients with infections. Multiple bacterial cultures were taken from the walls, equipment, and staff for any possible potential sources of infection. Anyone entering the suite was required to shower and change. No VIP visitors, such as politicians or visiting surgeons (or at least very few), were allowed in. This greatly reduced the risk of Dr Blaiberg developing an infection.

It amazed Chris how a considerable amount of money was readily made available for this to be done. 'Where, before, it took months or even years to get new equipment, now I only had to make a casual suggestion and it was done,' he remembered.

Immediately after the operation, Dr Blaiberg was transferred to this new facility. When he had recovered sufficiently to be taken off the ventilator (that was breathing for him), like Mr Washkansky, some of his first words were to express how he already felt better (as he was no longer in heart failure and so his breathing was much improved). 'As soon as I recovered from the anaesthetic,' he said, 'I knew the operation was worthwhile.'

In what must have been a blow, albeit perhaps mainly psychological, Professor Schrire told Chris that neither he nor the other cardiologists would be involved in the day-to-day care of Dr Blaiberg or of future heart transplant patients as they had too much routine work to deal with, although they would see the patient and give advice whenever required. This decision may have been the first indication of Professor Schrire's disenchantment with Chris's new 'love affair' with the media limelight. Chris and his surgical team were therefore very much on their own.

## Controlling the Media Circus

In view of the 'invasion' of the hospital by media personnel that had occurred after Mr Washkansky's operation, strict security measures were introduced in all areas of the hospital. Dr Blaiberg's progress was followed intimately by the media, but the hospital introduced tight control of access of the media people to the building, and even stricter access to the patient's suite. Uniformed guards were posted at each entrance of the transplant suite to ensure no unauthorised entry.

Initially, no press conferences were held as the medical superintendent of the hospital, Dr Burger, quite reasonably said he wanted the surgical team to be able to work unhindered and get more rest than had been possible after the first transplant. A hospital doctor was made responsible for providing bulletins on the patient's progress to the press and media twice daily, and also responded to other questions from the news agencies. Nevertheless, some members of the press again attempted to 'gatecrash' the operating theatre and Dr Blaiberg's isolation room before, during, and after the operation. The audacity of the press continued through several later transplants. One press photographer actually found his way into the surgeons' changing room, donned a scrub suit, and boldly entered the operating room in an attempt to photograph one of the early heart transplant operations.

Within a couple of days, a major controversy developed with regard to access to the major players in the drama. It became clear that, before the transplant—while Chris was in the USA—the Blaibergs had signed a contract with the National Broadcasting Company (NBC, one of the US's major television companies) that gave NBC exclusive rights to film the transplant operation and access to Dr Blaiberg and his family after the operation. The contract, worth US$50,000, stipulated that the money would be shared between the hospital, the Chris Barnard Fund, the Haupt family, and the Blaibergs. As the hospital authorities, apparently in consultation with Chris, had not allowed the operation to be filmed, the contract was evidently reduced to US$25,000.

When the South African press learned it would only be able to publish photographs and movies of Dr Blaiberg provided by NBC in America, there was an outcry, not only from the local press and public (who naturally felt the operation was a South African event), but also by the press from all other parts of the world who would be excluded by the contract. Chequebook journalism had arrived in South Africa. Even those who donated blood in South Africa, including, of course, for Dr Blaiberg's operation (without financial reward) objected to the principle of the contract. The situation was further confused by various rumours of photographers taking photographs in the operating room, and so on, with threats of legal action on all sides.

At this point, Dr LAPA Munnik felt obliged to step in and announce that GSH would ignore all instances of chequebook journalism, and that all information on the progress of the patient would be made available to all media companies equally. The regular press conferences were reinstated, but Dr Munnik explained that the hospital authorities were anxious to prevent a recurrence of the media circus that had occurred after the first heart transplant. It was not until six weeks after the transplant that the first photographs of Dr Blaiberg were allowed to be taken.

Nevertheless, it seems that Philip and Eileen Blaiberg remained under contract because, NBC pointed out, his long illness had reduced their savings and they needed the money. Despite the relatively minimal cost of medical care in South Africa at that time (particularly in contrast to the USA), it is fully understandable how Dr Blaiberg's long period of ill-health, with the prospect of a prolonged recovery from the transplant operation, had impacted his financial situation.

Dr Blaiberg's post-operative recovery progressed well, but was slow as he had to recover strength after his many months of inactivity before the transplant. On one occasion, Chris carried into his room a box in which was Dr Blaiberg's native heart, and he thus became the first man in the history of mankind to hold in his hands his own heart.

Seventy-four days after his transplant, Dr Blaiberg became the first patient with a heart transplant to leave hospital and lead a relatively normal life. An immense crowd surrounded the door from which he would leave (Figure 12.ii), and a great cheer went up when he emerged, a roar so loud 'that any soccer supporters' club would have been proud,' wrote Chris. Another crowd had gathered outside the Blaiberg apartment building to greet him when he arrived home. More than a dozen policemen were required to protect him from the enthusiastic and welcoming onlookers.

Dr Bosman, one of the department's surgical trainees, took personal responsibility for Dr Blaiberg's care, withdrawing from most other activities to ensure that his patient received the best possible attention. This included visiting him at home almost every day, which almost certainly contributed to the success of Dr Blaiberg's care. One might conjecture that this rather unusual, obsessive behaviour may have been a factor in Dr Bosman's tragic suicide some years later, while still a relatively young man, though I have no knowledge of the circumstances. Before this tragic event, however, he had been placed in charge of the hospital's kidney transplant program.

## The First Long-Term Survivor: Dr Blaiberg's Subsequent Progress

Once settled back in his own home, Dr Blaiberg began to make short visits to places of interest in the Cape Town area. On one occasion, he and his wife drove up to the Rhodes Memorial on the slopes of Devil's Peak, which overlooks GSH and the southern suburbs of Cape Town. Two men, recognising Dr Blaiberg from newspaper photographs, approached them and introduced themselves. One, Richard 'Bill' Heald, had been a contemporary of mine as a medical student in London, though a few years senior to me. Indeed, it was Bill Heald who had facilitated my brief sojourn as a ship's surgeon. He is now an internationally known professor of surgery. He was, by this time, a surgical trainee at Guy's Hospital, and was attending a surgical congress in Cape Town. They chatted with Dr Blaiberg for several minutes, asking him about his treatment and progress.

Such was the international interest in Dr Blaiberg's progress that, on his return to the UK, Bill Heald wrote a letter to *The Times* newspaper in London giving his impressions of the famous patient, as follows:

> There have been a number of wild and varied reports about the quality of life being enjoyed by Dr Blaiberg since his heart transplant. I met him, and a brief description by an essentially unbiased observer, like myself, may be of interest. He walks and talks normally with the exception of a slight residual weakness of the legs. At no time did I observe him to be breathless. 'I have had a hundred days of good life on borrowed time,' he told me, 'and if I die next week from rejection, the operation on me will still have been a success.' Having seen for myself that Dr Blaiberg is enjoying life, I can assure doubters that reports to the contrary are untrue.

Media attention continued unabated, and Dr Blaiberg's return to a relatively active life was followed intensely over many months. 'Photoshoots' were held to show him even taking a dip in the ocean, though I understand it was a very brief one.

By June 1968, about six months after the transplant, Dr Blaiberg's condition had deteriorated significantly, and he required readmission to GSH. At first, it was feared he may have developed an infection, like Mr Washkansky, but then Chris realised he had steadily been rejecting his heart. So great was his deterioration that Chris actually raised the subject of a retransplant with the patient and his wife. Indeed, for a few days, Chris was 'madly looking for a donor so that I could transplant a second heart into his body. In times of crisis, you grasp at straws.'

Dr Blaiberg was first administered extra cortisone, the standard treatment for rejection, but he failed to respond to this. As a last resort, Dr Bosman and Chris decided to try the relatively new immunosuppressive agent, anti-lymphocyte serum, some of which they had obtained from scientists in Europe. They had no experience with its use, but knew it could be associated with some serious side-effects. Nevertheless, if they were to save their patient's life, they had no choice. Fortunately, Dr Blaiberg tolerated the drug well; the rejection episode was rapidly suppressed and he recovered to an active life once again. He lived for another year.

As far as I am aware, this was the first time that this relatively new immunosuppressive agent, anti-lymphocyte serum (which Chris had seen administered by Tom Starzl in Denver) was used in a heart transplant patient to reverse a severe rejection episode. It had been used by others previously to prevent rejection, but not to show it would successfully reverse a severe rejection episode.

It was Dr Blaiberg's success, perhaps more than any other single factor, that led to guarded optimism that heart transplantation would eventually prove a valuable treatment option. He was the shining beacon while the vast majority of other attempts at heart transplantation worldwide that followed in the late 1960s seemed doomed to early failure. His courage and fortitude did much to establish heart transplantation as a realistic option for future patients with terminal heart disease.

However, he slowly developed the hitherto unknown complication of chronic rejection (or graft atherosclerosis, a form of low-grade, delayed rejection that results in narrowing of the coronary arteries, similar to that seen in regular coronary artery disease) from which he sadly died nineteen months after his heart transplant (on 17 August 1969). His autopsy demonstrated severe and widespread coronary artery disease, which came as a major shock to the medical profession, who had not anticipated that atherosclerosis could develop so rapidly. This was the first example of chronic rejection which now, almost fifty years later, dominates as the major cause of graft failure after the first post-transplant year. Today, however, with better immunosuppressve drugs, it does not always develop, and when it does, it may take several years to begin to develop and many more years to become problematic. When it becomes severe, the only realistic treatment is a second transplant (retransplantation), but only if the patient remains a suitable candidate.

Some patients may no longer be candidates because complications of the immunosuppressive drug therapy, as well as natural aging, may have rendered them no longer ideal. For example, some drugs increase the chance the patient will develop diabetes, others increase the risk of developing impairment of kidney function (possibly resulting in kidney failure), and yet others increase the risk of the patient developing certain forms of malignant disease. These conditions might possibly preclude the patient from undergoing a second transplant.

## Why was Dr Blaiberg so Important to the Future of Heart Transplantation?

Chris explained to me the importance of the relative success of Dr Blaiberg's operation.

> For two reasons, Blaiberg was responsible for other surgeons trying to get involved in transplantation. First, Blaiberg left hospital and, second, was the first patient to show that, after a human heart had been transplanted, you could live a normal life. He was on the beach, he was photographed, and he lived for one and a half years. So people saw there was a possibility, not only of living a normal life after transplantation, but of surviving longer than just a few weeks or months. He was the one who really got the transplant programme going. Immediately, there was an increase in the number of transplants world-wide.

Chris's first two heart transplants were therefore technical successes. The confidence and courage it took to undertake these procedures, when immunosuppressive therapy was primitive by today's standards, must never be underestimated. Chris picked himself up from the massive disappointment over the outcome of the first procedure and almost immediately went ahead with the second transplant which, considering his team's (and the world's) lack of experience, was a resounding success. This success did much to sustain some optimism that heart transplantation would eventually become a reliable therapy for patients in terminal heart failure, when most patients undergoing this procedure at other centres were dying at an early stage.

13

# Heart Transplant Fever

Norman Shumway carried out the fourth heart transplant in the world on 6 January 1968, just four days after the operation on Dr Blaiberg. Having led the research field for so long, Shumway must have been relieved and gratified to finally begin his own clinical programme. Despite the Shumway team's enormous experience in the experimental laboratory, the patient, Mr Mike Kasperak, did not do well. He suffered one major complication after another and died fourteen days after the operation. Perhaps Shumway's basic mistake was selecting a patient who had several other health problems, which greatly complicated his recovery—in other words, like many of the early patients who had undergone closed mitral valvotomy or early open heart surgery, he was too sick to get through the surgical procedure and the initial period of recovery, and to withstand the side effects of immunosuppressive therapy.

Mr Kasperak was fifty-four years old and was diabetic. After the transplant, he suffered widespread haemorrhage into the gastrointestinal tract, injury to his kidneys and adrenal glands, and pancreatitis, among other problems. He underwent three major operations in five days, mainly for intestinal bleeding. He required continuous ventilation (machine-assisted breathing) and dialysis, but became semi-comatose through liver failure. He died of septicemia, pneumonia (due to both a bacterial and a fungal infection), and continuing gastrointestinal haemorrhage.

As a former surgeon myself, I can readily imagine the mental agony that Shumway—ably supported by his right-hand man, Ed Stinson, of whom Shumway thought so highly—suffered during this two-week period. It is tragic enough when any patient is doing so poorly, but it must have been doubly so as Mr Kasperak was their first patient to undergo a procedure of which the Stanford team were considered the recognised masters. I would suspect that Shumway's disappointment at the outcome was equal to, if not greater than, that which followed Barnard pipping him to the post with the operation on Mr Washkansky. The operation on Mr Kasperak was Shumway's opportunity to demonstrate to the world the great expertise his team had developed, only to be faced by failure.

Three days after Shumway's first attempt, Adrian Kantrowitz did his second transplant, this time on fifty-eight-year-old Mr Louis Block, the world's fifth heart transplant. The donor heart was very small compared to the size of the patient, and struggled to support the circulation, failing completely within eight hours despite support given by a balloon pump (an external mechanical device designed by Kantrowitz to provide support to the heart).

Kantrowitz's undoubted mistake had been to believe that such a small woman's heart would support a much larger man. It is possible he was influenced by his eagerness to carry out a second transplant after the early failure of his first. Surgeons sometimes make errors of judgement from even subconscious desires or hopes. A surgeon's decisions must be based on facts and logic, and not influenced by less solid considerations. There is a surgical aphorism that says that 'there should be no hope in surgery.' Facts are preferable to hopes.

Whether this failure was too much for Kantrowitz to bear, or whether other factors (possibly pressure from the hospital administration to curtail his activities) affected him, I do not know, but he never carried out another heart transplant. This is very surprising when one considers the excellent research he had carried out over many years in the experimental laboratory, where he had performed approximately 250 transplants in dogs, compared to fewer than fifty in Barnard's lab (and almost 300 by Shumway's team). He devoted his subsequent career to his interests in the balloon pump and other forms of mechanical support of the failing heart. For reasons of which I am uncertain, he was relieved of his position at Maimonides in 1970, though he continued his research at a hospital in Detroit, where many of his former New York colleagues joined him.

The next surgeon to carry out a heart transplant was Dr Profulla Kumar Sen of Bombay (now Mumbai), whose patient died after only three hours. Of the first six transplants, therefore, only Dr Blaiberg was surviving, which heightens Chris's achievement.

Despite these generally very poor initial results, including failures by surgical groups with most experience in the experimental laboratory, from early 1968, there was enormous enthusiasm for heart transplantation for a period of about two years. Seemingly every heart surgeon in the world wanted to demonstrate that he, too, could perform a heart transplant. In 1968 alone, 101 transplants were performed in twenty-six different countries, but the results were generally very disappointing and sometimes disastrous.

I asked Sir Roy Calne if Chris's contribution was beneficial or detrimental to the field of organ transplantation or a bit of both.

> I think a bit of both. It was beneficial in showing it could be done, but detrimental in the celebrity attitude which he much encouraged. I don't think this was detrimental if you look at surgery in general, but it led to cardiac surgeons all over the world doing transplants without knowing anything about immunology or immunosuppression. I think they thought if Barnard can do it, we can do it. We're just as good surgeons.

Although many expected Dr Lower's team in Richmond to be among the leaders in entering the clinical arena, they did not perform a heart transplant in a patient until 26 May, the sixteenth such transplant. Despite Dr Lower's great experience in managing dogs with transplants, his patient was the first to die directly as a result of acute rejection, only seven days after the transplant. It is ironic that rejection should defeat the surgeon who had arguably contributed most to overcoming it in the laboratory.


## The UK Experience

I had personal experience of the initial transplants carried out in the UK, and so I will use this programme as an example of the many heart transplants worldwide during this period. At the National Heart Hospital, we had been carrying out research into heart transplantation for several months before Chris performed the transplant on Mr Washkansky, but there had been no indication of carrying out a transplant in a patient.

Not long after his second transplant in Cape Town, Chris and M. C. Botha visited London to take part in a television discussion about heart transplantation: a special edition of the BBC programme *Tomorrow's World*, called 'Barnard Faces his Critics'. One of my senior colleagues, Donald Longmore, a surgically trained physiologist at the hospital, had been invited to participate in the program. As I was a member of the research team, he kindly arranged for me to be in the audience. There was severe criticism of Barnard's work by one or two in the audience, notably the television personality Malcolm Muggeridge (also a journalist and author) and Dr Donald Gould (the editor of a medical journal). However, generally, the questions and comments were positive. Chris handled the criticisms with his usual incisive comments and sparkling personality.

Malcolm Muggeridge, the British author, asked, 'Why was it that this operation was first performed in South Africa? Was it because in South Africa there are more brilliant, more audacious surgeons? Was it because in South Africa there is better equipment, are better facilities? Or was it, as I suspect that because of the vile doctrine of apartheid in South Africa, life is held cheaper?' Barnard remained admirably calm.

> I think we have fairly good surgeons in South Africa. I think that my colleagues will agree with me that they have here in this country some very good surgeons who are South Africans [undoubtedly thinking of Donald Ross, but also several other cardiac surgeons working in the UK at that time]. Secondly, I feel that in South Africa we have excellent facilities to do this type of surgery. Thirdly, I think you should think that we hold a very high opinion of death and human suffering because we did this operation with the purpose of treating a sick man and relieving human suffering.

Chris later described this moment:

> [It was] the toughest encounter I'd yet had in open public debate. It was really kind of a match between some key players: M. C. [Botha] and I on the one side with Malcolm Muggeridge and Dr Donald Gould on the other side. Being South African—and one totally opposed to apartheid—I had faced, and would face many times again, attacks like this on my country. On this occasion, it was a relief when Professor Calne stood up and said, 'May I say, Sir, that I and most of my colleagues disassociate ourselves from the question put to you!' This was met with great cries of 'hear, hear!' foot-stomping and loud applause.

Roy Calne spoke in support of Barnard's effort, but questioned why the Cape Town team had allowed so much publicity. Barnard replied that it had been impossible to prevent the media people from overrunning the hospital and obtaining information (some correct and some incorrect) from multiple unofficial sources.

Towards the end of the program, from the front row of the audience, Donald Longmore announced that we were preparing for a transplant of the heart and both lungs. We were indeed investigating transplantation of the heart and both lungs in dogs (very unsuccessfully, I might add) but I was unaware of any serious plan to carry out this procedure in a patient, although I know that Donald Longmore had been trying to persuade his surgical colleagues—Donald Ross (Figure 6.i) and Keith Ross (not related, later Sir Keith)—to undertake this operation, which had never been attempted previously, on a patient he had identified. At that moment, one of my research colleagues entered the set pushing a wheelchair in which sat a gentleman who indeed would have benefitted from such a procedure.

This provided a dramatic finale to the program. I had been unaware that this denouement had been planned, and I personally felt this announcement was very premature in view of our relative lack of progress in the research laboratory. The patient never received a transplant and unfortunately died sometime later.

Before the patient's sad demise, Mr Longmore even briefly considered transplanting the heart and lungs from a large dog into him, which would have been highly experimental and would inevitably have led to a disastrous outcome. There was absolutely no evidence in the medical literature that such a procedure would have any chance of success whatsoever, but such was the misplaced euphoria at the time that this sort of approach was even discussed. Even today, it would be an immediate failure within minutes.

However, at the National Heart Hospital interest grew to enter this field and, in the spring of 1968, Donald Ross and Keith Ross came to the research laboratory one Wednesday to carry out two orthotopic heart transplants in dogs. I carried out both of the organ retrievals from the 'donor' dogs. The second procedure was the more successful and the transplanted heart functioned well. However, as the experiment had been planned simply as a technical exercise (as in Chris's early experiments), the dog was euthanised before being allowed to wake from the anaesthesia.

No mention was made of when a heart transplant might be attempted clinically, and my impression was that it was not imminent. I was therefore extremely surprised when I received a telephone call in the laboratory two days later from a member of the press asking me to confirm that a heart transplant was proceeding at the National Heart Hospital. As I had heard nothing to this effect, I denied the rumour. However, when a second call came through soon after, I checked with Mr Ross's staff at the hospital and found that indeed a transplant was planned and would be carried out that evening (3 May 1968).

Donald Longmore and one of the surgical registrars had gone to another London Hospital, King's College Hospital, to assess a potential brain-dead donor; the plan was to transfer the donor by ambulance to the operating room of the Heart Hospital where the heart would be excised and immediately transplanted into the selected recipient.

Naturally enough, as a member of the research group, I was disappointed (and indeed mildly irritated) that I had not been privy to these plans, although I understood the need to keep them as secret as possible to try to prevent a leak to the press. It was obvious, however, that this attempt at secrecy had failed miserably. I immediately went to the hospital to watch the surgical procedure. The security there, aimed at keeping out the press, was considerable. Very sensibly, no one except the members of the surgical team was being allowed into the operating room suite, both from fear of the risk of infection and from fear of media infiltration. Strict instructions had been given that no one was to be allowed even into the observation dome of the operating room. With Donald Ross's support, however, I managed to persuade the security staff to allow me to watch from the dome, only to find that blinds had been pulled down to obscure most of the view of the surgical procedure, presumably to prevent photographs from being taken. Although my view was necessarily severely restricted, I managed to see most of the operation through a gap in the blinds.

The surgery went well and the heart functioned very satisfactorily. It was the world's tenth heart transplant. At the end of the operation, I joined the surgical team in the surgeons' lounge in the operating room suite, where spirits were high. Dr M. C. Botha, the tissue immunologist from the Cape Town group, happened to be visiting London at the time and he joined us together with Dr James Mowbray, a transplant immunologist and renal physician from the nearby St. Mary's Hospital, who had been invited to collaborate on the immunological aspects of the care of the patient (as there was, of course, no kidney transplantation programme at the National Heart Hospital which, as its name indicates, treated only patients with heart disease). There was considerable discussion about the case and about transplantation in general. To a young surgical research fellow, as I was, it was an exciting experience.

While we were celebrating the success of the technical procedure, word came through that Dr Denton Cooley had performed his first heart transplant in Houston on the same day. As Dr Cooley had a reputation for rapidly performing a large series of cardiac operations, some wag at the Heart Hospital joked that Cooley would probably report his first twenty heart transplants within the next month. This did not prove to be so very far from the mark, as Cooley's group performed no fewer than four heart transplants over the course of that single weekend.

By the end of the evening, a relatively large group of reporters and photographers had formed outside the entrance to the hospital and it was felt that a representative of the surgical team should make a statement to them. It was decided that all of us present in the surgical lounge should participate and I can well remember (even though I had played no role in the operation) standing on the steps of the hospital entrance with many other members of the hospital staff while a short statement was read about the procedure and the patient's progress (Figure 13.i).

The following morning (Saturday), photographs of the group appeared on the front page of nearly every national newspaper, and I gained considerable prestige among my family and lay friends for being involved in this surgical triumph. I did not feel it necessary to shatter their illusions by mentioning that I had only watched the procedure from a crack between the blinds in the observation dome.

A full press conference was planned for the Saturday. I was tempted to show up in the anticipation that further photographs would appear in the newspapers and would again impress my family and friends. However, as I had already missed a key training session on the river at Thames Rowing Club on the previous evening, I reluctantly decided to forego further fame in order not to lose my place in the rowing crew. I therefore went down to the river and read about the press conference in the Sunday newspapers.

In retrospect, I was pleased that I had missed the press conference because it did not work out quite as everybody anticipated. At about this time, there had been a campaign to improve the economy in Britain (as ever in those days, and even today) and everybody was being urged to show pride in British products and achievements. It was fashionable to demonstrate that in whatever one was pursuing, one was 'backing Britain'. In the euphoria of the moment, and in an innocent gesture to show that British surgery could compete with the rest of the world, some of the members of the surgical team at the press conference were given cards on which were printed the Union Jack and the words 'I'm Backing Britain'. This subsequently backfired as it was incorrectly interpreted by some that the operation had been carried out for national pride rather than as an honest attempt to save the life of a patient. This was clearly not the case but the controversy initiated my painful education in how careful one must be in one's dealings with the press. Some weeks later, after the patient sadly died, the satirical magazine *Private Eye* mischievously embellished the photograph taken at the press conference and splashed it on its cover (Figure 13.ii).

I state that national pride was not the prime reason for performing the heart transplant in this patient but, in fact, I can see that the wish to prove that we too (in the UK) could perform this new operation successfully influenced the surgeons to begin the heart transplantation programme at that time. Although the transplant research programme had been underway for a year or more—and kudos to Donald Longmore for having this vision—to my knowledge, the initiation of a clinical transplant programme had not been seriously considered until Chris had started the ball rolling. I am certain that this was the case in most centres where heart transplants were carried out in 1968 and 1969.

The patient at the Heart Hospital, Mr Frederick West, initially did well. I played no role in his care, but was able to keep in touch with his progress through my colleagues. The British media followed his progress almost as closely as they had the first patient in Cape Town. Mr West was actually visited by Chris during a short stay he made in London to see his friend,

Donald Ross. After a couple of weeks of satisfactory recovery, however, Mr West began to develop respiratory problems, with deterioration in his lung function. The cause of his deteriorating lung condition was not fully understood until an autopsy was performed after his death.

This revealed that he had developed recurrent pulmonary emboli from a thrombus that formed in the residual native right atrial appendage that had been left *in situ* (multiple small clots formed in the remnant of his native heart, broke off, and were carried in the blood to his lungs, causing increasing injury). As a result, he died after forty-five days, having never left the hospital. A second heart transplant was performed at the Heart Hospital but was also unsuccessful.

One apocryphal incident that reputedly occurred at the time of either the first or second heart transplant at the National Heart Hospital (I cannot now remember which) caused considerable amusement among the junior staff. The brain-dead donor was being transported rapidly by ambulance from the donor hospital to the Heart Hospital. In the ambulance, one of the surgical team noticed that in the rush to change from his operating room scrub suit into his usual street clothes, his shirt tail had become caught in the zipper of his trousers (pants) and, even worse, the zipper had become jammed half open. It was known that a horde of press photographers and television cameras was waiting outside the Heart Hospital for the arrival of the ambulance. Most of the dash across London was therefore spent with one of the team making a frantic effort to free the zipper on his colleague's trousers. In the subsequent television broadcast, the dash across London was described in dramatic terms with details of the way 'the two surgeons fought courageously' to maintain the circulation of the donor and keep the heart pumping until they arrived back at the Heart Hospital; the truth would certainly have been less dramatic, but possibly far more entertaining.

Donald Ross performed a third transplant, this time at Guy's Hospital, which proved his most successful; the patient survived several weeks, but again still not doing well enough to leave the hospital.

Along with many other groups around the world, Donald Ross's team came to the conclusion that the immunological problems were too great, and no further transplants were performed at either the National Heart or Guy's Hospital. Surgeon Magdi Yacoub (now Sir Magdi) made one attempt at Harefield Hospital some time after Donald Ross's first three cases, but this patient did not survive the operation. Several years then elapsed before heart transplantation was resuscitated in 1979 as a clinical procedure in the United Kingdom. It was Terence English who led this programme at Papworth Hospital, just outside Cambridge. I had the great privilege of being a member of his team. This programme has continued unbroken ever since, and has had excellent outcomes.

This sequence of an initial largely unsuccessful rush to 'get in on the act', with subsequent closure of the programme for several years before its resuscitation a decade later, was typical of that of many programmes around the world.

## A Cautionary Tale

There is one other story that relates to heart transplantation that was recounted to me during my research into writing my previous book, *Open Heart*. For reasons that will be obvious, I shall not report who told me the story or where the event took place, although I will state that it was in a country where you would have expected medical care to be good (and, indeed, is good).

It was in the late 1960s during the initial great enthusiasm for heart transplantation, and groups all over the world were attempting this operation with very little or no research experience behind them. It was a time of relatively abandoned medical experimentation in this field.

Caught up in the excitement at the time, heart surgeons in one region of the world were planning their first heart transplant. A patient was identified who was in heart failure and who it was considered would not survive more than a few weeks. He was put on the waiting list to await a donor heart. A suitable 'brain-dead' donor was identified, and the operation was planned to be carried out within a few hours. The operating rooms and the surgical teams were alerted and prepared. For reasons that are now lost in obscurity, the operation did not take place.

According to my multiple informants, ten years later, the potential recipient remained alive and in reasonably good health (which was unlikely to have been the outcome if he had undergone heart transplantation in those early pioneering days). It was therefore fortunate for him that the operation had to be abandoned. Even though the news of his long-term survival came as something of a surprise and shock to me, since it had been presumed at the time that he had very few days of life left, it came as an even greater shock when my informants told me that, ten years later, the potential donor also remained alive and well. The tentative diagnosis of brain death had clearly been incorrect.

This story remains a lesson to us all that over-enthusiasm towards any new medical or surgical development should not be allowed to cloud the individual physician's judgment.

# 14

# Meeting of the Minds:
# The First International Conference

The South African government was, of course, delighted to continue to have some good publicity for the country, rather than the critical international (and some local) press about its iniquitous apartheid policy. Barnard and his team were given every support for the heart transplant programme and this included financial support from the government of the Western Cape for the world's first conference devoted to clinical heart transplantation. This international meeting in Cape Town, sponsored jointly by the Cape Provincial Administration and the University of Cape Town, provided the first opportunity for an exchange of views between the surgeons who had carried out heart transplants at that time. The total number of transplants performed in the world was then twenty-five.

'We had the first international heart transplant meeting in Cape Town [in July 1968],' remembered Chris, 'and the Province provided the money for it. It was a very successful meeting. We invited two members—a surgeon and an immunologist—from every unit in the world that was doing transplants' (Figure 14.i).

The proceedings of this meeting were subsequently published in book form as *Experience with Human Heart Transplantation*, edited by a South African physician, Hillel Shapiro. At the time, only thirteen surgeons in the world had attempted the procedure, with Dr Cooley having the largest experience with five patients. Among the attendees were Adrian Kantrowitz, Donald Ross, and Denton Cooley, but, notably, neither Norman Shumway nor Richard Lower participated, both of whom sent junior colleagues to represent them. By not attending personally, was this a small way of denying Chris recognition as the leader in the field at that time? I suggest it was.

Chris was disappointed that Shumway did not attend personally. He felt that Shumway regretted that he had not carried out the world's first heart transplant and not even the first transplant in the USA. Chris also claimed that Shumway remained professionally jealous of him for years (though whether this is true or not is uncertain). When Chris's operating room nurse, Pittie Rautenbach, visited Shumway's unit in Stanford sometime later, Chris recalled that Shumway's 'staff didn't want to show her around or extend any of the usual courtesies given to visiting foreign colleagues.' Whether this is an accurate opinion, I am uncertain. However, my impression was that one reason why Chris's contributions to the development of heart transplantation were not acknowledged by the International Society of Heart and Lung Transplantation was that its leadership at the time was heavily influenced by Dr Shumway's former or current trainees.

Shumway and Barnard did not meet again for twenty years until attending a medical meeting in Madrid. There is some evidence that Shumway took pains to avoid meeting with Chris, and would decline any invitation where there was a risk that this was likely to happen.

The July 1968 meeting in Cape Town extended over five days, each day being divided into discussion on major topics, such as 'Patient selection', 'Donor selection', 'Surgical technique', 'Rejection and its treatment', and 'Post-operative problems: results and the future'.

## Patient Selection

Professor Schrire summed up his opinion:

> I have learned that this procedure [the heart transplant] is technically possible; it is within the province of skilled surgeons; it can be performed at a very reasonable, acceptable surgical operative mortality ... I think all of us here are agreed that the only patients who should be subjected to operation at present are patients who are about to die, who have no hope at all, who very much wish to live and whom you can offer some sort of procedure, even on a temporary basis.

Others added that in the selection of the recipient, they should avoid, as much as possible, patients with other health problems that might complicate the patient's recovery, and that the recipient should have a stable personality. Furthermore, there should be unanimity of opinion that the patient's condition is irreversible and that there is no other treatment.

Dr M. C. Botha put forward the case for tissue typing, saying, 'I personally firmly believe that tissue typing does improve the chances of a recipient accepting a graft.' However, Dr Walt Lillehei, who by this time had carried out a heart transplant in New York, commented, 'I don't have the slightest doubt that tissue typing is extremely important, but I suspect that all immunologists would agree fully that we really don't know enough about what we are doing these days to make tissue typing, at this time, the significant determinant as to whether a dying patient should have cardiac replacement or not.'

In retrospect, Dr Lillehei was correct, as was so often the case. Tissue typing has improved immensely during the past fifty years, but a good tissue match is still not considered essential in heart transplantation.

## Donor Selection and the Question of Brain Death

Among the topics discussed by the attendees was the diagnosis of death of the donor. Was brain death acceptable as a basis on which to proceed with excision of the heart while it was still beating? Led by one of the Cape Town neurosurgeons, J. C. 'Kay' DeVilliers, there was much discussion on this topic.

Based on a careful clinical examination of the patient, French neurologists had already established a definition of brain death. The participants in the congress agreed that, with the advent of modern resuscitation techniques and devices, the old definition ('the apparent extinction of life' as shown by absence of heart-beat and respiration) could no longer apply. They also agreed that there was one sign that could be taken as irrefutable evidence of death: the brain ceasing to function.

However, to insure that a doctor does not 'pull the plug' on a dying patient simply to obtain a needed organ, the congress participants agreed that transplanters should not be allowed to attend the dying potential donor (as Chris's team had already agreed).

Donald Ross felt that 'the public has apparently developed some suspicion of organ transplant surgeons and this has led to difficulty in getting donors. The public ... should be educated to accept that it is surely wrong to bury a heart so that the worms can devour it instead of grafting that heart into a suitable recipient whose life can then be usefully prolonged.' Many years later, Dr Shumway told me of a donor, a victim of homicide, from whom he took the heart.

The case later went to court because the lawyers for the murderer said that the donor (or, at least, his brain) was 'okay until those guys came over and took out his heart.' The judge, of course, said it was nonsense, and validated the brain death criteria. That actually was the court decision, the judicial basis for the legislation that followed on brain death in the state of California. Prior to that, we had not really been legally justified in doing heart transplants.

It was not until 1974 that the State of California passed an act that allowed a donor's heart to be removed while it was still beating. This was allowed only if there was no evidence of brain function.

I mentioned to Dr Shumway that I had heard it rumoured in one case (maybe the same case) that a murderer's defense lawyer claimed that brain death [of the victim] was not sufficient and the heart had to irreversibly stop beating before the victim could have been considered dead; therefore, it was the transplant surgeons who had murdered the man. The lawyer looked pretty pleased with this specious argument, until the prosecuting counsel pointed out that the heart was still beating—in the transplant recipient—and therefore, by this criterion, the homicide victim, who had long been laid to rest, would still not be considered dead.

Dr Lower also outlined to me a $1 million law suit (in 1972) in which he had become embroiled when the family of his first heart donor, a man named Bruce Tucker, accused him of wrongful death since the heart had been excised from a brain-dead donor while still beating (in 1968). The family had not given their consent for the donation as it had not been possible to find any of them at the time of the transplant, though the effort to contact them had been admittedly limited. The deputy medical examiner (coroner in the UK) had given his permission for the surgical team to take the organ. Dr Lower recollected:

> Early in this case, which lasted in court for about ten days, it appeared that the judge agreed with the prosecution and thought we had done wrong. But, after hearing the opinions of several experts, including neurosurgeons, the judge instructed the jury to ignore the usual legal definition of death and accept the definition of brain death. That was the key turning point in the case. I gathered from talking to him afterwards that he studied the evidence long and hard before he made that decision. The evidence was that hearts get stopped and restarted all the time [in various medical conditions]. I was surprised myself to read later some of the legal criticisms subsequently directed towards the judge for his instructions to the jury.

Dr Shumway mentioned to me that, at one point in this trial, the judge, when calling upon Dr Lower to rise, had mistakenly said, 'Will the guilty please stand up?' Dr Lower's morale plunged to the depths.

According to Dr Lower, 'the newspapers made the most of the suggestion by somebody that I should be tried for murder by the World Court as I had removed a live heart from a human being.'

This court case had a major impact on the nascent heart transplant programme in Richmond because, once the donor family began the proceedings, the transplant programme was put on hold. At that time, Dr Lower had only carried out two transplants, the second patient doing very well, but it was four years before the programme could be resumed. The prosecuting lawyer, representing the donor's family, was Douglas Wilder, later to become governor of Virginia.

Barnard experienced a similar problem with his third transplant (in September 1968) in which he took a heart from an unidentified black woman to transplant into Mr Pieter Smith, a white man. There was a public outcry, which eventually died down, but the outcome was that it dissuaded (at least temporarily) many black and coloured people from attending GSH for treatment of any health problem; they feared their organs would be taken without their consent.

In Japan, in a similar legal case, a surgeon was accused of murder for removing a beating heart. Although the case was eventually dropped, it had a very negative effect on heart transplant programs throughout that country. Heart transplantation was not resumed for almost thirty years.

In 1968, the *Ad Hoc* Committee to Examine the Definition of Brain Death was formed at Harvard University, and included physicians, theologians, lawyers, and philosophers. Among the key recommendations made by the committee was one that previous definitions of death had either applied or hinted at—that a patient is dead when the brain is dead, or when the patient has gone into irreversible coma. Specifically, four grounds for the definition of death were recommended: 1. lack of responsiveness, 2. no movement or breathing, 3. no reflexes, and 4. a flat encephalogram (no electrical activity in the brain).

Many believe it was this committee's conclusions that formed the basis for the acceptance of brain death. However, Chris later pointed out that, two months before publication of the committee's conclusions, the surgeons at the Cape Town conference came up with very similar guidelines. Indeed, one month before the Cape Town meeting, the Council of the Organization of Medical Science, which met in Geneva, put forward guidelines very much like those worked out by the Harvard group. It should be remembered, however, that it was the innovative Belgian transplant surgeon, Guy Alexandre, who had removed the kidneys from a brain-dead donor as early as 1963.

Eventually, the United States passed legislation that allowed death to be defined by brain death, and South Africa adopted a similar legal definition soon afterwards.

Dr Cooley raised a topic that was considered controversial by other attendees:

There is another source of donors which could conceivably be tapped. Perhaps we in our clinic would have preceded you by several years if we had had the courage to ask for these hearts. This is in the States where capital punishment is permitted. In Texas, capital punishment is performed by electrocution. Why would it not be possible to utilise this source of normal young donors for cardiac transplantation? We use prisoners for other purposes on a voluntary basis, and if execution victims accepted this on a voluntary basis, why not use them for donors?

Dr Cooley's suggestion did not receive much support, presumably because the attendees realised this would be ethically controversial. To my knowledge, (with the exception of some in modern China) no surgeon ever proceeded to use executed prisoners as heart donors, though some kidney transplant surgeons, such as Tom Starzl, had previously used prisoners as voluntary living donors of a kidney, though they later discontinued this approach. Years later, in his final novel, *The Donor*, Chris introduced the idea of using hearts from prisoners being hanged; perhaps he had the idea from Dr Cooley's comments.

The other topics on the agenda—surgical technique, rejection and its treatment (which was very limited at the time), and post-operative complications—were discussed in detail.

## Alternative Approaches

The conference concluded with a discussion on the merits of mechanical support of the failing heart with devices such as ventricular assist devices, which were still in very primitive forms in those days. Chris believed:

> Mechanical devices today are for reversible heart conditions, because they can only assist the circulation for a limited time ... probably two weeks, and in that period they take the load off the heart, giving the heart time to recover ... Heart transplantation is for irreversible heart conditions and never for a reversible heart condition; the mechanical devices are for reversible heart conditions, except where in irreversible heart conditions they are needed to keep the patient alive until a heart transplant can be done.

That summarised the situation at the time. For many years, mechanical assist devices were used as temporary support until a heart transplant could be carried out, but improvements in design and performance have resulted in them now being used to permanently support or replace the failing heart (Appendix I).

In contrast, Donald Ross thought an auxiliary heart transplant should be considered as a temporary assist of a failing heart, an approach that both he and, particularly, Chris were to explore later (Chapter 19). The attendees even discussed the possibility of using non-human primate hearts (xenografts) to overcome the problem of the shortage of suitable human hearts. Chris was later to attempt this approach to support patients whose hearts could not maintain life but in whom recovery of the heart was anticipated (Chapter 19).

Dr Lillehei believed:

We can solve the problem of xenografts in the future, but it has been pointed out that currently there are only 500 chimpanzees in the world in captivity, and that this supply would be very quickly exhausted. Of course, there is certainly the possibility and even the likelihood that they could be bred in captivity, but this also is a relatively time-consuming endeavour.

Most attendees did not believe this was a very realistic approach.

## Criticism

A Cape Town psychiatrist, Francis Ames, was outspoken in her criticism of heart transplant surgeons.

When I turn to the needs of the surgeons I would like to take some of them up on the inference that surgeons are motivated purely by a desire to alleviate human suffering. I think, if one scratches long enough, all motivation is impelled by self-interest. This is very human and very natural and surgeons shouldn't feel guilty about it. The fact that a surgeon enjoys exercising his technical skill and enjoys a feeling of omnipotence, is very good and can be of service to the community.

Chris later expressed similar views to me.

She also reviewed the topic of 'the needs of the public'.

An indication of public uneasiness about heart transplants is the number of jokes there are about transplants [Figure 14.ii]. Joking is a well-known defensive mechanism, and although the transplant surgeons are riding the crest of a wave at the moment, the future is so uncertain that, if they put themselves in the position of promising too much, and not keeping the public fully informed of how little we really know about the future of these patients, they are laying themselves open to a lot of public opposition to their work ... I would strongly urge the members of this Panel to spread their responsibilities by involving psychiatrists, neurologists, neuro-surgeons and physicians because, although being a god is pleasant, it may also be lonely. I don't think, in this day and age, that the transplant surgeon needs really to take the omnipotent position of full responsibility for selecting patients, operating on them and predicting their future.

Dr Lillehei requested the surgeons in the room give Dr Ames a round of applause.

She certainly hauled us surgeons over the coals, but she did it so nicely that I don't think anybody has been very upset, except possibly Chris ... Most of us who have had some experience on committees realise that you don't get that much done in the way of positive action by a committee. In fact, it has been said that if Moses had had a Committee, the Jews would still be on the other side of the Red Sea.

In this regard, Donald Ross reviewed the difficulties of managing a post-transplant patient 'by a committee' as both he and Chris had done with their first transplants. 'Although the surgeon should take advice from other experts, it has since been shown that the management of the patient should be under the control of one responsible person, either a transplant surgeon or a transplant cardiologist.'

Chris, obviously upset by some of Dr Ames's comments, particularly those that related to a patient's psychological suitability to undergo a heart transplant, responded somewhat sarcastically:

Surgeons may not be as educated as psychiatrists, but as a surgeon I would never accept the statement that the patient must be allowed to die because he is not psychologically suitable to live. I think that would be a terrible statement ever to make and I, as a surgeon, would never accept that statement—because that is what Dr Ames is trying to say—that some of these patients are not psychologically suited to being treated by heart transplantation, and therefore they must be allowed to die.

I am not certain Chris was correct here. I have cared for several patients who were not psychologically suited to the demands and restrictions of undergoing a heart transplant, and of subsequently living under the disciplined requirements of immunosuppressive therapy. Some of these patients definitely contributed to their own demise by their lack of resolve

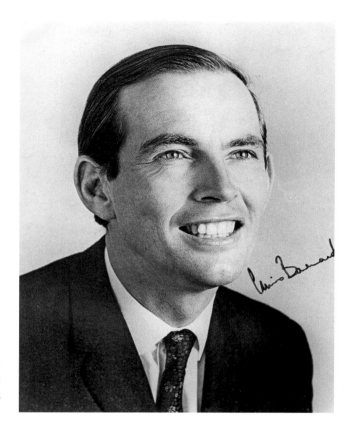

Fig. 1.i Chris Barnard at the time of the first heart transplant in 1967, when he was 45 years-old.

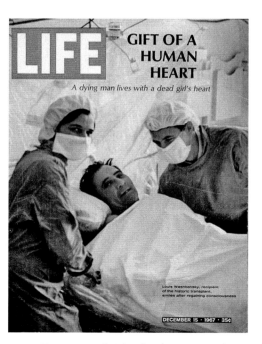

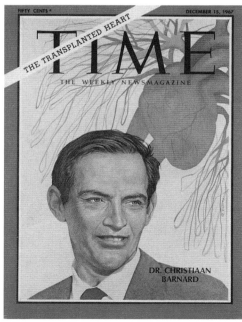

Fig. 1.iia & b The first heart transplant makes the cover pages of *Life* and *Time* magazines.

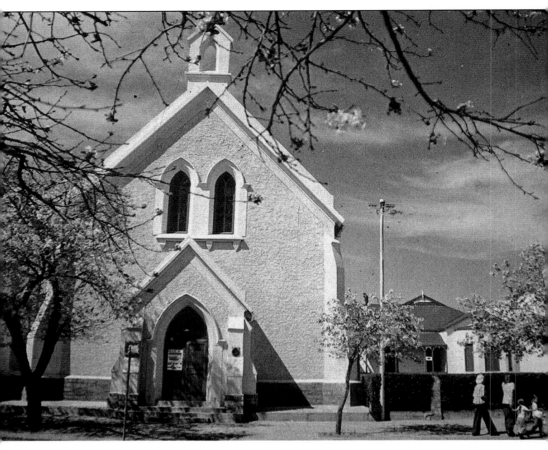

*Above:* Fig. 2.i. Adam Barnard's church in Beaufort West with the adjoining small house (to the right) in which the Barnard family lived.

*Below left:* Fig. 2.ii Chris strums a tune on his ukulele.

*Below right:* Fig. 2.iii The Barnard family on the beach during Chris's childhood. Back row left to right: his mother Maria, oldest brother Barney, father Adam, and a friend. Front row: Chris is second from the left. The state of their bathing clothes illustrates the family's relative poverty.

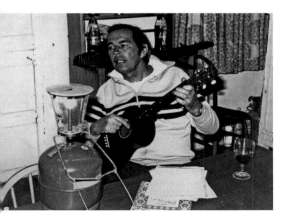

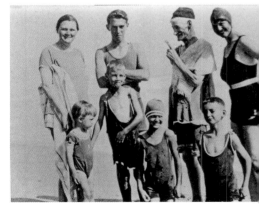

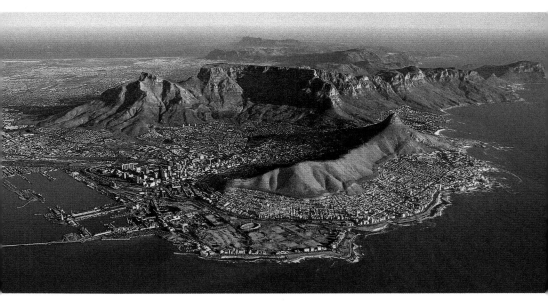

*Above:* Fig. 3.i An aerial view of Cape Town and the Cape peninsular extending south of the city. Table Mountain is in the center of the photograph with Devil's Peak to the left. As Cape Town faces north, Devil's Peak is to the east of Table Mountain.

*Below left:* Fig. 3.ii The University of Cape Town campus.

*Below right:* Fig. 3.iii Groote Schuur Hospital, as it was at the time of the first heart transplant.

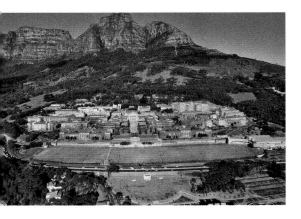

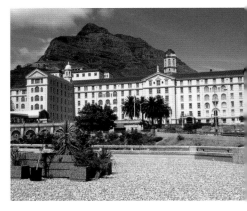

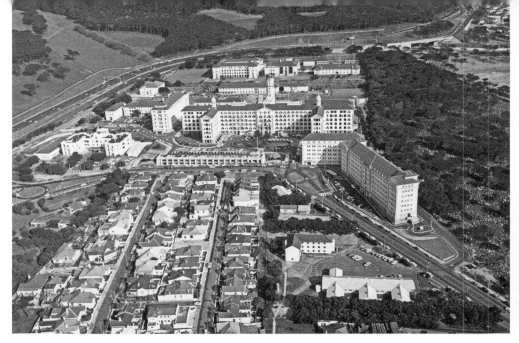

*Above:* Fig. 3.iv Groote Schuur Hospital, as it was in Chris Barnard's time, with Devil's Peak behind it. Wildebeest graze on the land behind the hospital. In the 1980s, the small houses in front of the hospital were demolished to allow construction of the current hospital. Fortunately, the original buildings have been retained, and continue to be used for many purposes.

*Below left:* Fig. 3.v Chris during his medical student days.

*Below right:* Fig. 3.vi Chris's wedding to Aletta ('Louwtjie') Louw in 1948, with his younger brother Marius as best man.

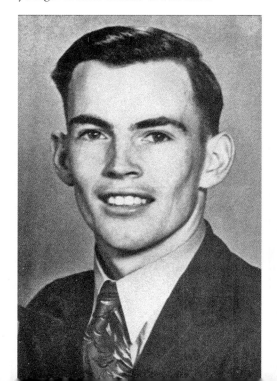

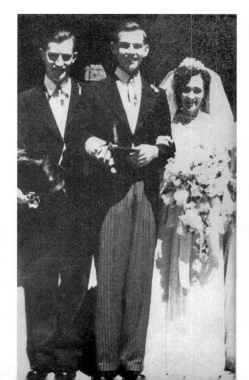

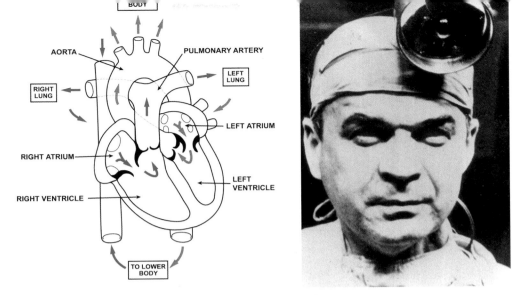

*Above left:* Fig. 4.i Diagram of the normal structure and blood flow through the heart and major blood vessels. 'Blue' blood (containing a low level of oxygen) (black arrows) returning from the body passes into a 'collecting chamber' (the right atrium), from which it passes through the tricuspid valve into a 'pumping chamber' (the right ventricle), which pumps it through the pulmonary valve into the pulmonary artery and thus, into the lungs. After picking up oxygen and releasing carbon dioxide in the lungs, 'pink' blood (with a high level of oxygen) (red arrows) returns to the left atrium, then passes through the mitral valve into the left ventricle, from which it is pumped through the aortic valve into the aorta and around the body.

*Above right:* Fig. 4.ii C. Walton 'Walt' Lillehei, Chris's major mentor in Minneapolis, who US heart transplant pioneer, Norman Shumway, described as 'the greatest surgeon in the world'.

*Below:* Fig. 4.iii Chris and Louwtjie with their children, Deirdre and André, in Minneapolis at Christmas, 1956. Chris's friend, John Perry, and his girlfriend, Genevieve (later his wife) are with them.

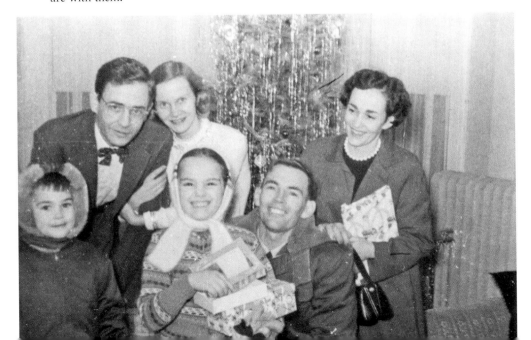

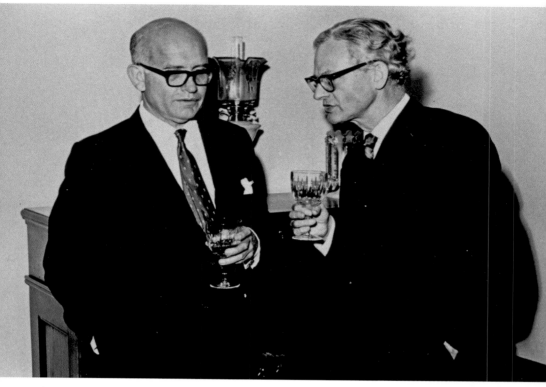

*Above:* Fig. 6.i Professor Velva 'Val' Schrire (*right*), head of the cardiology clinic at Groote Schuur Hospital, with Mr Donald Ross, FRCS, South African-born eminent London cardiac surgeon at the heart transplant congress held in Cape Town in 1968.

*Below left:* Fig. 6.ii Early open heart operation at Groote Schuur Hospital (1960s). Chris Barnard (with head obscured) is to the right of the operating table.

*Below right:* Fig. 6.iii Chris Barnard with a young patient, illustrating his empathy with children.

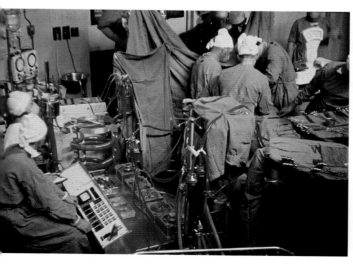

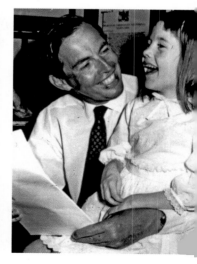

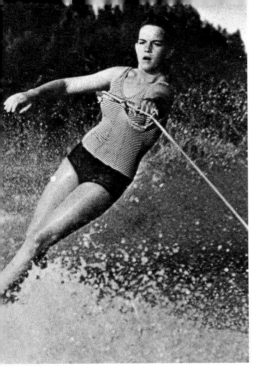

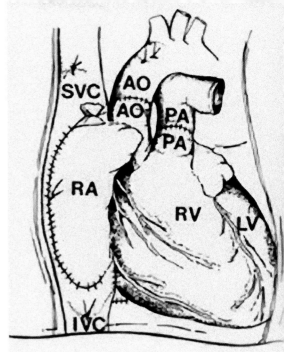

*Above left:* Fig. 6.iv Deirdre Barnard as a young teenager in her water-skiing days.

*Above right:* Fig. 7.i Surgical technique of orthotopic heart transplantation. The suture lines between the donor and recipient right atria, aortas, and pulmonary arteries are indicated. The suture line between the donor and recipient left atria is at the back of the heart and is not shown. Only the two ventricles and all four valves are replaced (see Figure 4.i). AO = aorta; IVC = inferior vena cava; LV = left ventricle; PA = pulmonary artery; RA = right atrium; RV = right ventricle; SVC = superior vena cava.

*Below:* Fig. 6.v Family picture of Chris and Louwtjie with their two children, Deirdre and André, and their housemaid, in their house at Zeekoevlei.

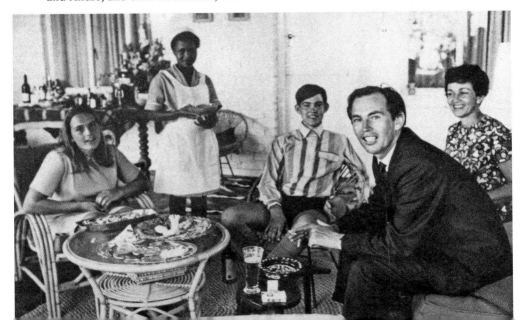

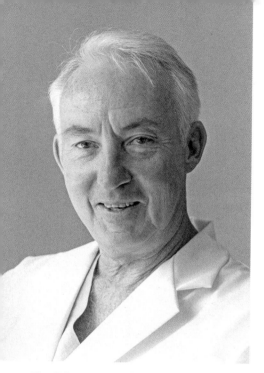

Fig. 7.ii Norman Shumway.

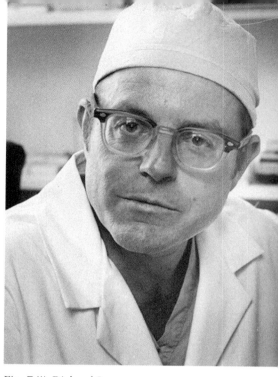

Fig. 7.iii Richard Lower.

Fig. 7.iv James Hardy.

Fig. 7.v Adrian Kantrowitz.

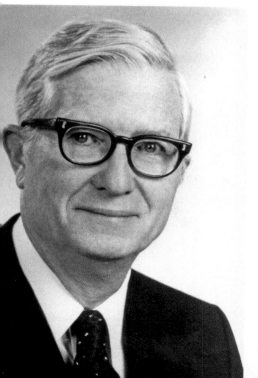

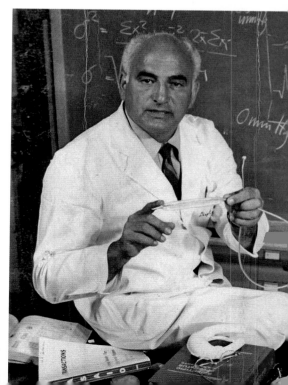

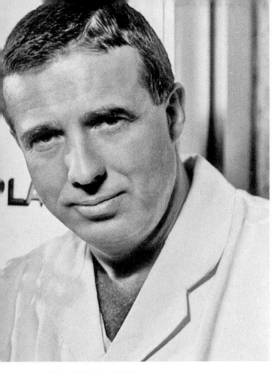

Fig. 8.i David Hume.

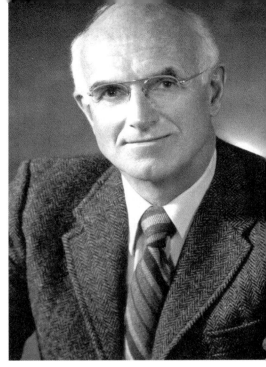

Fig. 8.ii Joseph (Joe) Murray.

Fig. 8.iii British transplant surgeon, Roy Calne (later Sir Roy) with Chris Barnard.

Fig. 8.iv American transplant surgeon, Tom Starzl.

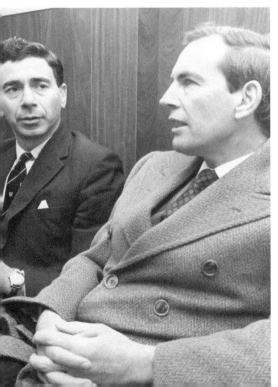

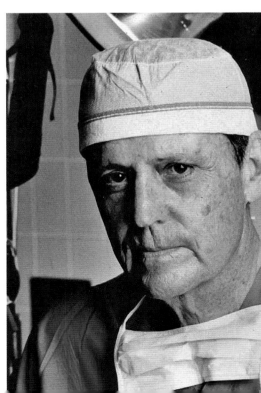

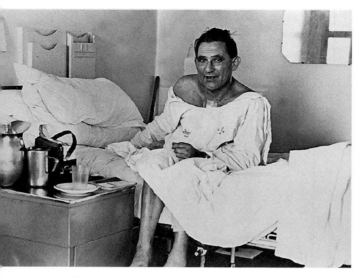

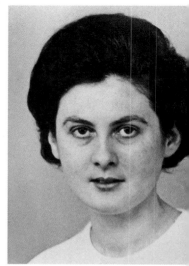

*Above left:* Fig. 9.i Louis Washkansky, the first recipient.

*Above right:* Fig. 9.ii Denise Darvall, the first heart donor.

*Below:* Fig. 9.iii First photograph of the surgical team taken on the afternoon of Sunday 3 December 1967.

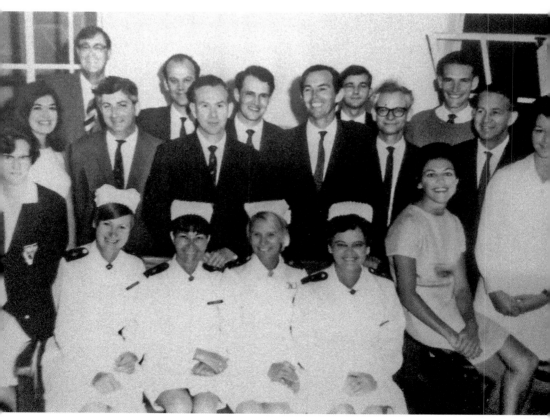

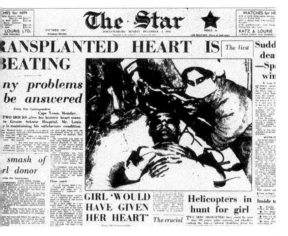

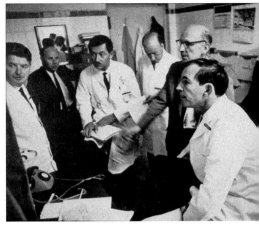

*Above left:* Fig. 9.iv  Front page of the South African newspaper, *The Star*, on Monday 4 December 1967.

*Above right:* Fig. 9.vi  Chris Barnard and his medical colleagues discuss Mr Washkansky's progress at a morning conference.

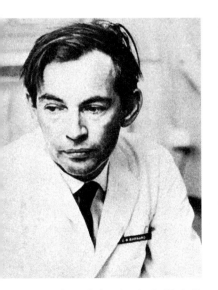

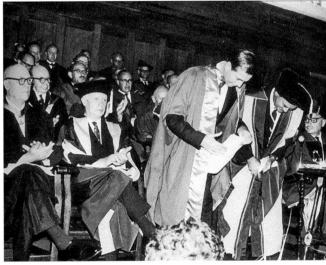

*Above left:* Fig. 9.vi  Chris Barnard showing the stress of caring for his patient as Mr Washkansky's health deteriorated.

*Above right:* Fig. 9.vii  Chris Barnard receiving the degree of Doctor of Science *honoris causa* from the University of Cape Town.

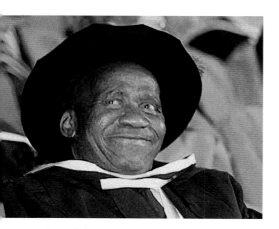

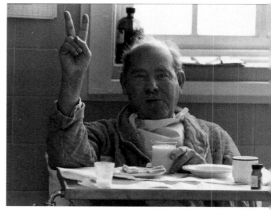

*Above left:* Fig. 11.i Hamilton Naki, at the academic ceremony when he received an honorary degree from the University of Cape Town.

*Above right:* Fig. 12.i Philip Blaiberg.

*Below:* Fig. 12.ii There was massive media attention when Philip Blaiberg was discharged home from Groote Schuur Hospital seventy-four days after his heart transplant.

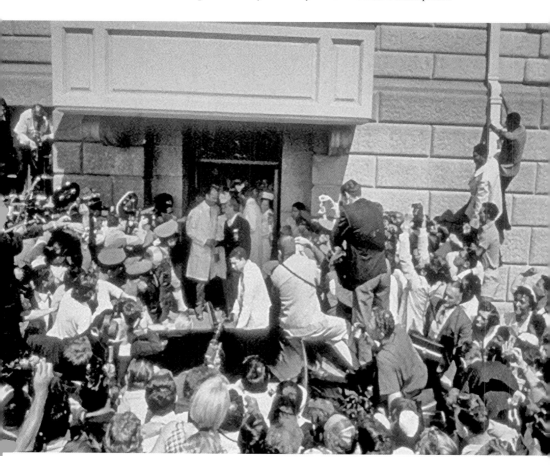

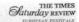

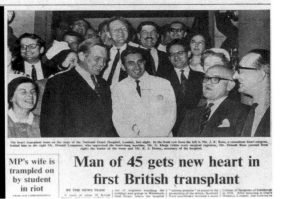

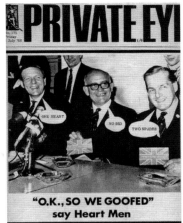

*Above left:* Fig. 13.i Front page of the UK newspaper, *The Times* (on 4 May 1968), showing the National Heart Hospital 'team' outside of the hospital on the occasion of the first heart transplant in the UK on 3 May 1968.

*Above right:* Fig. 13.ii Cover of the UK satirical magazine, *Private Eye*, in July 1968 when Britain's first heart transplant patient sadly died.

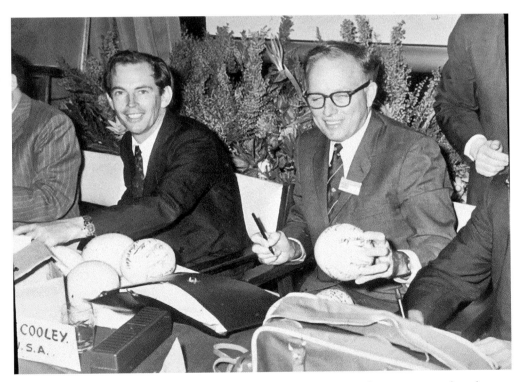

Fig. 14.i Denton Cooley (*right*) and Chris Barnard sign ostrich eggs presented to them as mementos of the first heart transplant congress held in Cape Town in July 1968.

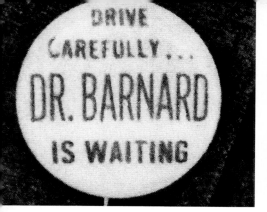

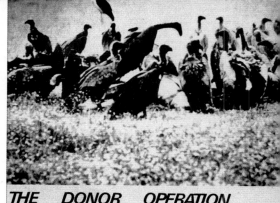

THE DONOR OPERATION

Fig 14.iia & b Two examples of the humour that came to be associated with heart transplantation.

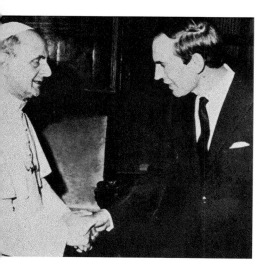

*Left:* Fig. 15.i A serious-looking Chris during his audience with Pope Paul VI in the Vatican.

*Below:* Fig 15.ii Chris Barnard with Italian film star, Sophia Loren, and Dr M. C. Botha. Chris joked that, after being in such close contact with the beautiful Loren, the smile on Dr Botha's face became permanent.

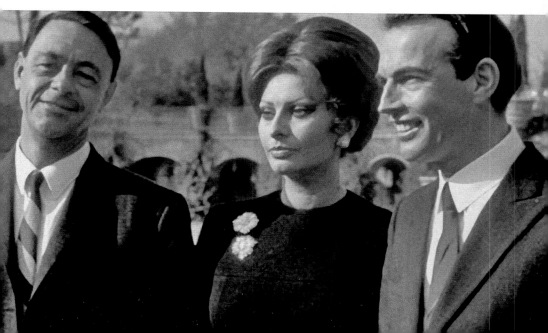

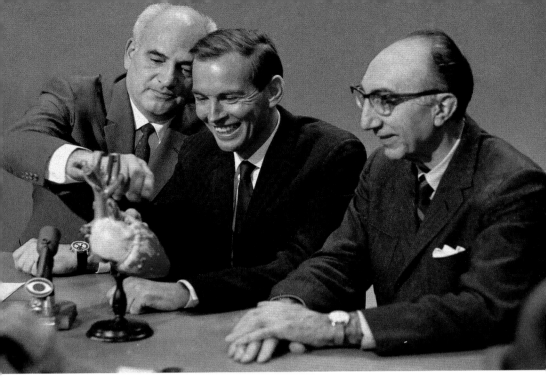

*Above:* Fig. 15.iii Chris, Michael DeBakey (*right*), and Adrian Kantrowitz (*left*) on the CBS program, *Face the Nation.*

*Below:* Fig. 15.iv Chris on his visit to the LBJ Ranch, face to face with President Lyndon B. Johnson. Claudia Alta 'Lady Bird' Johnson is on the sofa opposite. Louwtjie Barnard is holding the Johnson's baby grandson.

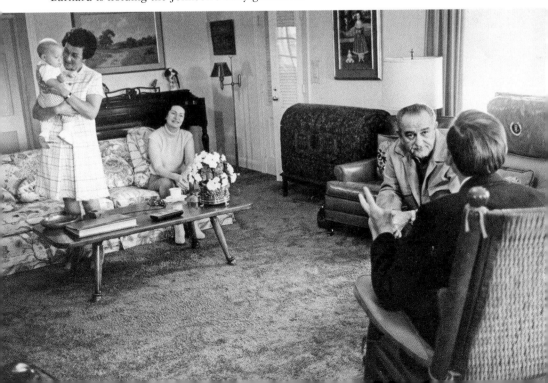

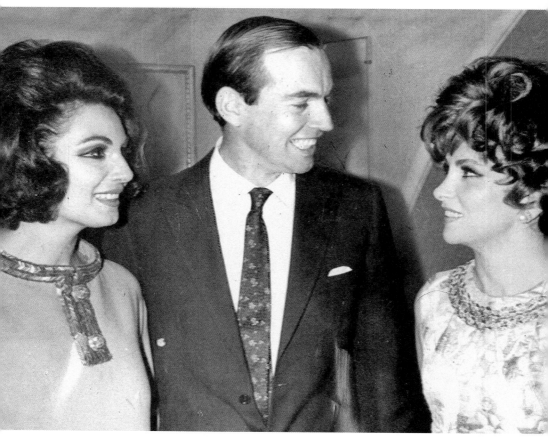

*Above:* Fig. 15.v Chris with Italian film stars Rosanna Schiaffino (*left*) and Gina Lollobrigida (*right*).

*Below left:* Fig. 15.vi Chris mobbed by autograph-seeking admirers.

*Below right:* Fig. 15.vii Chris (*seated, center*) about to address a typically-packed auditorium.

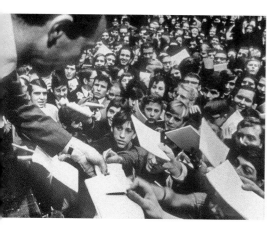

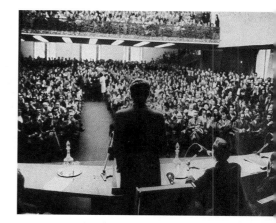

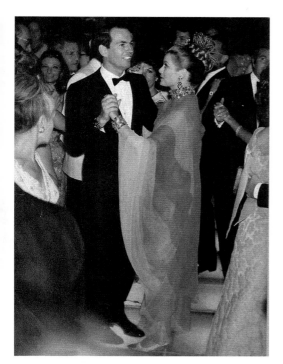

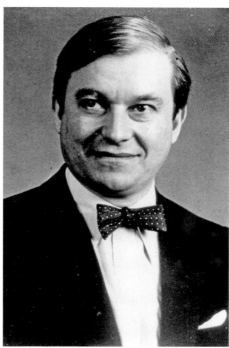

*Above left:* Fig. 17.i Chris dancing with Princess Grace in Monaco.

*Above right:* Fig. 19.i Belgian heart surgeon Jacques Losman who, with Barnard, developed the technique of heterotopic 'piggy-back' heart transplantation.

Fig. 19.ii The operation of heterotopic heart transplantation in which both the native left and right ventricles (pumping chambers) are provided with assistance by the donor heart (which is placed in the right side of the patient's chest, i.e., on the left of the diagram). AO = aorta; LV = left ventricle; PA = pulmonary artery; RA = right atrium; RV = right ventricle; SVC = superior vena cava.

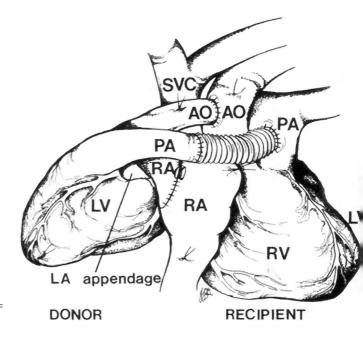

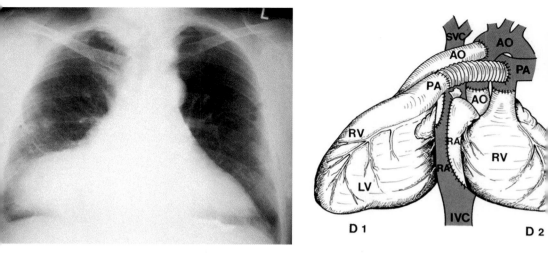

D 1                                                    D 2

*Above left*: Fig. 19.iii Chest radiograph (X-ray) of a patient with a heterotopic heart transplant. The donor heart is placed in the right side of the chest, i.e., on the left side of the X-ray.

*Above right*: Fig. 19.iv The operation of orthotopic heart transplantation following heterotopic heart transplantation. The original donor heart (D1) is left in place and the patient's own heart is replaced by the second donor heart (D2). The only remaining structures of the patient's own heart are indicated in dark grey. AO = aorta; IVC = inferior vena cava; LV = left ventricle; PA = pulmonary artery; RA = right atrium; RV = right ventricle; SVC = superior vena cava.

*Below*: Fig. 20.i Chris and Barbara before their marriage.

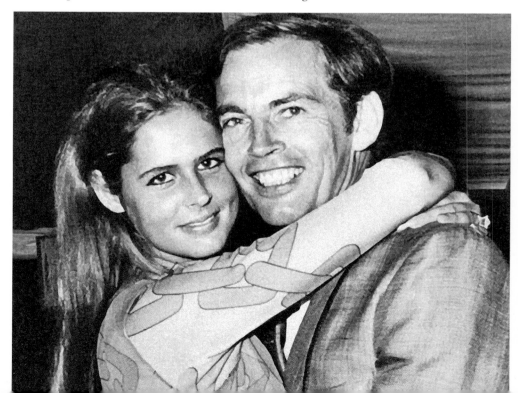

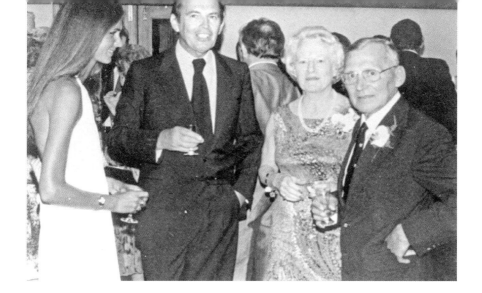

*Above:* Fig. 20.ii An elegant Barbara with Chris and Professor Jannie Louw and his wife.

*Right:* Fig. 20.iv The beach at Clifton, where Chris and Barbara made their first home.

*Below:* Fig. 20.iii Barbara, Chris, and their first baby, Frederick.

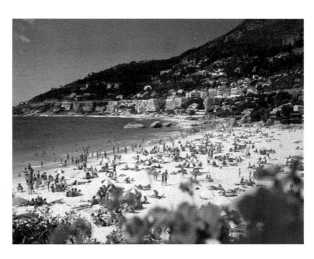

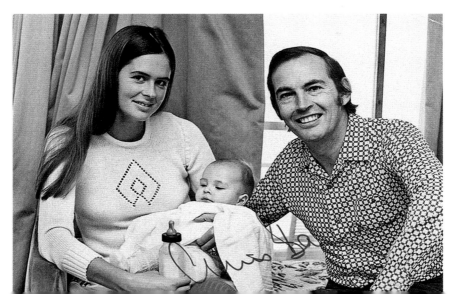

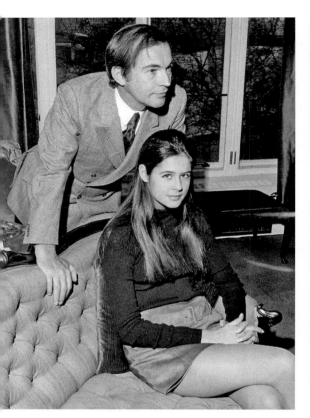
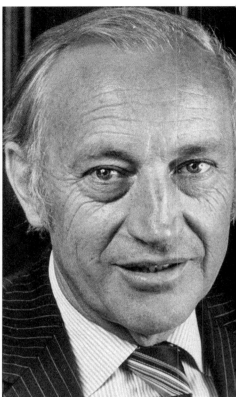

*Above left:* Fig. 20.v  Chris and Barbara at a press conference at the Savoy Hotel in London, 24 March 1970.

*Above right:* Fig. 20.vi  Marius Barnard, at about the time of his retirement from Groote Schuur Hospital.

*Below:* Fig. 21.i  Diagram of the technique of endomyocardial biopsy in a patient with a heterotopic heart transplant. Under X-ray guidance, the biopsy forceps is directed along a vein into the donor heart.

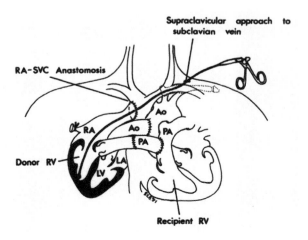

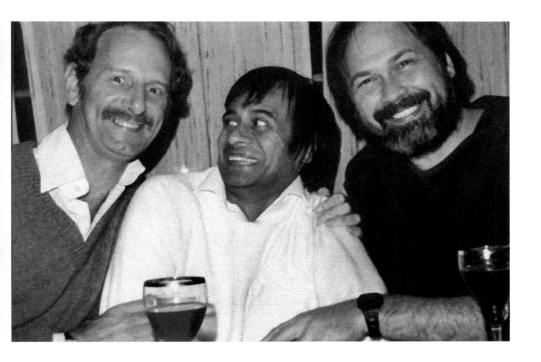

*Above:* Fig. 21.ii Winston Wicomb (*centre*), Dimitri Novitzky (*right*), and the author—an illustration of the great times they had working together in Chris's department.

*Below left:* Fig. 21.iii The first human heart to be stored by hypothermic perfusion is placed in Winston Wicomb's perfusion chamber.

*Below right:* Fig. 21.iv The perfusion machine (encasing the donor heart) is ready to be transported by air to Groote Schuur Hospital.

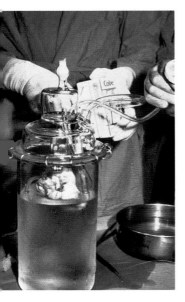

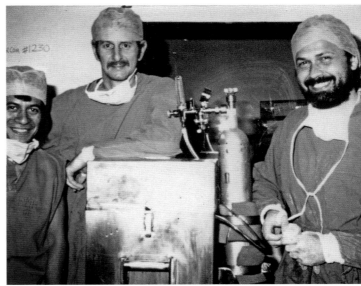

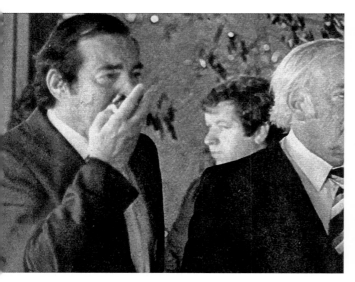
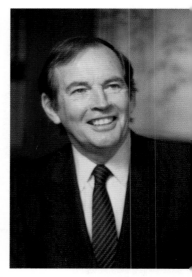

*Above left:* Fig. 22.i A distraught Chris, accompanied by Marius, at his son, André's, funeral.

*Above right:* Fig. 22.iii Chris at about the time of his retirement, when aged 61.

*Below:* Fig. 22.ii Chris with his two sons from his marriage to Barbara – Frederick (*right*) and Christiaan, Jnr. (*left*).

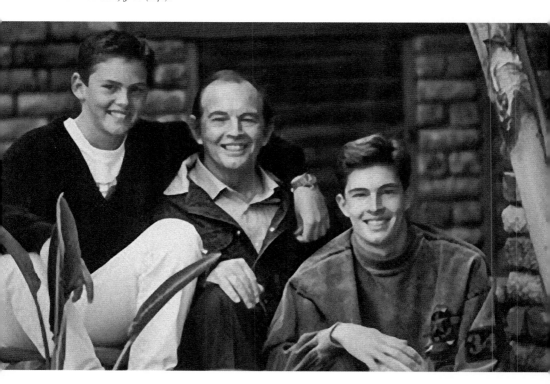

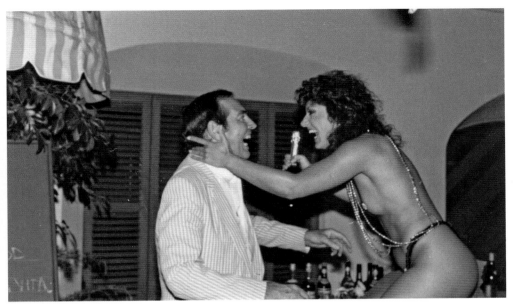

Fig. 22.iv Chris is surprised – pleasantly so – by the 'present' his junior colleagues gave him at a party to mark his retirement.

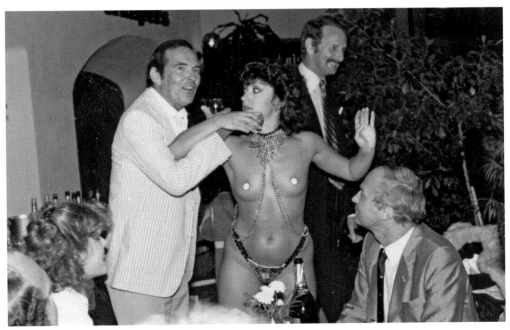

Fig. 22.v Chris and his 'retirement present' enjoy a celebratory drink together. (As an aside, as I was still a bachelor in those days, I tried to hit up a relationship with the young lady – without success, I might add. She proved to hail from the northern part of England and had been a primary school teacher there for several years before coming to South Africa. If I had had a teacher with her charms, I might have taken more interest in my lessons and mastered arithmetic and spelling more quickly. I am at the back in this photograph.)

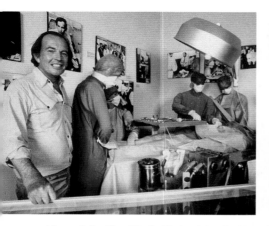
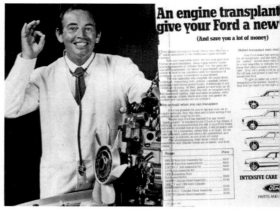

*Above left:* Fig. 22.vi  Chris visits the Beaufort West museum.

*Above right:* Fig. 23.i  An advert for the Ford motor company.

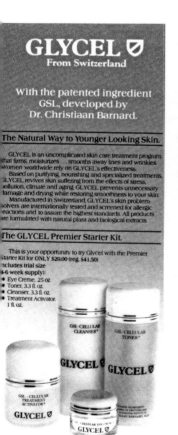

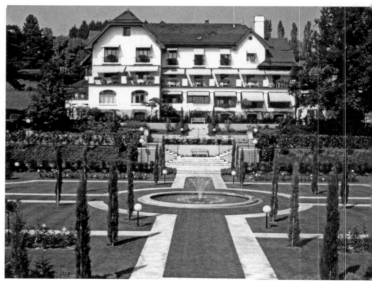

*Above:* Fig. 23.ii  Clinique La Prairie in Switzerland.

*Left:* Fig. 23.iii  Promotional information on *Glycel*.

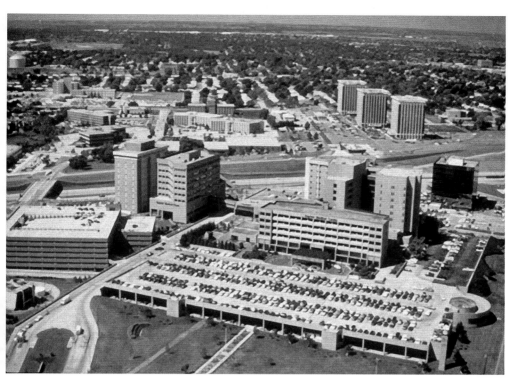

Fig. 24.i Baptist Medical Center in Oklahoma City as it was in 1987.

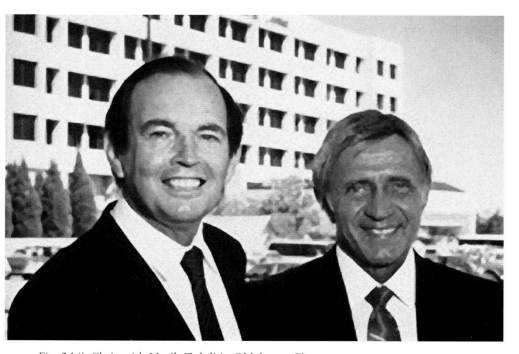

Fig. 24.ii Chris with Nazih Zuhdi in Oklahoma City.

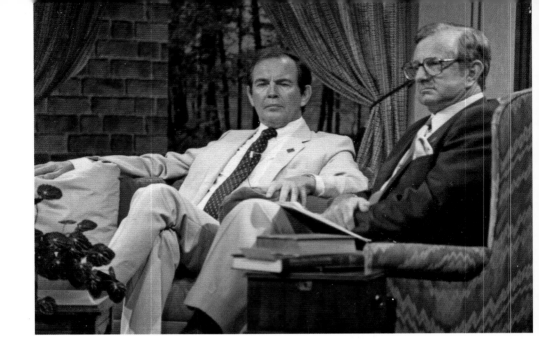

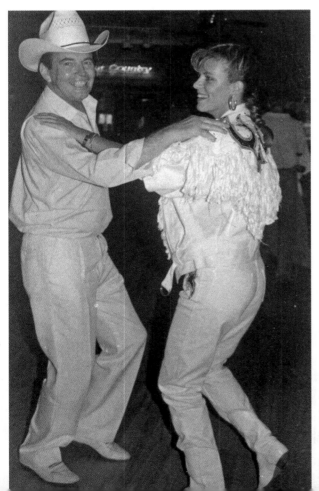

*Above:* Fig. 24.iii Chris preparing for a television interview in Oklahoma City.

*Left:* Fig. 24.iv Chris and his girlfriend, Karin (soon to become his third wife) enjoy a dance at a 'country and western' club in Oklahoma City.

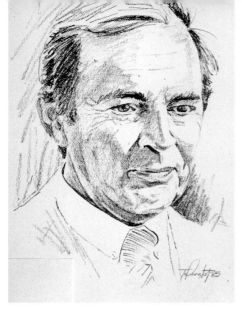

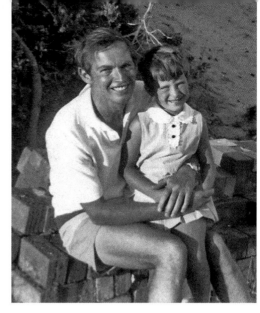

*Above left:* Fig. 24.v A drawing of Chris commissioned by Baptist Medical Center at the time of the 20th anniversary of the first heart transplant in 1987.

*Above right:* Fig. 25.i Chris with Karin when she was six years old.

*Below left:* Fig. 25.ii Chris with Karin when she was in her late teens.

*Below right:* Fig. 25.iii Chris and Karin at their wedding reception in 1988.

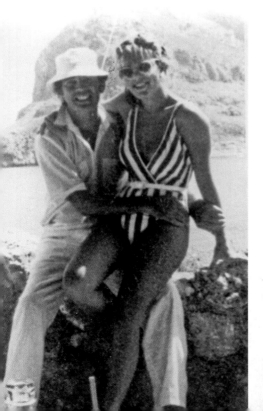

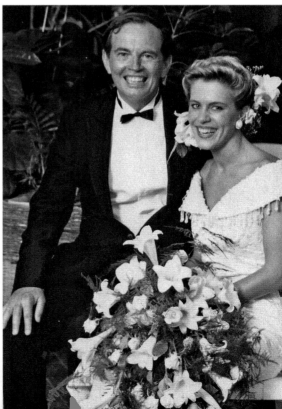

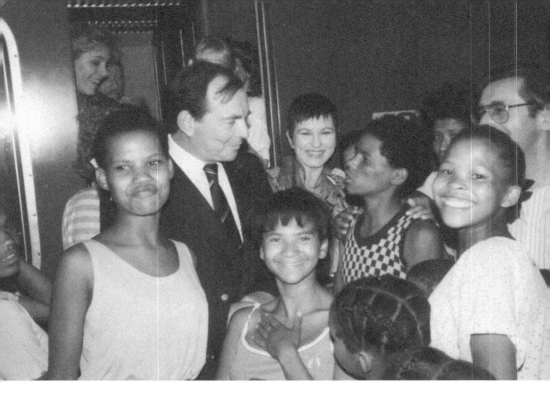

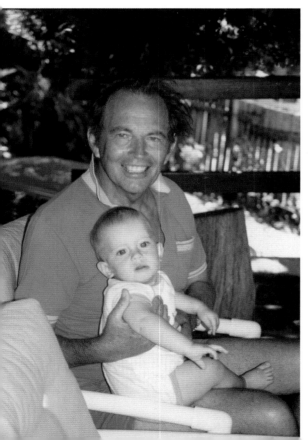

*Above:* Fig. 25.iv Chris is greeted by well-wishers at the Beaufort West railway station when he and his new bride, Karin, travelled from Cape Town to Johannesburg on the famed Blue Train on their honeymoon. Karin can just be seen at the top left, looking out of the coach door. The couple were accompanied by a few close friends. To Chris's left is Annette Zuhdi.

*Left:* Fig. 25.v Chris with baby Armin.

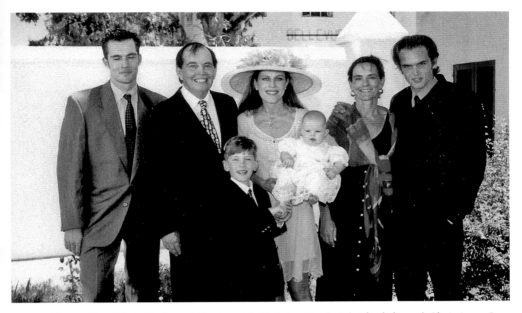

*Above:* Fig. 25.vi Chris and Karin, with Deirdre, Frederick (*far left*) and Christiaan, Jnr (*far right*) at the christening of their daughter, Lara.

*Below left:* Fig. 30.i Chris with Nelson Mandela.

*Below right:* Fig. 30.ii Chris in his late seventies looking tired, having had surgery to his face to remove the skin cancer.

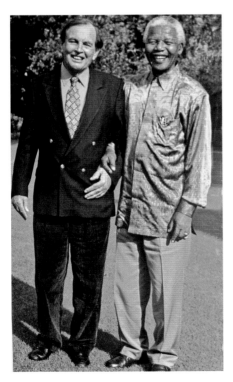

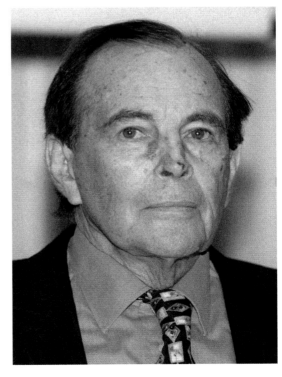

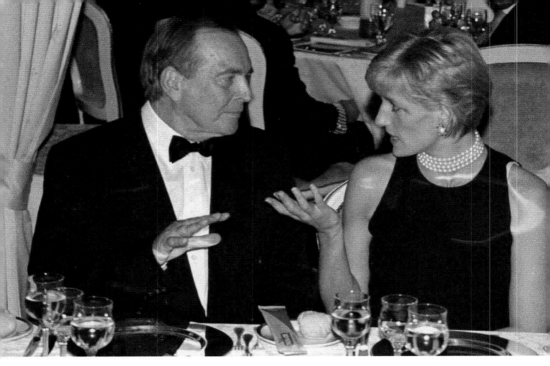

*Above:* Fig. 30.iii Princess Diana in conversation with Chris at a function in Italy in 1996.

*Below:* Fig. 30.iv Chris and Muhammad Ali on the occasion when Chris presented Ali with the sportsman of the century award.

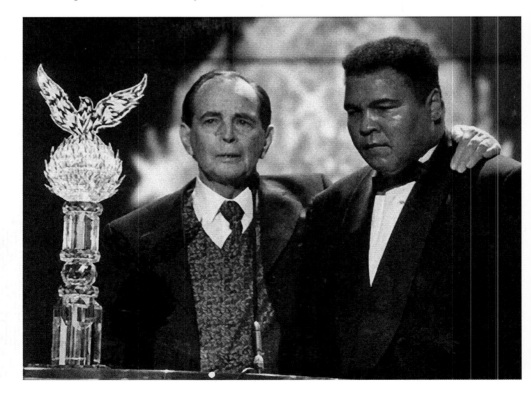

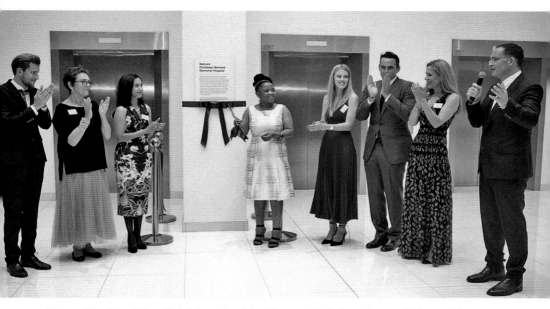

*Above:* Fig. 30.v The official launch of the Netcare Christiaan Barnard Memorial Hospital in Cape Town was celebrated on Saturday, 3 December 2016, to coincide with the 49th anniversary of the world's first human heart transplant.

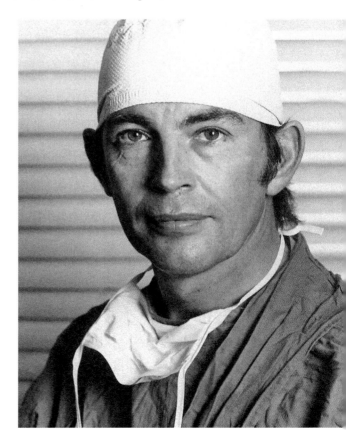

Fig. 31.i Chris Barnard as he will be remembered—the surgeon who carried out the world's first human heart transplant.

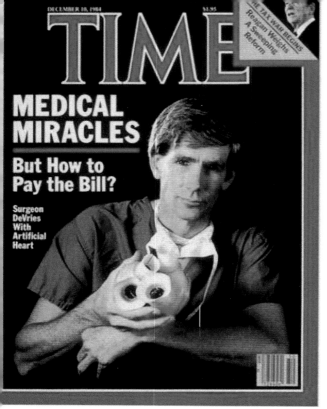

Fig. A1.i William DeVries, holding a Kolff-Jarvik total artificial heart, on the cover of *Time* magazine.

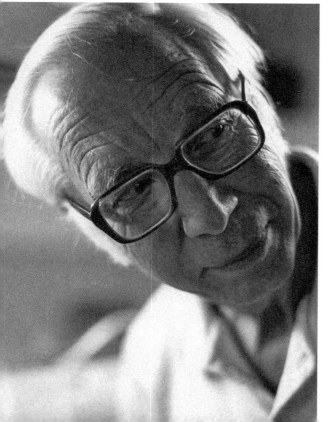

Fig. A1.ii Willem Kolff, the innovative Dutch physician who designed the first effective dialysis machine and the first artificial heart.

or self-discipline, and possibly should not have been selected to undergo the procedure. The donor heart given to them might have been better utilised—that is, cared for more conscientiously—by another recipient who was psychologically more suited to the demands of immunosuppressive therapy.

In the following months and years, the redoubtable Dr Ames was highly critical of Chris's womanising lifestyle, suggesting that he had remained emotionally an 'adolescent'.

## Summing Up

Chris summed up the meeting.

> I think this has been a very depressing sort of meeting, but I don't think it has shown anything that we didn't know before we started heart transplantation. It has shown exactly what our experience has been in the kidney [i.e. the experience in heart transplantation was very similar to that seen with kidney transplantation], and that we must accept heart transplantation as a palliative procedure at the moment, not as a curative procedure. Some of these patients we will keep alive for a few weeks, some for a few months and some for a few years until we can better control the immunologic attack of the recipient on the transplanted organs; so don't go away too depressed. This has certainly shown nothing new. The only thing it has shown to me is that the heart behaves very much like the kidney in rejection.

As we shall see, Chris's predictions proved entirely correct, with, during the next several years, survival of patients after heart transplantation ranging from only a few days in some to many years in others.

To end on a positive note, Donald Ross pointed out that, notwithstanding the death of his first patient, Frederick West, 67 per cent of the public polled in the UK were still in favour of heart transplantation. Of the younger age group (in the sixteen to twenty-four-year group), 80 per cent were in favour.

# 15

# The Consequences of Fame

The first heart transplant, in particular, and the subsequent ones performed in Cape Town brought Chris immediate public and professional recognition throughout the world. Public interest in heart transplantation and in Chris as a person was immense. As already mentioned, he rapidly found himself on the front pages of almost every newspaper and magazine in the world. For example, the Paris newspaper *France Soir*, and many other publications and organizations, voted him 'Man of the Year'. A gold replica of a heart was sent to him as a gift from the Society of Jewelers in France. A French popularity poll placed him third after President de Gaulle and Pope Paul VI.

The early success of the University of Cape Town heart transplant program, in particular the successful transplant on Dr Blaiberg, opened up the world to the forty-five-year-old surgeon, and this world was not confined to that of surgery. Rarely, if ever, has any surgeon been invited to speak so extensively worldwide, both to the medical profession and to the public. Chris's opinion was sought on every conceivable topic—not only on medical subjects, but any and all other topics. He later wrote how he had to evolve from the highly specialised field of heart surgery, where he felt he had been 'wearing blinkers which showed only the job I was doing and nothing else', to become an 'expert' and have an opinion on all matters.

In his autobiography, he wrote:

That's why it was such a shock when Chris Barnard the doctor suddenly became Chris Barnard the celebrity. While I had been training for one field, another was thrust on me. I, who was competent enough to handle a stethoscope, was suddenly required to show some dexterity with a microphone and perform with aplomb before a camera. From opinions on medicine I was required to have opinions on everything from apartheid to Zen.

The invitations came from almost every country. As interest both in heart transplantation and the man grew, Chris was provided with ever more opportunities to meet not only other major figures in medicine, but celebrities in almost every sphere of human achievement. In his extensive travels, he met with people from all walks of life, including statesmen and politicians, such as Indian Prime Minister Indira Gandhi, religious leaders, such as Pope Paul VI (Figure 15.i), and movie stars, such as Sophia Loren (Figure 15.ii).

His growing popularity as a guest at almost every type of function was not only because of the dramatic nature of his work and the almost spiritual qualities that have been associated with the heart in society and literature over the centuries, but also because of his attractive personality and his abilities as a speaker. He soon became a highly sought after and welcome guest almost anywhere in the world. He travelled widely and often. Once, when he landed at a New York airport, he had to telephone his secretary in Cape Town to inquire where he was supposed to be going.

Despite their interesting and attractive personalities, I do not believe that any of the other surgeons who participated in the early days of heart transplantation could have captured, even captivated, the public's attention as did Chris Barnard. None of them had his charisma, with the possible exception of Denton Cooley. However, possibly none of them would have wanted the attention Chris received; none of them would have been so attracted to being in the public eye.

To obtain an idea of Chris's appeal, the words of Peter Hawthorne, perhaps capture Chris's complex personality. Hawthorne, a freelance journalist who covered the period of the first heart transplant in Cape Town, subsequently put the story together in the form of a book *The Transplanted Heart*, published in 1968. Now fifty years later, it is of interest to read how Chris was perceived at that time. Hawthorne provided the following 'thumbnail sketch' of Chris Barnard:

At the age of forty-five, at the peak of his career, Christiaan Barnard is a fascinating character. More particularly so in that he is not such a perfect character at that. His consummate surgical skill is one thing, his personal characteristics, their qualities and their failings, are another. Within the bounds of his profession he is a genius. In human relationships he is frequently impossible. He is a man of human moods and passions, to be sure. His tall lean, slightly stooped handsomeness, is engaging—a hungry, boyish, buck-toothed look which promises a deep sense of humour and yet a serious view of life. He has an urchin charm that has people, especially women, eating out of his hand. Yet he can switch, with equally boyish impetuosity, to ill-temper. Like most men who live primarily for their work, he sets high standards of perfection and finds it intolerable if others fail to match his standards. He lives, eats, thinks and sleeps his work—and fully expects others to do the same. It makes him an extremely exacting man to work for.

Hawthorne added that men who live for their work are never easy to live with.

## First 'Post-Transplant' Visit to the USA

Chris's global travels began almost immediately after the death of Louis Washkansky. While Mr Washkansky was alive, Chris had accepted an invitation by CBS to appear on one of the most popular programs on television in the USA, *Face the Nation*, where he would be accompanied by two leading US heart surgeons: Dr Adrian Kantrowitz, who had carried out the ill-fated second heart transplant, and Dr Michael DeBakey, who did not enter the field of heart transplantation until later, but was perhaps the best-known cardiovascular surgeon in the world before Barnard appeared on the scene (Figure 15.iii). It is interesting to wonder whether Norman Shumway had been invited to participate—an obvious choice— but possibly had declined.

One day after Louis Washkansky's funeral, Mrs Barnard was informed that tomorrow afternoon, 'you leave for America on flight 313.' A big black car and escort drove her to the waiting plane. She notes in her memoirs:

> Kindness overwhelmed me … I was the first passenger in the first seat in first class. I waited anxiously for Chris to arrive. I had not seen him since early that morning. At last he made his appearance in another big black car, followed by an escort of reporters and photographers. At last we were on our way. At Jan Smuts Airport, Johannesburg, we were greeted by cheering crowds. Airport officials and dignitaries escorted us into the VIP room. We were cosseted as if we were the Crown jewels. We were now very important people. I felt proud, sad and bewildered. With these mixed emotions I left my country.

These flights were Chris's first experience of the 'good life'. He was plied with champagne and, for the first time in his life, he was presented with a menu on which were exotic dishes of which he had not previously heard. Louwtjie continued:

> Our plane touched down at Heathrow Airport, London, I looked out of the little window. There seemed to be a million cameras waiting to 'welcome' us. Slowly, I walked down the gangplank, but before I reached the bottom I became blinded and deafened by flashing cameras and a screaming mob of reporters. The next moment we were literally swept off our feet, pushed into a car and taken to a waiting plane.
>
> In America we were treated like kings. Kindness, consideration and admiration were showered upon us. This was a completely different America to the one I had lived in twelve years before. During our first visit, we had struggled to survive. Now everyone was at our beck and call, our every wish was their command. This visit to America was like a dream, a fairytale and sometimes like a nightmare.
>
> Soon after our arrival Chris appeared on his first television programme called *Face the Nation* [a programme regularly watched by millions of viewers]. With confidence, knowledge, wit and charm, he captured the hearts of millions and once more the world cheered and congratulated him. He accepted it with dignity and a smile. I thanked God for the privilege of being married to this brilliant man. Sitting among the audience of thousands, I admired and loved him silently. But little did I know that my husband would change beyond recognition in the next few years. Had I not witnessed it from start to finish, I would not have believed it possible.

The programme was a personal success for Chris. Few could have failed to be impressed by his charisma and passion. The subsequent newspaper and magazine reports, including that in *The New York Times*, were very positive. Louwtjie continued her account.

> We stayed at the luxurious Plaza Hotel in New York in a beautiful suite overlooking Central Park. There we spent an unfamiliar Christmas. It was bitterly cold. Our tour across the continent began. Hotels vied to outdo each other to welcome us. Flowers, fruit, champagne and exotic wines shimmered and glowed in their shiny translucent packaging. I enjoyed this film star treatment but when I looked into the depths of the capacious closets I smiled and thought to myself: 'We don't really belong here.' The closets were definitely not dripping with glamorous clothes, jewels or furs. Chris's three suits and my four dresses looked rather lost and homesick. But I said to myself: 'Woman, enjoy this while it lasts because this is an experience that only comes once in a lifetime.'

While in New York City, Chris met with his former mentor, Walt Lillehei, who was by this time working there. Chris also visited Dr Kantrowitz's laboratory, where he was impressed to see so many dogs surviving with heart transplants—something he had not been able to achieve in Cape Town, although he always claimed he was only interested in practicing the surgical technique and was not aiming to obtain long-term survival.

Louwtjie recounted a visit at President Lyndon Johnson's home on 29 December 1967 (Figure 15.iv), a visit that Marius claimed Chris had requested himself:

> We left in a big black car [before being whisked by plane to San Antonio]. It was a clear sunny day, the climate very much like our Karoo weather in winter. I became a little homesick because the countryside reminded me of South West Africa and my father's cattle farm. Our arranged half-hour visit was extended to about four hours because we were now invited to stay for lunch. There were six other guests. We enjoyed a tasty home-cooked meal around a very beautiful oval table. I had the place of honour next to the President on his right-hand side.

Chris, however, found President Johnson 'disappointing'. Although he admitted it was perhaps unfair to judge a man after such a short acquaintance, L. B. J. did not prove to be 'the formidable leader' he expected. He commented that although L. B. J.'s 'size and height were impressive; his intellect was not'. Perhaps President Johnson was not one of the most 'intellectual' of American presidents, but, in regard to the legislation he pushed through, he was certainly one of the most successful.

Chris appeared on a second television show, *Today,* and met the Mayor of New York, John Lindsay. He handled the press with skill, pointing out at a press conference that most of the surgical training he needed to perform the heart transplant had been gained in the USA, comments that would clearly please his American audience. 'When one gets to the top, one stands on the shoulders of many other people,' he said. 'I stand on the shoulders of many American doctors.' As Dr Kantrowitz's guest, Chris also attended the meeting of American surgeons organised by the NIH in Chicago.

On a later visit to the US, it would seem that Chris was not so tactful. Richard Lower made an insightful comment about Barnard to me.

> He came to a meeting in the US, probably in 1968, to give the honoured address. I felt terribly sorry for Chris because he was smart in a lot of ways, but he was really stupid when it came to this transplant thing. All the early pioneers of heart surgery and heart transplantation were in the

audience. Chris could have shown a little humility, and said, 'What we did was this and this, but we have really built on what a lot of you had done.' But he never once acknowledged anybody except himself. Every other word was 'I'.

After the lecture was over, I saw him sitting in a corner by himself, and I went over and talked to him. I don't think anybody else talked to him until he went out of the front door of the hotel and was mobbed by the press and the teeny-boppers. I thought, 'Gosh, how stupid he was.' He could have had the whole thing. Besides being so extraordinarily popular with ordinary people—young people and beautiful girls—he could have had the profession too, if he had just turned that corner. But he couldn't do it.

Chris's life as a celebrity began; he took to it like a duck to water. It was a lifestyle change of immense proportions that was to affect him, all of the members of his family, and his relationship with many of his colleagues at GSH.

Following the operation's triumphant success, Barnard embarked upon a series of extended international victory laps, which actually continued for several years. This placed an immense burden on the other surgeons in the Unit, which had been swamped with overseas patients following the publicity. At one stage, Terence O'Donovan operated each day for ninety-eight days. In addition, some of Chris's colleagues were not happy about giving priority to foreign patients when there were so many local ones awaiting operation.

It should be pointed out, however, that several of Chris's colleagues would have felt distinctly uncomfortable if attention had been directed to them equally. For example, Rodney Hewitson was a reserved, rather private man who eschewed publicity. Although Terence O'Donovan did carry out one lecture tour of the the USA, he was also not someone who sought publicity. It should also be remembered that it was Chris who virtually single-handedly pushed for the heart transplant programme to be established, and he alone who deserved any credit for this. None of the other members of the staff would have pursued this goal without Chris.

## First Post-Transplant Visit to Europe

Only three weeks after returning from the USA, the tour of Europe that Chris undertook after Dr Blaiberg's operation was perhaps the turning point in relations between Chris and his wife. Louwtjie later reminisced, 'As soon as the condition of the patient, Dr Philip Blaiberg, was fairly satisfactory Chris went off on his notorious European tour. This time he went alone. I was unable to accompany him because his sponsors were not prepared to pay my expenses. This tour was a disastrous one for the Barnard family and their future.'

There is no doubt that Chris's subsequent behaviour in both South Africa and overseas was humiliating to a conservative married Afrikaner woman, as Louwtjie was. The publicity his social life received greatly magnified the humiliation she had felt from his local infidelities before the transplant.

The trip took in Italy, the UK, France, and Germany. Chris was greeted at Rome airport by thousands. The welcome left him 'absolutely speechless. Never in my wildest dreams could I have imagined I would be so much in demand. It was impossible to believe the thousands of people there had come to see me. My first thought was perhaps the Beatles had been on the same plane.'

In Rome, Chris met the Italian President and the Pope (Paul VI), a meeting which would have appalled his late father, who had a very strong antipathy to the Roman Catholic Church. Chris, however, was very impressed by his visit to the Vatican. He told me once that this was perhaps the most memorable of his visits anywhere in the world. His visit, presumably like that of many who receive an audience with the Pope, was stage-managed to impress the visitor. Chris had been taken into a large palatial anteroom, where he waited by himself for several minutes. He was then escorted through large ornate doors into an even grander anteroom, where he again was left in silence for several minutes, during which period the exquisite surroundings impressed upon him the importance of the man he was about to meet. If I remember correctly, there was even a third (and grander) room in which he was left to sit and meditate before being taken through even larger doors for his audience with Pope Paul VI. It was an experience that impressed him immensely.

It was also in Rome that he signed a contract to write his autobiography for the publishing house, Mondadori. The newspapers showed him enjoying the social events with which he was tempted. Louwtjie recollected:

> Chris took Europe by storm. He was fêted and had many honours conferred upon him. But the newspaper reports that the children and I received indicated that more time was being lavished on social engagements than on medicine. We were disturbed and humiliated. We felt this was not the way a father and husband should behave.

She was referring to her husband's meetings with well-known film stars, such as Gina Lollobrigida (Figure 15.v), and reports on his activities in nightclubs and other social events. As a result, for the first time, criticism of Chris's behaviour began to surface in the conservative Afrikaans press in South Africa.

> When Chris came home, Deirdre and I waited patiently outside D. F. Malan Airport, Cape Town, protected by police. We were unable to leave the car to welcome Chris because a mad mob of reporters, photographers and an inquisitive crowd made it impossible. They all wanted to watch our reactions. How would we welcome this famous husband and father?

As time went on, life became more and more hectic for Chris, and sometimes Louwtjie. In *The Second Life*, Chris gave an example of how he tried to squeeze in every opportunity to travel and yet still attempt to continue his professional surgical life in Cape Town. On one occasion, after completing an operation, he left Cape Town in the late afternoon, flew 9,000 kilometers to Frankfurt during the night, and arrived the next morning. He immediately attended a conference and 'gave a talk to a most excited and enthusiastic audience.' He then took another overnight flight back to Cape Town, arriving on the following morning, and completed another operation in the afternoon. This lifestyle was certainly not good for his rheumatoid arthritis, which flared up constantly, forcing him to take large doses of non-steroidal anti-inflammatory drugs, which were also not good for him. However, he must have thought the rewards worthwhile. Perhaps the public acclaim had become addictive.

One of the 'Barnard-watchers' of that early period was Roger Williams, a journalist on the staff of the *Cape Times*, the main morning English language newspaper in Cape Town. He followed Barnard during those heady days after the first transplant, and interviewed others who were close to Chris at the time. In an article published on 24 February 1968, soon after the first two transplants performed at Groote Schuur Hospital, Williams gave some idea of the already hectic pace of Chris's life during those weeks. The article, entitled *What's Driving Prof. Chris Barnard?* also quoted comments from Don MacKenzie, a Cape Town photographer who accompanied Chris on some of his overseas travels and became a good friend, and from 'other close associates of Prof. Barnard'. I quote from this article:

> What is driving Chris Barnard? By the time he gets back to his waterside home at Zeekoevlei early next month from a tour of the Americas, the young surgeon will have travelled some 50,000 exhausting miles since he gave Louis Washkansky a new heart in early December. [It is estimated Chris travelled well over a quarter of a million miles during

the twelve months after the first transplant.] He has lived in a constant blaze of publicity, much of it favourable, some of it not. His tremendous personal magnetism has drawn admirers from all over the world, while in the insularity of his home-base Cape Town, it has become almost fashionable to say, 'I'm sick to death of all this Barnard business: haven't the newspapers got anything else to write about?'

Don MacKenzie is reported as saying, 'This man is building a tremendous store of goodwill towards his country, and particularly towards the medical profession in South Africa through the lectures, discussions and public appearances he is making.'

Another 'close associate' of Professor Barnard is quoted, 'If you want the answer to why he drives himself the way he is doing, it is because he has a very real sense of mission in all his. He feels he hasn't the right to withhold knowledge and information that can be vital to the preservation and prolongation of human life ...' He added prophetically 'and let me assure you, we have by no means heard the end of the Barnard story yet!'

'If there is any criticism of the publicity, then it is that it tends to be unbalanced,' continued Williams. 'Pictures of Sophia Loren [a beautiful and well-known Italian film star at the time], with whom he had a hurried lunch along with many other important people, seem to have been preferred by the newspapers to pictures of him being mobbed by Italian doctors and medical students, or facing 3,000 members of the medical profession in one of the addresses he gave.'

Louwtjie reported:

Invitations from all over the world were still pouring in. I accompanied Chris on four more trips. Then I dug my heels in. I could not stand the false hero-worship any longer. They were treating Chris like a super-being. I lost my temper only once. A representative of the Mondadori publishing house [that published Chris's first autobiography, *One Life*] visited me. Clasping his hands, he said in a suave voice: 'Mrs Barnard, if you ever decide to write a book, please do not say anything bad about Professor Barnard, because he is a god.' I looked at this man in disgust. I shouted: 'People like you will destroy Chris. There is only one God and he lives up there.' For the first time in my life I threw someone out of my house.

The frequent traveling and life as a VIP gave Chris increasing opportunities to meet beautiful women. He recounts some of his romantic 'adventures' and 'one-night stands' in his second autobiography, *The Second Life*. A couple of stories that stick in my mind relate to his relationship with the other Italian film star of the era, Gina Lollobrigida. Chris met Lollobrigida on one of his travels in Europe, and they were mutually attracted to each other. He told me that, on one occasion, when he had to catch an early plane in Italy, she drove him from her home to the airport dressed only in a fur coat she had thrown on after getting out of bed.

She begged him to visit her whenever he was in Europe. Once, when he was in Portugal, Lollobrigida sent her young secretary to him with an urgent message for him to come to Italy before returning to South Africa. He was unable to do this, but took the opportunity of sleeping with the young secretary.

He later regretted this lifestyle, writing, 'I feel I made one mistake—and that was to accept too many invitations.' There is little doubt that his frequent absences abroad were detrimental to the functioning of his department.

## Celebrity Status

Barnard became a 'phenomenon' and soon a 'celebrity'. Wherever he went, he was mobbed more like a rock star than a distinguished surgeon (Figure 15.vi). He received invitations to lecture worldwide, and huge numbers came to listen to him speak (Figure 15.vii). He was a stimulating and entertaining lecturer, and did not disappoint those who had come to hear him. He rapidly became a media favourite and, on television, he had a quick mind, was highly articulate, and had a sense of humour that appealed to the masses.

He recollected that he was receiving 'about two hundred letters a day from all over the world with all kinds of offers from women offering me their hearts in marriage to others giving me their hearts as a donor. At that stage, I was listed in the *Guinness Book of Records* as the person receiving the most fan mail—whether that was true or not I can't say—but my name was in the book anyway.'

At various times during his celebrity life, for charity events, Chris and Sophia Loren or other women were persuaded to sing (or mime) the Peter Sellers comedy song 'Goodness Gracious Me', which he did very well.

Cape Town physician and politician, Dr LAPA Munnik, remembered a trip with a colleague to Rome.

> In very broken English, the taxi driver asked us where we came from. On hearing that we came from South Africa, he let go of the steering wheel, turned right around in his seat and shook hands with us vigorously, repeating time and time again, 'Chris Barnard! Chris Barnard! Chris Barnard!' This was the impact that the heart transplant had made on the ordinary man in Europe.

British transplant surgeon, Roy Calne, summarised the situation in a nutshell.

> Being naturally good looking and enjoying the limelight of the media, his public appearances tended to be similar to those of a film star rather than a surgeon. All his dealings with non-medical people were highly successful, well publicised and brought him much criticism from colleagues who felt that public adulation of a surgeon is not appropriate.

Chris had undoubtedly become a success. Years later, I met with the kidney transplant pioneer, Joe Murray, who commented on this aspect of Barnard's life:

> I think the human being can stand anything except success. That's really true. Barnard and I were at a Transplant Congress dinner. He said, 'I didn't know how to handle success. I had no mentor. I didn't know.' It's sad. It's the story of Dorian Gray.

Ben Cosimi, a distinguished transplant surgeon at the Massachusetts General Hospital in Boston commented to me:

> With regard to Chris Barnard, there are people who are daring—daring for a variety of reasons—and they expect to be celebrated, otherwise they wouldn't carry out the daring procedure. People who do things in a dramatic way want to be dramatic and seen as such. It's amusing to see them taken over by the fame that they want, and then they don't quite know what to do with it.

This must clearly have been a fascinating time for the 'small town boy' from the 'boondocks' of the Karoo. As a child in Beaufort West, I doubt that he ever anticipated that one day he would be entertained by presidents and royalty, would have an audience with the Pope, or would be honoured by citizens and states the world over.

A good example of the society in which he mixed is a visit he (and his second wife) made later to the Philippines as guests of President and Mrs Marcos. During the visit, Mrs Marcos decided they should accompany her to the wedding of the King of Nepal, which, after they were provided with clothes suitable for the occasion, they did. Dr Munnik followed Chris's global travels at that time.

> In a relatively short period Chris Barnard had not only spoken at surgical symposia at various universities throughout the world but he

had met more kings, heads of state and prime ministers than any person living or dead. One of his most treasured invitations came from the Pope. On his return from one overseas visit, he [Chris] told me how he had been entertained by the Shah of Persia. A few hundred guests—all kings, princes and other heads of state—were present, and the cutlery and plates were all made of gold. I asked Chris, 'What were you thinking about when you sat there?' 'I thought about the days when I walked barefoot in Beaufort West.'

At first, it appears that Chris felt a little uncomfortable in the company of others who were accustomed to life in 'high society'. Distinguished American cardiac surgeon John Oschner, who had interacted with Chris at several social events, told me that occasionally these proved stressful to Chris. He was worried about his social skills, such as table manners, and so on. He would frequently invite a lady in the group to dance as this gave him a break from the social interactions of the group.

Bob Frater remembered the time when Chris first began to behave as a 'celebrity'.

In the spring of 1968, the American Association for Thoracic Surgery had its annual meeting in Pittsburgh. I met Chris for a cup of coffee and he talked about how unfair the press had been, how they had criticised him for making a record [I believe the one with Sophia Loren], the proceeds of the sale of which were going to charity, how they had photographed him in a Parisian night club in an awkward position, and how they were interested only in the sensational. I paid for the coffee and we stopped off at the men's room where there was a little old gentleman who had a saucer full of quarters and the odd dollar bill, and a brush in his hand. He promptly proceeded to brush down our jackets and, as he finished, Chris turned to me and said, 'Bob, tip this man will you, I don't carry money anymore.' I thought he was joking, and laughed. It turned out that he was serious. It was clear that the hype and the media attention had at least partly captured Chris.

This was sad because a truly remarkable physician-scientist was, I thought, likely to have his productive career limited in the future by this fact. There is no doubt that this did happen and it was a pity, but it was also the inevitable consequence of the extraordinary complexity of the character of a most unusual man.

## The Red Carpet

An example of Dr Denton Cooley's excellent sense of humour is the following story told to me by Chris, which also illustrates how Chris was treated during this era.

Soon after the first heart transplant, I was in the United States on a lecture tour and being treated very royally by my hosts. After a busy schedule, there was fortunately one day free of speaking commitments, and the United States Air Force kindly put at my disposal a plane that would take me anywhere of my choosing. I asked if I could be flown to Houston to see some of the work of Dr Cooley's group. The flight was organised and arrangements were made with Dr Cooley for my visit.

The following morning, I was flown in a large Air Force jet to the airport at Houston. Word of my arrival had obviously preceded me, as the airport terminal was packed with a large cheering crowd—it was at a time when there was great interest in heart transplantation. A red carpet was laid out from the plane to the terminal and, waiting in the terminal, I could see Dr Cooley and some of his associates. If my memory serves me correctly, the organisers had even laid on a military band to greet me.

As I walked down the red carpet flanked on either side by senior Air Force officers, each literally sparkling with gold braid and medals, with the band playing and the crowds cheering, I must say I felt, momentarily at least, like 'a very important person'. The walk from the plane to the airport building seemed to be interminable, but finally, among all this pomp and splendor and acclaim, I eventually arrived at where Dr Cooley was standing. As he stepped forward to greet me with outstretched hand—and a twinkle in his eye—he said, disarmingly, 'Hi boy! What's your name?'

If there were any risk of the splendor of my arrival 'going to my head' or giving me any undue sense of self-importance, it was immediately abolished. I burst into laughter, and have never forgotten the incident.

Dr Cooley, well-known as he was in medical circles, was also impressed by Chris's celebrity status. He remembered how he always enjoyed Chris's personality:

[He was] friendly and intelligent ... and his honest approach to surgical technique. He seemed most humble and appreciative of any information that he could gain. I felt an immediate warmth between us which has existed and increased throughout the subsequent years.

My first opportunity to meet him after the transplant was in March 1968, in Lima, Peru, at an international cardiovascular meeting. We were staying in the same hotel, and one evening my wife and I were on our way to a planned social event. In the lobby of the hotel, we were met by an expectant crowd of people and reporters with their bright lights and television cameras. When I arrived, several people applauded, I think believing that I was Chris. One woman asked me for an autograph, which I supplied. She looked at the paper and then quietly turned to my wife and asked, 'Who is this doctor? It is not Dr Barnard?' My wife replied, 'Dr Cooley is just a simple surgeon from Texas,' whereupon the woman crumpled up the paper and waited for the star to arrive. Outside the hotel, a throng of people were also waiting for Chris's arrival; the police had to hold them back. Throughout that entire meeting, people anxiously hoped to get a glimpse of Chris. His next stop on that trip was Buenos Aires, where he was again met by an enormous reception. Such was the recognition given to this individual.

As a complete aside, I just have to relate a story that captures Denton Cooley's own panache. He had been subpoenaed to court to provide testimony as an expert witness in a case in which a heart surgeon was being sued for malpractice. The opposing attorney wanted to cast Dr Cooley in a bad light to minimise the strength of his testimony.

'Tell me, Dr Cooley,' began the lawyer, with a slight sneer in his voice. 'Some would say that you are the best surgeon in the world. What would you respond to that? Are you the best surgeon in the world?'

Dr Cooley thought for a moment, and then replied, 'Yes, I probably am.'

'Isn't that rather arrogant of you?' accused the attorney, with a greater sneer in his voice.

'Yes, it probably is,' responded Dr Cooley. 'But remember, I am under oath.'

I think this is a wonderful story about a very gifted and extremely pleasant man.

# A Change of Clothes

Before the first transplant, Chris was well-known in Cape Town for his lack of interest in clothes. His appearance was plain and simple, sometimes bordering on the 'scruffy'. When dressing for his first trip abroad after the transplant, he admitted 'I had never been particularly fussy about clothes. They just didn't interest me at all. After our divorce Louwtjie even said, truthfully, that she [had] insisted I wear underpants! So, dressed in my least-frayed shirt and a blue suit I'd bought fifteen years before when my daughter, Deirdre, was baptised, I joined my wife in the lounge.'

Presumably, his lack of interest (even for underpants) was a hangover from his childhood when he was lucky to have any clothes at all.

On his first visit to Rome, however, when he was due to meet with the Pope, he was contacted by a tailor, Angelo Litrico, who admonished him for the poor cut and styling of his suits, and offered to make him a new suit free of charge. According to Chris, Litrico ripped the jacket off his back, threw it on the floor, and stepped on it to show his disdain for a suit that Chris had purchased off-the-peg in Cape Town.

'*Professore*,' he said, 'this "soot" is not good for *Il Papa* [the Pope]. You cannot have an audience with *Il Papa* dressed in this "soot".'

When Chris put on the new outfit that Litrico made for him (literally overnight), it was an epiphany. 'Putting these clothes on was one of the most sensual experiences I'd ever known,' wrote Chris, 'and very new to me. I would never have believed clothes could feel so good, almost orgasmic. They were absolutely perfect and I preened in front of the mirror.'

These remarks reminded me of those that the British film star, Michael Caine, made in his entertaining autobiography. He also came from a very poor background, claiming that as a boy, his mother insisted he had one bath a week 'whether he needed it or not.' He remembered that, very early in his career, when he began to make a little money from his acting activities, the first extravagant step he took was to purchase perfumed bars of soap and bottles of men's cologne, items he had never been able to afford before but had always wanted to enjoy. It would seem that in many of us, there is a need to fill the previous void. Thereafter, Chris had a 'love affair' with good clothes, enjoying their quality and showing them off to friends.

At the time of the first heart transplant, Hannah-Reeve Sanders had been a junior medical superintendent at GSH and later rose to become chief medical superintendent of the hospital. She was in a position to follow Chris's love affair with his appearance. She later wrote:

His transformation from, as one of his staff put it 'someone who slept in his clothes' to the meticulously and fashionably dressed jet setter took place quite suddenly when he visited Italy after the heart transplant, and we all reveled in his new image. When I bumped into him in the hospital one day, and admired his appearance, he twirled around and unbuttoned his jacket to show off its red silk lining. On another occasion, we shared our love of Italian shoes. Complaining about the very casual clothing and uncared-for shoes of the students, he said, 'Of course, not everyone can wear Guccis,' and he showed off by displaying well groomed feet, to which I responded by displaying my feet, equally well groomed in Ferragamo shoes. I believe we both enjoyed a good laugh.

Chris's new interest in his appearance increased his wife's concern as much as his interest in women.

> But the change I saw in Chris worried me more than the women his name was being linked with. Clothes had now become an important factor in his life. Chris had always had a complete disregard for clothes and his appearance was always bordering on the shabby. Throughout our married life, I was the one who purchased all his clothes. He would never allow me to give away even his oldest possessions. Now he preened in front of the mirror. He glared at his reflection. Although belying his age by fifteen years, it still showed thinning hair. His image—the one he had suddenly acquired—had to be constantly nourished and pampered. Was Angelo Litrico's suit well cut? For this fashionable Italian tailor now had a new client on his impressive list. Now, most of his faithful clothes were cast to one side, in the same way he had cast us, his family, aside. The age-old desire of man to be free got the better of him. I have often wondered what would happen if the old, humble, carefree Chris Barnard met with the new sophisticated, worldly, well-dressed Chris Barnard. Would they recognise one another?

Marius Barnard, who we must remember had never seen 'eye-to-eye' with his older brother, also observed what he perceived as a significant change in Chris's attitude to life.

> Chris, at first, could not get enough of the publicity. Strange characters, journalists and others entered his life as great benefactors and loyal friends, but most of these so-called friends had a very bad influence on him. He craved praise and adoration but was, regrettably, blind to the consequences. This later led to unhappy and disastrous events that would come back to haunt him. Chris was changing in front of my eyes. Though never having been a concerned dresser before, he now wore tight-fitting white polo-neck jerseys, white shoes and specially cut trousers, and the grey in his hair disappeared overnight. The saddest part, however, was that my brother underwent a total personality change. He was no longer the casual, unsophisticated country boy whom I knew so well, but had become a self-opinionated and intolerant person. He changed his friends and the new ones were people who used and abused him. As long as he was praised, he remained totally oblivious to this.

The Team he so lavishly praised just after the transplant disappeared, and the word 'I' replaced 'we' and 'them'. His real friends and those people to whom he owed a lot—Hewitson, Schrire and others—were slowly pushed aside. These unfortunate transformations obviously caused problems at home.

Some years later, however, when Marius himself experienced being at the centre of attention and admiration and had the opportunity to enjoy the 'good life' on one or two occasions (first-class travel, staying in luxury hotels, and generally being treated as a VIP), he began to have some insight into the allure to which Chris succumbed. He wrote:

I now had some understanding of why Chris very seldom refused an opportunity to leave the reality of cardiac surgery for the fleshpots of overseas to experience the most addictive 'drug' of all: applause and adoration. I think very few people in his position and from his background could have resisted such opportunities. Unfortunately, it changed him, his values, his integrity and his personality, and contributed greatly to his final, lonely days on earth.

## Opportunities

After the first few transplants, Barnard was offered several jobs in the USA. He told me:

One offer included a salary of a quarter of a million dollars a year, plus private practice. That was a lot of money in those days. I never even considered it. I was so really in the flood of going around talking, publicity, and things like that, that I didn't think about anything else. I decided that I was not going to leave South Africa. I thought about it this way. I'm not a youngster anymore [although he was only in his mid-forties at the time], and I'm like a tree who has grown and become mature and is bearing fruit. When you transplant a tree like that, it takes a long time before it gives fruit again because it's got to find its roots again and start growth. Only then will it produce. I didn't have the time. If I had been a young man, I probably would have moved to the USA.

It is interesting that he suggests one of his reasons for not moving to the US was that he was so wrapped up with his 'celebrity' activities. It was as a result of the adulation showered on Chris and the obvious rewards of being a celebrity that some 'cooling' of the relationship between Mrs Washkansky and Chris and the hospital took place. I have heard that she believed that too many of the rewards were going to Chris and GSH, and not enough to her and her family. She felt that her late husband was being forgotten in the euphoria of the time, and this is understandable, and possibly true.

In contrast to the opinions of Louwtjie, Marius, and several others who believed they saw a change in him, Chris was of the opinion that, at heart, he did not change. Chris told me:

> I want to stress one thing: after I did the transplant, I decided I'm not going to change myself. I'm not going to be what other people want me to be. I'm going to continue to be myself. I could have become a very high and mighty professor who doesn't speak to anybody, but I didn't. Why shouldn't I be myself, because that's what I have been all my life? The only difference was that when I did things before, I didn't get publicised and didn't get in the newspapers. Before, when I was with women, they didn't take pictures of me but, after, they started taking pictures of me. One thing that I really tried to be and continue to be is myself.
>
> I was asked to give a lecture in Heidelberg, Germany. When I came on to the stage, I said, 'I remember a song that I loved. It's called, "I've Lost My Heart in Heidelberg", and you can sing this song.' The students said, 'OK'. I chose a beautiful girl to come up with me on the stage, and we conducted the song, and they sang. And then I gave a talk, and really talked to them on their level, and they enjoyed it. It was a tremendous success. When I came off the stage, a reporter came to me, and said, 'Dr Barnard, in Germany you're not going to be well-accepted because this is not the image that we have of a professor of surgery.'
>
> So I said to him, 'Let me get one thing clear. I don't want to project the image of a professor of surgery. I want to project the image of Chris Barnard. This is how I am and, if you don't like it, I can't do anything about it because that's me.'

## Chris and Bureaucracy

In theory, Chris had to request—and be given—permission for all of the travels he took abroad. After all, he was being paid by the Cape Provincial Administration (CPA) to see patients and perform cardiac surgery at GSH, not to be spending so much time away from the hospital on other activities, even if they were often related to his work. The hierarchy at GSH and the CPA could have denied him the opportunity to travel whenever it wished. In the event, however, at first the South African government authorities were keen for him to remain in the international public eye, as he and his activities helped change the image of the country abroad. Chris therefore did not feel the need to seek permission for his travels, and his secretary would often just inform the GSH administration that he had left town. Dr Hannah-Reeve Sanders commented on this aspect of Chris's relationship with the hospital.

I do not believe Chris Barnard was ever a conformist; it surprises me when I think back on how he actually functioned all those years, within such a tight bureaucratic system. Perhaps it was the Calvinistic environment of his childhood, together with the superb disciplined clinical training of the University of Cape Town Medical School, and his own incredible will to succeed, that kept him in line.

In the administrative area, and especially when it came to dealing with the authorities, he found it impossible to conform. During the years following the heart transplant, one would need to talk to him on one or other issue, and then find he was somewhere abroad, and that no leave forms had been completed. This caused very serious repercussions with the powers-that-be, who insisted that such requests were made six months in advance. This was an impossible demand to meet when Chris was traveling constantly—and many times on the spur of the moment, or so it appeared. I remember many times when his secretary would phone my secretary and say, 'Please tell Dr Sanders that Professor Barnard will not complete the form—and that the administration knows why.' And I would get my office to process the papers—it kept the peace.

The travel programmes were vast—guest speaker, memorial lectures, interviews, honorary citizenships; he became an international celebrity. On 29 February 1968, the entry in his overseas leave request was 'Lunch with Governor Reagan of California.' Groote Schuur Hospital, with its staff of 7,000 other people, could not accommodate Chris Barnard within the normal regulations. These frequent absences disturbed not only the administration—I believe his own department suffered more and more from the lack of his leadership. And many felt deprived because he was not there to teach and initiate the research areas in which he had proved to be so superb.

The enormous influx of visitors for at least fifteen years' post-heart transplant—at times Groote Schuur Hospital was like Grand Central Station—was handled reasonably effectively by the hospital, even though no public relations unit existed. Many times Chris Barnard would join a planned programme—many times one had to apologise for his absence. Coming across him in the hospital unexpectedly was always an experience, and he would respond warmly and appear interested in a way that I like to think was his natural personal way.

Dr Sanders concluded, however, that eventually 'the hospital and his department became irrelevant. He thought we had rejected him, but I believe he rejected us.'

Although his travels proved a distraction to his work at GSH, for several years, Chris remained on top of his game—that is, he remained on top of the field of cardiac surgery, providing an excellent and skilled service to his patients. Due to his excellent reputation, and his new-found fame, patients were referred to him for routine cardiac surgery from all over the globe. It was rare for him not to have at least one or two in his unit at any one time. Chris's clinical acumen remained well-regarded by many members of the medical profession, especially by those in cardiology and cardiac surgery.

The distinguished British surgeon, Sir Terence English, remembers being a research fellow under John Kirklin—by this time chairman of the department of surgery at the University of Alabama in Birmingham, Alabama—when Barnard was invited as a visiting professor.

> He came to Alabama when I was there in 1969. This was just a year and a half after his first transplant. He was coming to receive the Freedom of the City of Birmingham. Kirklin asked him to join him in Grand Rounds on Saturday morning. For days beforehand, the chief resident and the residents were all searching through the recent cases to try and find the most difficult cases imaginable to show to Barnard. They wanted to make him look a fool because they thought he was a 'lightweight' cardiac surgeon. He acquitted himself amazingly well, and showed a depth of clinical skill which I don't think any of them could approach.

Indeed, I would suggest that no other heart surgeon of that era was as good a clinician, or as good a cardiologist, as Chris Barnard, with the possible exception of Donald Ross, who had also been trained at UCT, where the staff were clinically outstandingly good.

Chris's colleagues did not participate much in the overseas trips, largely because Chris was the 'draw' and outshone the others. Some of his colleagues, however, such as Rodney Hewitson, were not at all interested in being in the limelight. Dr Hewitson remained a stalwart member of the GSH team until his retirement in the 1990s. After he retired to the attractive coastal town of Hermanus, about one hour's drive from Cape Town, tragedy struck him when his wife was murdered during an attempted robbery at their home. Rodney died in 2013.

Terry O'Donovan did make one tour of the US, speaking at several cardiac surgical centres and even appearing on television. He fully realised that, without Chris's 'drive and ambition, we would never have taken the plunge.' He soon moved from GSH into private practice at other hospitals in Cape Town, and was subsequently appointed to the chair of cardiovascular surgery at the University of the Witswatersrand in Johannesburg, a top job in South African surgery. However, he remained there for only four years before accepting a senior position at Tulane University in New Orleans, where his salary and lifestyle increased significantly. Tragedy struck him also after retirement when he was killed in an automobile accident in 1998.

The other prominent member of the first heart transplant team was, of course, Marius Barnard, who remained at GSH until 1981 before following other career avenues.

# 16

# A Way with Words:
# Chris as a Public Speaker

As a speaker at both professional and public meetings, Chris proved himself to be most articulate and entertaining, and could always pitch the lecture at exactly the level that was ideal for the audience, whether learned physicians or school children. He was stimulating, serious, and humourous, a speaker who could immediately capture his audience's attention and hold it seemingly effortlessly for the next hour. I never saw him using notes to remind him of what he wanted to say, although to medical audiences, he would illustrate his talk with slides (which we all use as a prompt).

Several of his surgical peers commented on this aspect of his travels abroad. Well-known heart surgeon Larry Stephenson remembered Chris's visit to his medical school in Milwaukee when he was a student in May 1970.

> The auditorium was so packed that people stood outside in the hallway. Some could not actually see Dr Barnard, but could only hear him speak. Although the main theme of his talk was on heart transplants, he covered many other subjects. He felt that exercise in itself was not a cure for heart disease, and quoted Chauncey Depew, who stated, 'I get exercise acting as pallbearer to my friends who exercise.'

From Dr Stephenson's vivid memory of the occasion, it is clear that Chris's lecture made a great impact on his audience.

David Bregman, a pioneer in the development of the balloon pump, wrote:

> Chris and I spent about three days together in Iowa, and this proved to be my first experience in humility … I lectured immediately before

Dr Barnard. My lecture was well received and politely applauded. Dr Barnard then proceeded to give his lecture on cardiac transplantation, and this was immediately followed by a coffee break. I do not have to tell you that the entire audience swarmed up to Dr Barnard immediately after our lectures for autographs, handshakes, etc., while I was left standing at the podium virtually 'naked'!

When you meet the man, you see someone who is virtually bubbling with life. He is enthusiastic, extremely intelligent, and a gentleman to the tee. He is polite, highly inquisitive, and constantly searching for new ideas and answers to complex questions. I have always found him to be a charming gentleman with, of course, not only an excellent fund of medical knowledge, but also very streetwise in worldly matters. Chris Barnard certainly is an extraordinary human being who in the test of time will be recognised as one of the true innovative pioneers of the twentieth century.

## An Example of a Barnard Presentation

Some years later, Jay Kesler, the President of Taylor University, a Christian evangelical liberal arts college in Indiana, invited Chris to address the student body. When I asked him for his recollection of the occasion, he wrote the following report:

Greeted by a long round of applause, Barnard quickly sliced into his topic, the value of life, by defining the boundaries of his views. 'I'm only qualified to talk about the value of life as a surgeon values life,' he said. 'I'm unable to talk about what value the guards in the concentration camps during the Nazi regime placed on life. I'm also unable to tell you of the value the soldier, who shoots his enemy in cold blood, puts on life. Neither have I the ability to tell you what value the doctor who performs twenty abortions a day puts on life. Or the lawmakers, who spend billions of dollars on creating machines to destroy and kill people when there are millions of people dying of hunger and malnutrition, what value they put on life.'

And with those few words, Barnard captivated his audience for the next half-hour, pinning them with pathos, peppering them with humour, and piercing them with thoughts, philosophies and ideas that have been battered and shaped by the trials of his profession like a castle of sand by the waves of the ocean. The surgeon's remarks became the basis for hours of stimulating discussion in classrooms and residence halls for the next weeks—discussions that drew students, faculty and staff into timely issues and helped them to define their thinking on those issues.

Before discussing the value of life, Barnard took several swipes at his own profession and society in general. 'Do you know what is the most important disease in the world?' he queried his audience. 'Malnutrition and starvation. I worked out that in ten years I had operated on about thirty patients, trying to help them through cardiac transplantation. And in that same ten years, 250 million children died from starvation and malnutrition. But because cardiac disease is a disease of the wealthy and the rich, this is the most important disease. The most important heart disease is not coronary heart disease. The most important heart disease is rheumatic fever, because the most important heart disease in the Third World is rheumatic heart disease. Rheumatic heart disease is a preventable disease; starvation and malnutrition is a preventable disease. We cannot prevent coronary heart disease, and yet what do we do about those diseases we can prevent? We've got our sense of values totally wrong.'

Later in his address, Chris introduced a favourite topic of his, that of the quality of life and the potential role of euthanasia. Kesler wrote:

Just as he had asked his audience to define life, Barnard indirectly asked them to define death. 'If there is the presence of a heartbeat and the presence of respiration, without that individual's being able to make any communication with his surroundings, or get any pleasure from his surroundings, or emit anything that gives pleasure to his surroundings, is that God's idea of life?' Barnard asked. 'I don't think so.'

Finally, Chris described a hypothetical patient for whom no quality of life existed. He told his hushed audience that the patient had suffered enough. 'During the night,' he explained, 'with the strength he had left, [the patient] managed to disconnect the respirator himself. But before he died, he wrote a note to his doctor. It said: 'Doctor, the real enemy is not death; the real enemy is inhumanity.'

Kesler remembered that Chris urged his audience to think about that.

Death is not the enemy of the doctor. If he values life, then death is not the enemy. It's strange to think that the doctor should prevent death. Death is often good medical treatment, because death can achieve what all medicine cannot do; it can stop the suffering of that individual.... Cutting to his topic's heart, Barnard challenged his Taylor University audience to define what life is before placing a value on life. He then related a tale that established his personal definition of life.

The scene was a children's ward, and Barnard told how two youngsters had commandeered a breakfast trolley. It became their grand prix racer, and the corridor became their track. The trolley had two sections; at the bottom sat the driver, steering the trolley with his legs, and behind ran the mechanic, head down, propelling the cart down the hall. 'Unfortunately, the driver didn't maneuver the trolley well enough, and they ended up going into the wall, and of course the cups and saucers ended on the floor and broke,' Barnard said. 'That was not very popular with the attending nurse; she put them both to bed and scolded them. I walked into their room and looked at the mechanic and the driver. The driver had only one arm; I knew him quite well, as I had operated on him because he suffered from tetralogy of Fallot (a congenital heart disease). We corrected that surgically, then sometime later we saw him again, and he had a sarcoma of the humerus, which is a very malignant disease. Unable to help him, they had to do a forequarter amputation—they had to remove the whole arm, plus the shoulder girdle.

'He was the driver. He was laughing and telling me it was not his fault that they had the crash; it was the fault of the mechanic, who didn't put on the brakes when he told him to. The mechanic was a little boy I did not know, but at that time he was really a picture of horror. He grew up in a very poor home; his mother and father came home drunk one night and had an argument. The mother threw a paraffin lantern at the father, but it ended on the boy's head and burst. The boy developed third-degree burns of the whole head, and both his eyes were burned out—he was blind. At that stage, he had a big tube grafted to his nose to try to reconstruct the nose. He was squinting, like somebody who is blind, but he argued that it had been totally unnecessary to stop the race, because a few cups didn't matter very much—and he did believe they had won the race. And I realised all of a sudden that life is the joy of living; that is what it is.'

Barnard continued quietly. 'It is really a celebration of being alive. You see, what they taught me was that it's not what you've *lost* that's important, it's what you *have left* that's important. But I qualify this. There must be a *joy* in living. There must be still enough left so that there can be a celebration. You can't celebrate *nothing*; there must be *something* to celebrate. So I think one must realise that, as a doctor, if you value life, your goal must not be to prolong life; your goal must be always to provide something for that patient that he can celebrate— provide something so that life can be the joy of living.'

Perhaps the most remarkable point about this recounting of Chris's lecture is that, like Larry Stephenson, President Kesler remembered it so vividly.

## The 'Chauffeur Story'

Chris could relate the same stories to different audiences and yet what he said always seemed fresh and new. I heard him tell his famous apocryphal 'chauffeur story' many times, but I always laughed at the punchline. I record it here because it illustrates not only how well he could tell a humourous story, but also gives a glimpse into his excellent sense of humour.

Apart from his lectures abroad, Chris also accepted speaking engagements in South Africa. For this purpose, the South African government provided him with a limousine and a chauffeur. According to Chris, 'The chauffeur was a tall fair-haired young man [not unlike Chris himself] who took great pride in his new and prestigious appointment. He bought himself a smart grey jacket and a peaked cap so that he looked the part [personal chauffeur to the famous Dr Barnard].'

Together, the professor and his chauffeur visited various cities and towns within South Africa, Chris giving a rather standard, well-organised and reproducible, twenty-slide 'canned' lecture. Chris would explain that 'the young driver, clearly intelligent and interested in the topic, always sat at the back of the lecture hall and listened intently.' On the way home from these lectures, he frequently asked Chris for more details regarding heart transplantation. 'After a few weeks, he became quite knowledgeable about the subject, at least for a chauffeur.'

On one of these occasions, as the limousine was approaching a small town where Chris was booked to give a lecture, he said to the chauffeur, 'Driver, I am very tired this evening. Since you have heard this talk of mine many times, I wonder if you would like to give the talk yourself today.' The driver looked somewhat perplexed, but Chris added. 'Look, the talk is rather standard, and you have seen all the slides many times. There will be no doctors in the audience tonight. I think it would be quite alright for you to give the talk while I sit and rest at the back of the room.' Still, the chauffeur hesitated. 'The people here do not know me,' continued Chris, 'and you and I look very similar. I am sure they will not suspect a thing.'

Outside the small town, the chauffeur and Chris exchanged clothing; Chris took off his handmade Italian suit and put on the chauffeur's outfit, with the chauffeur putting on Barnard's suit. Chris took over the wheel of the limousine, and the chauffeur sat elegantly in the back seat.

When they entered the town, there was a large crowd waiting to greet 'Dr Barnard'. The chauffeur, dressed as Chris, emerged from the limousine and was immediately ushered into the lecture hall where he was directed on to the podium. Dressed as the chauffeur in the smart grey jacket and peaked cap, Chris sat at the back of the room. According to Chris, the lecture proceeded uneventfully and he was actually quite impressed with how well the chauffer had delivered it. Indeed, it made him feel slightly insecure to know that a chauffeur could give the lecture almost as well as he could. The driver had started rather hesitantly, but as his confidence increased, he had become quite articulate and informative. The young man clearly enjoyed being the centre of attention, and when he had concluded his remarks, he gracefully acknowledged the applause. Chris remembered:

> At the end of the lecture, the chairman asked, 'Dr Barnard, would you mind answering a few questions?' I began to feel a little nervous. It was one thing to give a lecture, parrot-like, but quite another to answer unrehearsed questions. But the young driver, now full of confidence, immediately said, 'Of course.' All went well for a while. The questions were simple and the chauffeur, from his many discussions with me in the car, was able to answer them without difficulty.
>
> But then a distinguished gentleman stood up in the middle of the room and announced that his name was Dr DeBakey and he was a visitor from Houston in the United States, and he would like to ask a question. I immediately recognised the well-known American heart surgeon, and my nervousness started turning into panic. What on earth was Michael DeBakey doing in this small town in South Africa?

He was the last person Chris had expected to see there. Now, his chauffeur's lack of knowledge would be exposed, and it would appear as if he, Professor Christiaan Barnard was unable to answer the question correctly. Dr DeBakey would return to the States believing Barnard to be an ignorant fool.

Chris continued with the telling of his story.

> Dr DeBakey then proceeded to ask 'Dr Barnard' an extremely complex and difficult immunologic question about heart rejection. There was no way the young chauffeur would know the answer—we had never discussed such a complex topic in the limousine. On the podium, the chauffeur, who also recognised the great Dr DeBakey from the photograph he had seen in my office, was clearly at a loss for an answer. He looked very agitated and began to sweat profusely. At the back of the room, I became increasingly anxious.
>
> But after a short pause, the chauffeur broke into a confident smile, and said, 'I recognise you, Dr DeBakey. You are certainly one of the most famous heart surgeons in the world. Your reputation is impeccable and your knowledge extensive. I therefore cannot understand how you can possibly ask me such a simple question. In fact, to show you how simple

it is and how easy to answer, I am going to ask my chauffeur at the back of the room to answer it for me.'

Needless to say, the answer from the 'chauffeur' at the back of the room received tumultuous applause from the very impressed audience, and the crisis was over.

I should add that this apocryphal story was never told with the aim of belittling or making fun of Dr DeBakey. Indeed, his name had obviously been chosen to represent the highest possible knowledge and achievement in the field of heart surgery.

In one of his later books, *Chris Barnard's Program for Living with Arthritis*, Chris stated that, as a young man, until well after the first heart transplant, 'lecturing to any kind of audience never worried me at all. In fact, I enjoyed it immensely. I would go to a lecture virtually unprepared, and the words would tumble out as I talked.' However, as he became older, by which time he had gained an excellent reputation as an entertaining speaker, 'I get more tense about having to lecture, and I prepare myself for it. If your reputation is as a good lecturer, then you have got to be good.'

Chris was equally at ease when interviewed for radio or television, or when giving a press conference. Honest and direct, sometimes dangerously so, Chris was a reporter's dream. His personality came to the fore; his engaging smile, his sense of humour, his charisma, won him many admirers. His honesty on occasion landed him in 'hot water', sometimes with his wife or friends, more often with the authorities. He said things that others, be they hospital or university administrators, the medical profession, or the South African Government, had not wanted to hear. At one press conference, he insisted he had 'killed' a patient through inept surgery. The hospital's public relations people quickly tried to explain what the professor 'really meant', but their efforts were undermined when Chris commented bluntly, 'They're talking crap.'

This facility to respond to an interviewer's questions was a natural gift, and had shown itself early in Chris's career. Leading heart surgeon, Sir Brian Barratt-Boyes, remembered a visit Chris made to his home country of New Zealand.

As part of the programme publicity, New Zealand television interviewed a number of the speakers and these included Chris. My wife and I well remember watching him perform on television and deciding among ourselves that he was clearly a most experienced performer. The next day we chided him about his TV performance and were surprised to hear that this was possibly his first TV appearance and that television was not then available in South Africa. Looking back on these events it is clear that Chris Barnard had natural abilities in communication, particularly with the media and that this ability was to stand him in good stead when he succeeded in performing the world's first heart transplant.

Chris's sense of humour often came to the fore. I well remember when he was interviewed on a Saturday late-night television chat show in the UK. With skill equal to any stand-up comedian, he told an amusing story about a patient who had come to see him at Groote Schuur Hospital asking for a testicle transplant. The mere subject, of course, raised laughter from the studio audience.

'But who will be the donor?' asked Barnard.

'My father,' replied the patient.

'But then your son will be your brother,' pointed out Barnard, with a broad grin. Although certainly not the sort of story one might expect from a leading member of the medical profession during an interview broadcast to millions, it brought the house down, and added greatly to Barnard's popularity with the public. I never asked him whether the anecdote were true or not.

Perhaps surprisingly, however, Chris was not at ease reading from a script or a prompt card. He admitted to me that his introductions to a BBC television series based on one of his books were eventually cut almost entirely due to his inability to read from the prepared script in a natural and fluent manner. He was clearly at his best as an ad-lib man.

# 17

# Fame over Family

There is no doubt that Chris's lifestyle rapidly evolved. As we have seen, his suits were handmade for him, he grew his hair trendily long, and he mixed with the fashionable and famous. His penchant for being in the company of beautiful women made him a favourite of the paparazzi. Photographs of him with them appeared frequently in the world's periodicals and magazines. He realised that he had become a public figure and that he would remain under surveillance by the media, but he believed that, as time passed, he would be able live the life of the average man. This proved not to be the case, at least not for many years. For years, he was 'hounded by photographers … any girl I was seen with was a photograph and a story. This, to the newspapers, appeared to be vitally important news that the public just had to know about.'

The lifestyle engendered by his success as a surgeon and his sudden celebrity took its toll on his family, whose lives underwent upheavals of major proportions that had lasting consequences. For the home-loving and more reserved Louwtjie, it soon became a nightmare.

She wrote:

People, known and unknown to us, came to our home to look, to talk and to listen. Suddenly, we were overwhelmed with bouquets, baskets of fruit, cases of whisky and presents of all kinds. Our private life had vanished overnight. We were like some rare animals in a cage. Admired, praised, criticised and, in the end, condemned.

The telephone rang incessantly. These calls were from friends, genuine people, sadists, hypnotists and astrologers. Intruders invaded our home by day and by night. Without even asking, they entered our private property, walked round my precious garden, trampling the flower beds, relaxed on the lower end of my lawn which overlooks the lake. One man actually came right up to our sun-porch window and photographed us. Then there were the sightseeing buses full of tourists who looked at our little house as if it were some ancient historical castle. And on Sundays, there was the endless procession of motor-cars that crawled past, filled with curious sensation-seekers' eyes.

But worst of all were the news-hungry reporters, the television companies and the photographers. They descended on us from all over the world determined to 'get their story' at all costs. Some were downright nasty. If you granted them an interview, they shamelessly twisted the facts for the sake of sensation. And if you refused to talk to them, they simply invented their own stories.

For a while, Louwtjie tried to fight back by taking an unusual interest in the things that Chris seemed to find glamorous.

Dinners, parties and the latest fashions consumed me. I started to spend far more than I really could afford on clothes and cosmetics. All I lived for was the next trip to somewhere. How soon could I leave the dull confines of my home? Fame and glory had begun to catch up with me, and the honest truth is that I started to attach too much value to worldly things. My powers of resistance became less and less. I could not even find the time to read my Bible.

She accompanied Chris on several trips abroad. She found Tehran in Iran (or Persia as it then was), still ruled over by the Shah, the highlight of their visit. However, during this visit when they were being overwhelmed by throngs of admirers, she claims Chris turned to her and said in Afrikaans, 'Louwtjie, you will have to get used to the idea that people are interested in me and not you.' Even though this statement was undoubtedly true, this is not the sort of comment you would make to someone you truly love. She wrote:

In the beginning, I also enjoyed the fame, glory and artificiality of our new life, but slowly, as the whirlwind of publicity became a hurricane destroying everything in its path, I realised that this new exciting world was destroying the real and true values of our lives. There was no time for the ordinary day-to-day little tasks. Everything became one mad rush, from one country to another, from one social engagement to the next. All these things were exciting and fascinating but I was to realise that they paid no real dividends.

But now the world had lost sight of Chris's achievement and was only interested in Chris the man. And Chris, blinded by the brilliant glare, and egged on by two new friends, reveled in his role.

According to her mother, Deirdre became unhappy and disturbed whenever her father's private life made the headlines. Both children were constantly reminded of his flamboyant activities by magazine stories and newspaper reports.

Deirdre remembers wondering why it was that her father, whom she had known all her life, was suddenly being made such a big fuss of. She comments on how the press attention and the unending questions she was asked about her father and family affected her personally.

> I could have let it upset me and sometimes it did. I could have let it bother me and sometimes it did that too, but in the end, I decided the old ways were best and I might just as well do what my parents taught me and be as polite and as helpful as I could. After all, it didn't take too long after my father made his first headline before I began to learn that for a great deal of the rest of my life this was likely to go with the territory. Sometimes the territory is not very much to one's liking.

Deirdre realised that Chris was not focused on family life anymore and that, 'as his career pressure increased … those old carefree days became a thing of the past … and that he wouldn't ever come back again.'

The impact of Chris's new status on Deirdre was considerable. GSH physician, Peter Jackson, pointed out that before the first transplant, 'Chris had apparently only one big ambition, which he pursued with the utmost ruthlessness and single mindedness, namely to make his daughter the world champion water skier.' This situation changed dramatically.

Bob Frater commented:

> You must know about his daughter, and the way he trained her to be a very good water skier. It was the typical young female sports star with a father coach. At her first competition in South Africa, she won the South African championships. She came third in the European water ski jumping championships. He would schedule his trips to be close to water ski meets. Do you know when the last time he ever took her water skiing was? The Thursday night before the first heart transplant. For her, it was quite devastating. For awhile she just couldn't understand what the hell had happened to her.

In her memoirs, Deirdre comments on the abrupt change in her life.

> Despite my success at water skiing, [our ordinary life] didn't change until my father 'went public'. Once his life changed, that particular partnership broke up. There were other people who could do the things

that he'd done for me, but it could never have been the same. If I can make a comparison, it's like two dancers, say Fonteyn and Nureyev or Fred and Ginger. They could have danced and did dance with others, but without each other the magic was never really there. Now, if I wish to, somewhere inside myself, I can always go back to those two people who don't exist anymore. The small-town doctor at the wheel of the boat and the little water skier, skimming over the water on a day that never changes somewhere in timelessness where conditions are just right and the moment is perfect.

When I once asked Chris when Deirdre gave up competitive water skiing, he replied, 'When I stopped training her.' She did, in fact, continue for a while after this. He did not appear in any way distraught or guilty that he had seemingly abandoned her in this way, perhaps reflecting that his effort to push her towards achievement was largely self-centred rather than directed solely towards her success. He later wrote:

> From America, I went to Copenhagen to spend a few days with Deirdre who was preparing to take part in the European water skiing championships. My heart went out to my daughter. She was not with her father any more, she wasn't skiing well and, worst of all, she was considerably overweight. I realised then how a physical defect visible to others caused much more suffering than one that was hidden from view. I would never again criticise people who resorted to plastic surgery. I took Deirdre shopping and bought her some clothes that would hide the bulges. She pleaded with me to stay on because she needed some security. But I was drawn like a magnet to St. Tropez.

In this passage, Chris is quite honest in stating that he put his own wishes (to attend a social gathering in the south of France) before those of his daughter (competing in the European championships), who was clearly suffering psychologically from the sudden change in her relationship with her father. He damns himself with his own words. Deirdre did, however, go on to ski professionally for a year with an 'aqua star' group (who entertained the public with an exhibition of top-quality water skiing), which gave her the opportunity of traveling in South Africa and even several other parts of the world.

Chris's flamboyant lifestyle not only resulted in strains in his marriage and in his relationships with his children, but also led to problems with some of his colleagues. Marius reported that 'Professor Schrire strongly disapproved of Chris's behaviour, and their hitherto close and friendly relationship deteriorated to the extent that they seldom spoke to one another.'

It appears that Schrire was more upset than most by the change in Chris's lifestyle and priorities. He and Professor Jannie Louw, Chris's long-time surgical mentor, were upset because they felt Chris was not taking his professional responsibilities as seriously as he should have been. Chris told me:

[Before the first heart transplant] the number one man in my life in Cape Town was Professor Val Schrire. He was very supportive. This man was like a god to me. You see, he had taught me when I was learning cardiology. There was not a day that I didn't go to speak to him, just to talk to him. We were very, very close. He was absolutely 90 per cent of the success that I had. It's so sad that afterwards [i.e. after the first few transplants] he became strange and sort of jealous, and started working against me. I wanted to really fly into him because he was doing a lot of things behind my back, but I changed my mind. I said, 'We have really worked together so well. The progress we have made and the success we have had is due to this combination between cardiac surgery and cardiology, and I think we should make peace and forget the past.' Val Schrire said, 'No. I'm prepared to cooperate, but I will never forget,' or something like that. The next day, the general surgeons operated on him and found he had inoperable cancer of the pancreas.

It was not long before Professor Schrire died.

Chris's weakness for beautiful young women was well-known both before and after the first transplant. For example, Sir Brian Barratt-Boyes mentioned to me that 'when Chris visited Green Lane Hospital [in Auckland, New Zealand], he kept trying to meet the nurses. We literally had to lock the doors of the Nurses' Home to keep him out.'

John Kirklin commented that 'we participated in an international symposium in Auckland, New Zealand, where I was once again reminded of his brilliant mind, his warm personality, and his wandering eye.' Denton Cooley wrote that Marius, whom he had helped train in surgery, was less flamboyant and outgoing than Chris, and 'less interested in the nurses in the operating room.'

I asked Chris whether he felt he alienated other people in Cape Town by his flamboyant lifestyle. 'Of course, I did. When they see somebody enjoying life—young girls and beautiful women and all that—they are jealous because they want to do the same thing. But they are not capable of doing it. That's the point. That's why they criticise you because they feel they can't do it themselves.'

Chris's friend, Father Tom Nicholson, and Deirdre's friend, Dene Friedmann, felt that a factor in the allure of nightlife to Chris was the fact that in some respects he had 'missed his youth' because of his need to largely forego a social life as a student to ensure he did not fail his exams, which would have meant losing his scholarship. He liked to be with young people, possibly because he had missed his youth. In his forties and fifties, he was always keen to visit night clubs, which he enjoyed very much.

## Crisis Point

Chris's marriage had long had some problems, and it now suffered further by his frequent absences from home when he travelled abroad, and from his increasing opportunities to mix with the glamorous jet set. Wherever he went, he was followed by photographers and journalists. Published photographs of him with many beautiful young women led to increasing problems with his wife. The emotional turmoil she went through, particularly as Chris's popularity increased, when his social activities were vividly reported in the newspapers the world over, is well-described in her aptly named autobiography, *Heart Break*. There is no doubt that at times she suffered mental anguish, even agony. The tension between them was already at a high level.

One particular incident (in March 1968) that Chris once told me about and subsequently recounted in his follow-up autobiography, *The Second Life*, still puts shivers down my spine. Chris had been invited to lecture to the American College of Cardiology, and the invitation had allowed for his wife to accompany him. They were staying in the plush Hilton Hotel in San Francisco.

Chris was in the lecture hall preparing to give his presentation when he realised he had left some slides in their bedroom. He phoned Louwtjie and asked her to look for them while he came up to collect them. In looking into his attaché case, she came across a letter from one of his lovers.

Their marriage was already almost at breaking point and the discovery of the letter led to a blazing row during which Louwtjie threatened to throw herself out of the twenty-third floor bedroom window. Chris was forced to break off the argument as the time had come for his lecture and so, promising to change his behaviour, he left her in the bedroom and went down to the congress auditorium. In the middle of his lecture to the distinguished audience, he heard the unmistakable sound of an ambulance's siren outside the hotel. The thought inevitably crossed his mind that Louwtjie had fulfilled her threat to jump, and he had visions of the hotel management or the police rushing into the lecture room to apprise him of the shocking news. Fortunately, the ambulance was in the vicinity for a different patient, but how Chris finished his lecture with that on his mind I will never understand.

The lecture, however, proved a great success. Chris, nervous after his encounter with Louwtjie and realising that his audience of American cardiologists included several who might be antagonistic towards him, began with his 'chauffeur story', which won over most of his audience, and then proceeded to discuss the potential of using animal hearts for transplantation into patients in the future. He received a standing ovation.

Louwtjie described the same incident in the San Francisco hotel as follows:

Alone in our suite, I discovered concrete evidence of his denied love affairs in Europe. Chris had asked me to find some documents in his briefcase. While rummaging through its contents I found love letters from an internationally renowned actress. Was she also 'mad' (as Chris had claimed a previous young lady was)? Shattered and terribly alone I decided I must give Chris his freedom. I thought the best, and only, thing to do was to get out of this now famous man's life. In a daze, I walked to the window. Suicide was the quickest way out of this terrible mess. The only sound that broke the awful silence was the opening and shutting of the lift doors. A gentle hand on my shoulder restrained me. I had not heard anyone enter our suite. I turned around. There was no one there. From a picture frame on the dressing table, the two radiant faces of my children smiled at me. That was what saved me from taking my own life. I could not hurt them.

When confronted by Louwtjie about his infidelity, Chris had promised to change his ways, but according to her, 'at the banquet, only hours later, his promise was already forgotten. This sudden fame was too much for Chris. His social and personal image excluded everything else. He was a man obsessed.'

The 'terrible moment in San Francisco' left her for many months 'in a dumb misery before the shattered fragments of my life. Painfully, and slowly, I began to build a new future for my children and myself.'

It should be kept in mind that Louwtjie wrote her short autobiography at a time when she was still suffering emotional turmoil from the break-up of her marriage, which she blamed largely on her husband's romantic indiscretions. She pointed out that her book was written 'for those who do not know what really happened to Christiaan Barnard and his family when he became the first man to transplant a human heart.' The picture she paints of Chris must therefore be viewed in the light of these comments and the state of her mind at the time she put pen to paper. The tribulations of life with him had clearly forced her opinion to sour. 'I will always admire Chris's work, achievements and determination,' she wrote, 'but I have lost all respect for him as a man and I will never trust or believe him again.'

Louwtjie Barnard's message is that Chris's character and behaviour changed markedly following the unprecedented attention and adulation he received after the first heart transplant. She makes a strong case for her message, at least with regard to his attitude to his wife and family, although it may just have been that his infidelity was now in the public eye rather than in private, as it was before he became famous. His behaviour may not have changed markedly, although perhaps the opportunities for affairs had increased exponentially. Whether Louwtjie's views changed in the years that elapsed after their subsequent divorce, during which time the pain she experienced during the break-up of her marriage may have been relieved to a degree, I do not know.

## Divorce

In her memoirs, Deirdre wrote that she and André could hardly fail to notice that their parents were 'living like strangers', that there were 'tensions' and an 'apprehensive feeling', but little talk of divorce. When her father was in Cape Town, he was living at 'home' in their house in Zeekoevlei. Deirdre clung on to her hitherto happy childhood and close relationship with her father as long as possible. 'He still had a front door key and there was no sound in the world as wonderful to me as to hear that key turn in the lock when my father came back from wherever it was he had been. It meant Pappa's home, the circle's complete, we are still a family; but it couldn't continue.'

She also states, 'He made mistakes but he never tried to deny them. Perhaps he will not be remembered for being the perfect parent, but I really do believe he loved his children and did his best for them.'

When Deirdre was in her final year at high school and her mother told her that her parents were considering a divorce, her first response was to ask, if this indeed had to happen, who would be there to take care of her father. Her concern for his welfare demonstrated the special bond that had developed between father and daughter.

After struggling with her domestic situation for months, Louwtjie decided she would have to seek a divorce. The humiliation of her position became too much to bear. Louwtjie explained in her own words what made the situation particularly sad:

What was so unbelievable was that all this was so unlike the Chris we had known. This was the man who over the past twenty years had always been a good and loving father and who had devoted most of his free time to his children, especially to Deirdre by training her to become a champion water skier. He had helped them with their homework, encouraged them to do well at school and to face the daily obstacles of a child's world. He was a good father, husband, and friend.

For his part, Chris undoubtedly appreciated Louwtjie's good qualities. In *The Second Life*, he wrote:

> She was a wonderful mother and a good wife—in the true Afrikaner tradition. She liked to sew and cook and keep house. She never wanted to be anything more than a 'boeremeisie' [farm girl] and, being married to someone like me who wanted much, much more from life, the marriage never really stood much of a chance. Of course, when the world opened its doors to me, with all the fanfare and bright lights, it was probably her worst nightmare.
>
> Louwtjie wasn't to blame but nor was I when I think about it. We just sort of drifted. I'd grown with my career and she was still married to the medical student. The first few sips of success were so sweet and I wanted to enjoy every last drop—but that very success and publicity we were now enjoying … had every prospect of bringing our marriage to a very painful end. She knew it and I knew it.

The differences in their personalities and goals in life are perhaps illustrated by a comment Louwtjie made in her memoirs. 'When Chris phoned me early in the morning from the hospital after the first transplant to tell me the patient was okay I said "congratulations—that's wonderful" and I went back to sleep.' To her, as to be expected, the first transplant was nowhere near as important as it was to Chris. She perhaps could not even begin to understand just how important it was to him. A discrepancy in goals in life between an ambitious husband (or wife) and his (or her) unambitious spouse must be common, but perhaps was extreme in the case of Chris and Louwtjie.

Chris did not blame her for doing anything wrong. He told her, 'You've been a wonderful wife and you've sacrificed a lot to help me get where I am today, but what you have not done is you haven't tried to be a companion to me. You've been willing to share the bad times with me—why can't you share the good times too? Why must everything always be so miserable, why should we be wary of people—and unfriendly, why can't we just have fun?' When asking her this, he didn't think he was asking, or expecting, too much.

Although it was painful for him to admit later, Chris realised that he had lost interest in his family and old friends. 'The glitter of the new world I was living in had intoxicated me. I'd become addicted to all it had to offer and wanted more and more of it. My appetite for the good life seemed insatiable.'

His words appear to give credence to Louwtjie's opinion that, 'Chris had become a completely changed man. Fame, and hero-worship had gone to his head.' Elsewhere, she commented, 'There are two tragedies in life—not to get what the heart desires, and the other is to get it.' In her opinion, Chris had obviously achieved his heart's desire: fame and hero worship.

The ultimate break with Louwtjie was now inevitable. Perhaps the final nail in the coffin came when he was invited to attend the Red Cross Ball in Monaco. Louwtjie made it very clear that if he went, the marriage would be at an end. He was determined to attend this glamorous event, and went ahead with his plans. He danced with Princess Grace of Monaco (Figure 17.i).

The final break-up was, at least from Chris's perspective, sudden and unexpected. He recounted to me that, on his return from a visit to the USA, he was met at Cape Town airport by the car and driver provided for him by the South African government. When Chris had settled into the passenger seat, and they were pulling out of the airport driveway, the driver looked over to him and asked where he would like to go. Chris, surprised by this odd question, replied, 'Home, of course.'

'You can't,' replied the driver. 'Your wife doesn't want you back. I've all your belongings in the boot (trunk) of the car.' In the back of the car were all of Chris's clothes, packed in cardboard boxes. Without prior warning, he was being ignominiously kicked out. Years later, he could look back and laugh at the incident, but at the time, his driver's words must have come as an unpleasant shock. Louwtjie deserved full marks for bringing off such a convincing *coup de grâce*.

Chris went to stay at a friend's beautiful apartment in La Corniche in Clifton, one of Cape Town's most luxurious beachside suburbs. As Deirdre noted, he moved not only to a different address, but also into a different, far more luxurious world. 'He now had a far more glittering arrangement in Clifton, the millionaire strip of the Atlantic seaboard.'

The end came on Friday, 23 May 1969, approximately eighteen months after the first heart transplant, when Louwtjie appeared in Court. 'Chris was also notified,' she wrote, 'but he did not defend the case.' He was not required to attend by law; indeed, he was abroad at the time.

Neither my children nor my parents or family knew when I had to appear in Court. That Friday, only four close friends accompanied me.

It was a soul-destroying experience, but only lasted about five minutes. The sordid public part was over, but the divorce was only finalised on 23 July 1969. As soon as I left the Court Room, my children, parents and family were told. The last thing I wanted was for them to read it in the newspapers.

At the time of the divorce, Deirdre was in Bloemfontein water skiing in the South African Games, and unfortunately appears to have read about it in the newspapers. She found it a very painful experience.

The settlement between Chris and Louwtjie was very much in her favour. According to Marius, Chris found it intolerable that he had to pay Louwtjie maintenance. Whether this is true or not, I do not know, but Chris did later write in his second autobiography that it appeared that Louwtjie and her lawyer wanted him to 'become as impoverished as they could make me.'

All I would be allowed to take from my house in Zeekoevlei were my clothes. Louwtjie would continue to live there until she died, or got married again. I would pay for the rates, taxes, insurance and maintenance of the property. She also asked for an allowance of R500 a month—and I had to pay for the education of our two children as well. This placed an awesome financial burden on someone like me. At that stage, I was earning only R1,200 a month—before tax [at a time when the rand was worth about $3].

However, as he did not want the divorce to drag on, he agreed to all of Louwtjie's demands 'against advice given me from many quarters'.

From my conversations with Chris over several years, it is my belief that he had few sustained regrets when his first marriage failed. With regard to his divorce, Chris realised the harm it could do to his children. He is quoted as saying:

How sad that it all had to end like this. André told me that he had heard about it for the first time when he was coming out of school one afternoon. He read about our separation on the newspaper poster in big bold print. Who can ever quantify the effects of such shocking news to a boy that age? The children of divorce are frightened and frequently depressed. Even though the parents may be concerned, they are seldom able to provide sufficient help or emotional support. In our children's case, it was made much worse by the wide publicity the proceedings attracted.

The first heart transplant, which had originally been a happy event for the members of the Barnard family, had eventually led to them being torn apart. Whether Chris's marriage would have survived intact if he had continued as just a very good heart surgeon, but not a famous surgical innovator and a celebrity, is, of course, unknown, but there is little doubt that the fact that the family had to face their problems in the glare of worldwide publicity placed an immense strain on all of them.

## The Mid-Life Crisis

What Chris Barnard had undergone, of course, was a massive, and very public, midlife crisis, not unlike many successful men, including many doctors and surgeons known to me personally. In the USA, in particular, the story of the medical student who marries a nurse, who works to help him pay his way through medical school and subsidises the costs of their growing family while he trains as a poorly paid surgical resident, is far from uncommon. When he is established in practice and financially secure—at the height of his professional powers—he becomes the centre of attention for many much younger women, often nurses themselves. His head is turned from his now relatively humdrum family life to the attractions of a younger woman with whom he is thrust into contact on a daily basis, and with whom he can attempt to recapture his youth and fill his life with excitement again. He succumbs to the need for a 'trophy wife' (as did Chris later), and abandons the first wife—now perceived to be dull—who helped him succeed professionally and brought up his family.

Louwtjie clearly understood this. With regard to Chris, she stated that 'the undoubted attractions of young and glamorous women were too strong to enable his marriage to continue.'

During this period of time, Chris said words to reporters that would have been better unsaid. When discussing the attraction of young women to middle-aged men, he made disparaging and hurtful remarks about 'older' women—that is, women of his own age—commenting on their wrinkled skin and loss of youth. Dumping a wife of twenty years for a 'new model', someone ten or twenty years younger with the full bloom of youth still in her, is not uncommon for successful middle-aged men, but Chris's remarks, made publicly and reported in the mass media, must have been particularly hurtful to his ex-wife. They were clearly unnecessary, and would not have been said by someone with more tact and a deeper sense of kindness. However badly the break-up of their marriage had affected him, to make such comments, which were clearly directed to the mother of his two children, reflected very poorly on him.

Walt Lillehei also believed Chris had undergone a midlife crisis.

> I think he adopted what is generally known as the hedonistic lifestyle. He lived for pleasure. That's not bad—I mean, after all, the exact opposite would be an extreme pessimist. That's not a very pleasant way to live. Chris allowed his pleasure-seeking instincts and disposition full rein … Let's say you're talking about a mid-life crisis, which is a well-recognised syndrome. It can be faced in any endeavour where people are intensely dedicated, doing something to the exclusion of even families and personal life—and suddenly, a mid-life crisis! Some escape into alcohol or drugs, others straighten out later, and others change careers. It's frequently seen in surgery, but I don't know that it's any more frequent than in any other walk of life. Certainly, I think in a way that's what happened to Chris in his mid-forties. That's when his crisis hit. It's usually in the late forties or early fifties, if it's going to hit a person at all—this mid-life crisis to change your endeavour or work. I think he did that quite obviously.
>
> He didn't change radically, but some of his characteristics became more firm. For example, I think his self-confidence increased. He frequently gave opinions on things entirely divorced from medicine. That's one of the great things, they tell me, about winning the Nobel Prize. Instantly, overnight, you become an expert both in your own field and in every other field, of which you may have no knowledge whatsoever! People listen to what you say. I suppose he enjoyed having these unconventional opinions—he wasn't inhibited about expressing them. The press hung on his every word. Sometimes, of course, they didn't necessarily write it up to his credit, but he certainly had a forum to speak out on any subject that he desired. And he wasn't speaking in silence—people were listening and reporting what he said. I suppose that got more pronounced as time wore on.

I asked Dr Lillehei whether Chris's sudden fame went to his head.

'No. I don't think so. He possibly became more selfish in regard to what was good for him and what he wanted to do. For example, I never recall that he did any significant philanthropic work—but maybe he didn't really have time.'

As we shall see, Dr Lillehei was forgetting, or possibly did not know, that Chris's donation of the royalties from his first autobiography was philanthropic. If he had kept the royalties himself, it would have made him personally a very wealthy man.

# First Autobiography: *One Life*

His early fame encouraged Chris to take the opportunity of the global interest in him and his work to pen an autobiography, *One Life*, which he wrote with the help of a professional writer, Curtis Bill Pepper.

'The idea was that we would generate money for the Chris Barnard Fund (the charity set up in Cape Town to provide grants for local research into heart disease and organ transplantation).'

Chris told me that Bill Pepper 'came to Cape Town, and I didn't like him very much because he had long hair and looked like a hippie. Then he became my closest friend. He became like Val Schrire to me, such a good friend. I absolutely idolised this man because I recognised his tremendous skill and potential. He was a very good human being. He looked after me and cared for me. He knew how to write a book. I think he wrote that book [*One Life*] very nicely.'

The book traced Chris's life from his childhood in Beaufort West, through his studies at UCT and in Minneapolis, until he had carried out the first heart transplant. It was fast-moving and readable. It proved very popular and was eventually translated into thirteen different languages, and published throughout the world. Chris travelled globally, promoting and publicising the book, and he generously donated the royalties to The Chris Barnard Fund, from which many subsequent researchers, myself included, benefited significantly. Royalties from the book provided more than R500,000 to the Fund. In the days when the rand was worth considerably more than the US dollar, and the price of an average house in South Africa (even in the white areas) was R15,000, this was a great deal of money. Chris once told me jokingly that, if he had known the book would make so much money, he might not have donated the income to the Fund.

Importantly, and generously, the Fund was not just used for Chris's own research. All applications from Cape Town physicians and surgeons working in research into heart disease or organ transplantation were considered on merit. His colleague, Lionel Opie, an internationally known researcher into heart metabolism and drug therapy, expressed his gratitude that 'Chris not only allowed but encouraged the Fund to support me heavily.'

At this early stage after the first few transplants, Chris had visions of building a major centre for the treatment of heart disease at the University of Cape Town. Bob Frater stated:

The centre was very important to him. He was rather starry-eyed in those days, and I think he had a vision of Cape Town and Groote Schuur being some kind of mecca where specialists and researchers from all over the world could come to pool their knowledge and exchange ideas. If he had not allowed himself to be distracted by the lure of the 'high-life', I believe Chris could have achieved this goal, and UCT/GSH could have become one of the great academic research centres in the world, at least in the fields of cardiology and organ transplantation. The South African government was more than willing to fund this enterprise, and organizations such as the mining houses and other South African philanthropists would have contributed further financial support.

Unfortunately, Chris was distracted from establishing this lasting legacy, and, as a result, UCT was not destined to become one of the world's truly leading heart or organ transplant centres.

The veracity of *One Life* in relation to the stresses and strains of the Barnard marriage was subsequently questioned by Louwtjie. In her memoirs, she wrote:

> I cannot understand why Bill Pepper, in writing about my life with Chris in *One Life*, never interviewed me or the children. Part of the first draft which Chris invited me to read was fairly impartial. Even if the facts were not entirely correct, at least it was not cruel fabrication. But, I understand that Bill Pepper was asked to come to Cape Town after the divorce was finalised to re-write many of the incidents in the book concerning our life together. The version of *One Life* which finally sold to the public was a different matter altogether. I read through it with increasing horror because many of the parts relating to me had been changed. Suddenly I had become the terrible wife with whom Chris had been condemned to live for twenty years. No wonder everybody felt sorry for Chris!
>
> A strange incident that took place on 12 February 1970, confirms this. On that day—the day before Chris married Barbara Zoellner [who was to become his second wife]—Bill Pepper paid me a short visit at my home. Sitting opposite me on the sun porch overlooking the lake, he told me, with tears in his eyes: 'Louwtjie, I am truly and deeply sorry for the terrible things I wrote about you in *One Life*, but it was beyond my control.'
>
> I replied: 'Yes Bill, there are many things that were distorted. It hurt me deeply.' Bill was genuinely upset and became emotional again. He asked me to forgive him and told me: 'I discovered only lately that Chris did not make you happy and I realise now that your life with him must have been hell at times.'

According to a biographer of Barnard, Chris Logan, Bill Pepper evidently denied that the book was rewritten or that he had anything for which to apologise to Louwtjie.

# 18

# Keeping Up With the Pack: Subsequent Heart Transplants in Cape Town

After the first rush to 'join the club', the number of heart transplants carried out each year declined to a handful. Fulton Gillespie, a British journalist, reported that, within a year of Barnard's first transplant, '100 heart grafts were carried out by sixty-four different teams of surgeons.'

However, in the late 1960s, many of the patients with heart transplants around the world started dying, which obviously generated bad publicity for the operation. Most of the surgical teams gave up their programs just as quickly as they had jumped in originally. For example, Denton Cooley carried out twenty transplants between 3 May 1968 and 29 September 1969, but soon after, he abandoned his programme and put a moratorium on further transplants when only two of the previous nineteen patients remained alive.

Marius Barnard recollected that, within two-and-a-half years after the first heart transplant, all but twenty-one of 150 transplant patients worldwide had died. 'The number of transplants dropped to forty-seven in 1969 ... In 1971 only seventeen transplants were performed worldwide.' However, this did not detract from the dramatic result that was obtained in a few patients, who were saved from a miserable early death.

Nevertheless, heart transplantation became established during the decade after 1967, but only on a limited scale and only through the persistent efforts of four groups: two in the USA and one each in France and South Africa. These four persistent groups were the real pioneers of clinical heart transplantation and deserve our great respect and thanks. During the 1970s, the University of Cape Town program, together with those at Stanford (Shumway), the Medical College of Virginia (Lower), and Hôpital La Pitie in Paris (Cabrol) were the only centres performing heart transplantation continuously, and thus the only centres where experience was being gained. It is interesting to note that three of the men who led these groups (Chris, Shumway, and Cabrol) were trainees of Walt Lillehei, and the fourth (Lower) was a trainee of a Lillehei trainee (Shumway).

The results were only modest and, at times, dismal, with only about 40–50 per cent of patients surviving the first year after the transplant. However, several innovations and modifications to surgical techniques, management of the potential donor and of the patient, and immunosuppressive therapy slowly brought about an improvement in outcomes (Chapter 21). The slowly improving results eventually consolidated heart transplantation as a realistic treatment for patients with terminal heart failure.

Of the four groups that 'carried the banner' of heart transplantation during these relatively bleak years, it was the Stanford group that was the most active. After Chris's initial successes and Shumway's disappointing results, Shumway was to become not only the leading figure in the experimental development of heart transplantation but, in the formative years of heart transplantation in patients, his group led the way forward, generally just a little bit ahead of the other three groups.

## Subsequent Heart Transplants in Cape Town

Chris's team performed only eleven heart transplants between 1967 and 1973. There was one year when it did not do a single transplant.

'I never had any idea of stopping,' Chris told me. 'The reason we only did a few is because no patients were referred to us. It's funny, but the cardiologists started not referring patients. The neurologists were the worst; they didn't want to refer donors. At first, they were all on the bandwagon to get better facilities, better post-operative care units, because they were going to be involved in cardiac transplants. But as soon as they got all this stuff, they just fell out.'

According to Chris, on one occasion, when a member of the heart team asked one of the GSH neurosurgeons to sign a form confirming that a potential donor was brain-dead, the neurosurgeon 'stormed out of the hospital, determined to be as uncooperative as possible,' warning that, 'if you come to my house and disturb me, I'll put my dogs on you!' This story was confirmed to me by one of the junior surgeons in Chris's team at the time. However, the Province (of the Western Cape, the regional government) and the University 'went out of their way to facilitate matters and to get us better facilities.'

In one of the articles Chris later wrote for the *Cape Times* ('Dying by Inches'), he commented on the lack of donor hearts his group was experiencing.

In two months the Groote Schuur heart team lost three out of six heart transplant candidates or 50 per cent of such patients who had come to us in the belief that we could help them. They died not because there were no donors but because red tape has so ensnarled the process of obtaining donor hearts that by the time all requirements were met the organs were unusable.

Worse still, the regulations force qualified medical specialists to act as touts, putting through endless phone calls to police to trace relatives, pleading with district surgeons or state pathologists who seem less concerned with dying heart patients than with adhering to the rules, and, at last, explaining to relatives of the donor why the heart is needed.

There were technical problems and mishaps from time to time that had to be overcome. Terry O'Donovan remembered one incident.

The heart-lung machine pump broke down in the middle of the operation and, as an emergency, the arterial line pump had to be turned by hand. I rushed across to Red Cross Children's Hospital to get a lead from the machine there … I returned with the lead and the pump was reconnected and functioned satisfactorily for the rest of the case.

The early results in Cape Town, although poor by today's standards, were exceptional when one considers the primitive nature of the immunosuppressive therapy available at the time (basically azathioprine, corticosteroids, and anti-lymphocyte serum), and the team's lack of experience in diagnosing and treating rejection episodes. For example, the first four patients survived an average of more than 200 days, which was markedly in excess of those at any other centre worldwide. Dr Blaiberg and the third patient, Pieter Smith, both lived for more than eighteen months. Even more remarkable than the results in the first four patients, Chris's fifth and sixth patients lived for more than twelve and twenty-three years, respectively.

The fifth patient, Dorothy Fisher, whom I personally came to know well, was a coloured woman who, if I remember correctly (the records being no longer available) received a heart from a white donor, demonstrating Chris's—and indeed, to some extent, Groote Schuur Hospital and the University of Cape Town's—independence from the government's party line on apartheid. She became something of a celebrity in Cape Town and led a very full and active life for almost thirteen years.

The sixth patient, Dirk Van Zyl, was remarkable in that his ischemic (coronary artery) heart disease was so bad that he had a cardiac arrest when he was being anaesthetised for the transplant operation. While being given external cardiac massage (attempted heart resuscitation by compression of his chest), he was urgently connected to the heart-lung machine and the transplant was performed, even though it was uncertain whether his cardiac arrest had resulted in brain damage.

He made an uneventful recovery from the transplant operation, and returned to work after three months. Since I saw him on his visits to the hospital for several years in the 1980s, I can personally vouch that he did not miss a day's work through illness for the next fifteen years, at which time he retired. Mr Van Zyl never received a new and improved immunosuppressive drug, cyclosporine, which was introduced by Roy Calne in the late 1970s (Chapter 21) and became available in South Africa in the mid-1980s. As he was doing so well, he was maintained only on the original azathioprine and prednisone (a steroid) therapy.

Following Mr Van Zyl's retirement, his underlying vascular disease began to trouble him, that is his atherosclerotic disease (that had been the cause of the coronary artery disease that resulted in his heart failure) began to narrow the blood vessels in his legs so that not enough blood reached the muscles and skin. He required vascular reconstructive surgery to both legs, which was only temporarily successful, and eventually, he had to undergo amputation of both legs. He died in his twenty-fourth post-heart-transplant year from a stroke (injury to his brain from atherosclerotic disease in the blood vessels supplying the brain).

At autopsy, although he had severe graft atherosclerosis (narrowing of the arteries in the transplanted heart, like Dr Blaiberg), the disease in his native vessels in the rest of his body was, if anything, more advanced than that in his heart. His transplanted heart had thus outlived the natural progression of his underlying atherosclerotic disease that had been the cause of his original native heart failure and which continued to affect arteries throughout his body and ultimately cause his death.

Chris's quite phenomenal initial results, unmatched by any other group, could be considered beginner's luck, but are more likely due to an innate judgment that certain physicians and surgeons have to know what is the right approach to follow. In addition to considerable intelligence and an ability for extremely hard work (by him and, importantly, his entire team), Chris had this enigmatic judgment to a considerable degree, as vouched by his one-time surgical colleague, Bob Frater (Chapter 6).

During this same period when Chris had carried out only six transplants, Cooley had performed twenty-one and Shumway a remarkable forty-three. Although Cooley discontinued his programme for a number of years, Shumway's group was steadily amassing valuable experience that was to keep them in the forefront of this new medical field.

The results of Chris's next four transplants were distinctly less successful, and I suggest this might possibly be related to the distractions provided by his frequent travels so that he no longer spent so much time at his patient's bedside. For some years, Chris always happened to be in Cape Town when a suitable donor heart became available, but for the eighth transplant, he was away and Marius carried out the operation.

In 1971, Chris attempted to transplant the heart and both lungs into a patient, Adrian Herbert. This was the third such procedure in the world, following previous attempts by Denton Cooley (1968) and Walt Lillehei (1969). The patient survived only twenty-three days, but this was the longest survival at that time. The patient's post-transplant progress was complicated by an air leak from the bronchial tubes of the lungs, and pneumonia. Air leaks were related to inadequate healing of the recipient and donor bronchi or trachea (airways) due to the detrimental effect of one of the immunosuppressive drugs, the steroid cortisone. Mr Herbert remained the longest survivor of a heart-lung transplant until the discovery of cyclosporine, which made it possible to reduce the dose of cortisone (Chapter 21).

Due to the persistence of these four groups, heart transplantation slowly became established, but for almost a decade, it could realistically be offered at only this handful of centres worldwide, where the necessary expertise and experience had been developed. Although hanging on by its fingertips, heart transplantation was not fully established until cyclosporine was introduced by Roy Calne in the late 1970s.

## Obtaining Donor Organs

Just as the kidney transplant surgeons had been struggling to obtain suitable kidneys from deceased donors for the past couple of decades, so the heart surgeons had difficulty obtaining suitable hearts. Public education of the need increased and, of course, gained welcome publicity from the initial dozens of heart transplants that were performed between 1968 and 1970. However, the subsequent deaths of many of these patients reduced the public's enthusiasm to consider donation. Various advertising campaigns were initiated, and many 'catchy' phrases were used to draw attention to the need. One of these was 'Don't take your organs to heaven; heaven knows we need them here.'

At first, a donor heart was usually directed to the sickest patient, the one closest to death. The families of some patients made special efforts to make the public aware of their need and possibly 'attract' a donor organ more rapidly. Occasionally, this took an unusual approach. In the relatively early days, one leading physician told me of a patient referred to him who needed a heart transplant. The patient was evidently a well-known senior member of the Chicago Mafia. When his name was added to the waiting list, it was explained to him and his entourage that the surgical team would have to wait until a suitable donor heart became available. How long this would take was uncertain; the team, of course, had no control over when a potential donor might be referred.

The Mafia boss and his henchmen listened carefully. Not many days later, my colleague was woken in the middle of the night by a telephone call from a man in the Mafia boss's hometown of Chicago, who, in a gruff and vaguely threatening voice, said, 'Doctor, we have a donor.' Rather shaken, my colleague had to explain that this was not how the system worked; donor referrals had to go through the official channels.

This anecdote reminded me of an experience of my own. When I was with Chris in Oklahoma City, I flew one night to remove a heart from a donor in Chicago, which I was to take back to Oklahoma for transplantation into one of our patients. When examining the brain-dead donor (a well-built young man) before taking him to the operating room to excise his heart, I was struck by the fact that he had a bullet hole right in the middle of his forehead just above his eyes. The siting of the hole was so accurately placed that the bullet must surely have been shot at very close range. I commented on this to the attending nurse, who told me that the young man had been caught on a previous occasion by his girlfriend in a compromising position with another woman. On that occasion, the girlfriend had warned him that, if she ever caught him again under these circumstances, she would kill him, and she did.

There are other remarkable stories regarding donors. For example, I have read of one man in Britain who was on the waiting list for a heart transplant when his teenage daughter was tragically killed, and her heart was transplanted into him.

## Routine Cardiac Surgery

Despite the restrictions and demands his traveling made on him, it should not be assumed that Chris did not continue to work hard (often very hard) when he was in Cape Town. For several years, he continued to run a very busy cardiac surgical service and he personally carried out complex and demanding operations on a regular basis, although less frequently than earlier in his career.

Indeed, Chris's very high profile attracted patients, particularly children, from throughout the world for open heart operations, especially from Italy, Greece, Mauritius, and parts of Africa. Chris and, particularly, Marius were also referred patients from Romania, where heart surgery was very limited at that time. Perhaps surprisingly, occasional patients even came from countries in which heart surgery was already as well developed as in South Africa, such as Australia and the USA.

Journalist Bob Molloy wrote, 'Those kids [Chris's patients] come from everywhere—from poor Black Africa, from the rich West and even from the Eastern bloc where the Barnard name had penetrated far behind the Iron Curtain. Of all creeds and colours, each received the most advanced medical treatment possible at a cost tailored to the parents' pocket—in many cases, *gratis*.'

Many of these patients had been declined an operation in their own countries, usually on the grounds that their heart condition was 'inoperable'. If there was no alternative therapy available, however, Chris was reluctant to deny anybody the chance of a better quality of life, even if the risks of the operation were high. Molloy wrote:

> Privately, I wondered why a successful surgeon with the world at his feet should accept patients who had been turned down elsewhere by equally competent surgeons. Surgeons perhaps who didn't want their record spoiled by no-hopers. It was a facet of Barnard of which I was to see more—a man who quite frankly didn't give a damn for the conventions, whether medical, social or political. A doctor who cared for his patients with an almost naïve honesty ... He demanded, and got, high standards from his heart team—anything less than perfection was regarded as inept.

## Barnard as a Doctor

The following passages explore how Chris was viewed by his juniors and colleagues during this period.

Patrick (Pat) Commerford, who was later to become professor and head of cardiology at GSH, worked in Professor Barnard's department as a very junior doctor, and interacted with him throughout his career as a cardiologist. He therefore had the opportunity of assessing Chris from varying perspectives over a number of years. In 1992, he recorded for me his experiences and impressions of Chris.

> Chris Barnard, because of his immense popularity and achievements, became something of a hero to many medical students. Strangely, however, rotation through his department during internship was not popular and a lot of maneuvering went on among the interns to avoid spending part of the surgical time in cardiac surgery. I soon learned why

when I ended up spending two months of my internship as Professor Barnard's intern in cardiac surgery. He proved to be a hard task master and made an intern's life miserable. At the time, his demands and objections seemed petty and irrelevant. In retrospect, however, it is clear that his absolute clinical honesty and requirements for the accurate determination and recording of the patient's course were what provided the excellent results obtained by his unit.

The times of his appearance in the ward were unpredictable. He always attended scheduled ward rounds but was as likely to appear at 11 p.m. after a social event, dressed in a dinner jacket [tuxedo]. The standards expected of staff at such unscheduled appearances were the same as he demanded at formal ward rounds. Interns, registrars or nurses who were not completely familiar with the most recent details of their patient's clinical course, or who had failed to document a recent event, were treated to a humiliating tongue-lashing which was usually well-earned and served to stimulate improved attention to detail in the future.

He worked hard and expected that others should work at least as hard. All junior staff were expected to be available as necessary for emergencies. His attitude was uncompromising and he clearly believed that medicine [or cardiac surgery] was best learned by constant exposure to patients and their problems. After some six weeks I timidly asked if I could leave Cape Town for a weekend during which I had no scheduled clinical duties. His response, 'You may as well go because you do nothing anyway,' seemed unjust, unfair and was, I hope, untrue. Irritated by what I thought was an irrational approach, I did go away and returned to find I had missed the opportunity of witnessing and possibly assisting at some exciting surgery.

Some years later as a registrar in cardiology I was privileged to train under Professor Wally Beck [who had succeeded Professor Schrire as head of cardiology]. The highlight of the week was the Saturday morning conference at which the clinical details and results of cardiac catheterization and angiography of each patient scheduled to undergo surgery in the coming week were presented to a joint meeting of cardiac surgeons and cardiologists. Barnard and Beck clearly respected each other's knowledge and abilities but did not always agree on the particulars of patient management. Discussions were often heated, but always open and fair.

The meeting ended with a recounting of the results of the previous week's surgery. Surgical failures were reported as openly and as honestly as the successes, with a critical re-examination of the pre-operative data and an honest open-minded ability to admit mistakes and determine their cause to ensure they were not repeated. All lucky enough to be involved in those meetings learned an enormous amount and remember them with pleasure.

Later still, as a consultant [member of the faculty] it was a delight to refer patients to Chris Barnard for surgery. He was always prepared to discuss difficult issues with patients and relatives and advise them personally of his recommendations. An endearing quality was his inability to remember names and thus, when publicly complaining about a cardiologist's diagnostic error, he was quite likely to blame the wrong member of the department.

Not only did Chris continue to work hard, but he also continued to innovate new approaches when this became necessary.

# 19

# Another Innovation:
# The Piggyback Heart Transplant

The heart transplant programme at Groote Schuur Hospital progressed steadily, but relatively slowly, at least in part due to the difficulty in obtaining donor hearts. After performing only eleven orthotopic heart transplants (in which the patient's native heart is replaced by the donor heart) between 1967 and 1973, Chris decided to give up this approach after experiencing a tragic failure because a donor heart did not function after implantation.

He performed a heart transplant on a man, Martin Franzot, who had been very close to his eldest son, André, who had virtually lived with him and his wife when he was at school in Pretoria. In some respects, the man was a surrogate or 'adopted' father for André, in the relative absence of his true father, Chris. Tragically, immediately after the transplant, the donor heart failed to beat satisfactorily, which was not that unusual in those early days, and the patient died on the operating table. When Chris came out of the operating room to break this sad news to André, the young man replied, 'Then why didn't you put back his old heart? At least that had kept him alive.'

This struck Chris as a reasonable approach. If the patient's own heart had been left in place, and the transplant inserted as an auxiliary pump, failure of the donor heart may not have resulted in the patient's demise. Furthermore, with the support of the patient's native heart, perhaps the donor heart would have been given time to recover its function. Why a heart that had been beating well in the donor before being excised and transplanted might not beat strongly in the recipient will be discussed in Chapter 21.

Chris set a young Belgian surgeon, Jacques Losman (Figure 19.i), a junior faculty member of his team, to develop a surgical technique by which the donor heart could be inserted as an auxiliary (or additional) pump—the 'piggyback' heart transplant, as it became popularly known—where the second heart is placed in the chest and the two hearts have the opportunity of working in parallel. The technique is officially known as heterotopic heart transplantation, heterotopic signifying that the donor heart is not in the usual position of the heart in the chest.

This was not a new concept: the Russian, Vladimir Demikhov, who had performed the controversial head transplant in a dog that had fired Chris's interest, had developed several such surgical techniques in the experimental laboratory previously. However, the design of Losman and Barnard's surgical procedure was original and efficient. It had at that time certain advantages (and some disadvantages) over orthotopic transplantation, in which the patient's own heart is removed and replaced by the donor heart.

Using Chris's suggestions, Losman developed two techniques in the laboratory, in one of which the donor heart assisted only the left pumping chamber (left ventricle) and another in which assistance to both pumping chambers was provided (Figures 19.ii and 19.iii). The first operation in a patient, Ivor Taylor, was performed on 25 November 1974. In the first two patients, the first technique was found less than satisfactory (even though one of the two patients lived for more than ten years), and so the second technique was used in all subsequent patients. As with the original heart transplant program, the second patient did much better than the first.

Pittie Rautenbach remembered:

On 31 December 1974, we were summoned for a transplant on a Mr Leonard Goss [the second 'piggyback' heart transplant patient]. Of course, having to work that particular night was not our idea of celebrating a New Year's Eve. But afterwards Professor Barnard, who was his usual disciplined self while operating [I am not sure whether Pittie was being sarcastic here], opened champagne, and we all toasted 1975 together. At times like that early morning of 1975 he was relaxed and happy—all the stress and strain of the past operation behind him, and just a member of his team.

As with orthotopic heart transplantation, Chris's early results were encouraging, again demonstrating that his team's judgment in selecting patients and in managing the post-operative complications were good. Two of the first five patients survived more than ten years, and a third for more than eight years, all of whom I had the privilege of caring for as outpatients during my time in Cape Town. Nevertheless, overall one-year survival remained at approximately 50 per cent and five-year survival approximately 20 per cent.

No one can claim that these results were perfect, but they compared favourably with the results for the transplantation of many other organs, and they were certainly as good as the results obtained when some patients with other life-threatening diseases, such as cancer of the stomach or lung, were operated on in those days in a desperate attempt to prolong their lives.

Apart from enabling the patient's native heart to help out if the donor heart took a day or so to recover good function after the transplant, the main advantage of piggyback heart transplantation in the 1970s, when it was introduced, was the fact that if the donor heart suffered from severe rejection (damage by the patient's immune system) as frequently occurred in those days, this was not necessarily fatal. The patient might remain alive supported (at least in part) by his own native heart, even if it was beating relatively feebly. This allowed time for either the rejection in the donor heart to be reversed by increased drug therapy or, if that failed, to obtain a second donor heart and carry out retransplantation, thus giving the patient a second chance.

One memorable young man, Jack Smith, was such a patient. He had an admirable independence and wish to enjoy his new life to the full, but sometimes he took what can only be described as reckless risks with his own health. He was not the most compliant of patients with regard to taking his immunosuppressive medication or in attending the follow-up outpatient clinic. On one such occasion (before I joined the team), when he had not been seen in the clinic for some time as he had been traveling, he actually came to the hospital with features of severe heart failure. Urgent investigations demonstrated that the donor heart was in ventricular fibrillation (because of a serious rhythm disturbance it was not pumping out any blood) but he was being kept alive, just, by his very diseased and barely beating native heart. His donor heart was undergoing a severe rejection crisis. Intense immunosuppressive therapy (to reverse the rejection) and electrical defibrillation (to start the donor heart beating regularly again) eventually rendered him well enough to leave hospital and resume his eventful life—Lazarus, if ever there was one. He lived for nearly ten years with his two hearts, but unfortunately, he stopped taking his anti-rejection medication regularly again and, on this occasion, sadly died.

One other potential advantage of piggyback heart transplantation was that, in patients with an inflammatory disease of the heart (known as acute myocarditis, possibly due to a viral infection), the support given by the transplant might enable the myocarditis to resolve and the patient's own heart to recover. Indeed, this occurred in one patient, making it possible to remove the transplanted heart when it developed a moderately severe rejection episode. The patient was, therefore, not committed to a lifetime on immunosuppressive therapy, with its potential complications.

Another small but significant advantage was that a pulse trace, taken over the carotid artery in the neck, for example, could provide information on the contractions of both the recipient and donor left ventricles. A change in the ratio of the strength of these two pulses, with the donor pulse declining in relation to the recipient pulse, suggested that rejection was occurring. Increased immunosuppressive therapy could then be administered. This is obviously not possible after orthotopic heart transplantation where there is, of course, only a single pulse. Later, in cases of doubt, an endomyocardial biopsy could be carried out in order to examine a small sample of heart muscle under the microscope, but this was not available during Chris's first series of heart transplants (Chapter 21).

In one early patient, his own very diseased heart permanently ceased beating, but he remained alive because of his transplant. Chris later commented that he had 'had the dubious honour to be the first man to drive his car without his own heart beating inside his chest'. When the native heart stopped beating, there was a risk that, despite anticoagulant therapy, clots of blood would form in it and break off and lodge in the brain causing a stroke. This was an indication to surgically remove the dead heart.

## Ingenious Variations

UCT pathologist, Alan Rose, provided me with further evidence of Chris's 'gift for original thinking and innovation', and illustrated this by the following incident.

One of the heterotopic [piggyback] heart transplant patients had developed a serious infection of an artificial valve prosthesis in his own heart, and this virulent organism was resistant to all the known antibiotics. The prognosis was particularly grim since the patient was receiving heavy immunosuppressive drug therapy to prevent rejection of the donor heart. The cardiologists' collective opinion was that the patient was doomed, but Chris Barnard immediately claimed that he could cure the patient. This remark was met with not unjustifiable skepticism, but grabbing hold of a piece of chalk, Barnard outlined an ingenious operation whereby he would excise the infected valve together with one entire wall of the heart and close off the area using a leaflet of another valve and a patch. [The patient would therefore be kept alive by part of his own heart and part of the donor heart—a very unusual 'hybrid' situation not seen before or since. He now had one and a half hearts.]

The operation was a resounding success. The patient, who subsequently worked as a salesman for almost ten years, probably never realised how close a shave he had had with death.

It was at the beginning of 1980 that I joined Barnard's team, having the privilege of working with him at Groote Schuur Hospital for four years until his retirement at the end of 1983, and subsequently (in 1987–1988) in Oklahoma City. During this time and in the few years that followed, it became clear to my excellent surgical colleague, Dimitri Novitzky, and me, together with our new colleague, Bruno Reichart, who took over from Barnard on his retirement, that, if irreversible rejection and failure of the donor heart developed, removal and replacement of the donor piggyback heart was not only technically difficult, but could be associated with significant complications. The heart might be tightly adherent (stuck) to the right lung, and removal might be associated with considerable bleeding. At the retransplant operation, therefore, it was preferable to replace the patient's native heart by performing an orthotopic transplant, leaving the original donor heart in place (Figure 19.iv), even if it were no longer functioning. This prevented the necessity of dissecting the donor heart from the right lung.

Led by Dimitri, we operated on two fourteen-year-old boys, both of whom had initially received piggyback transplants. Like Dr Blaiberg, both boys had slowly developed chronic rejection (graft atherosclerosis) in the donor heart, leading to its failure.

Both boys underwent a second (orthotopic) heart transplant, and were therefore the first patients in the world to have two donor hearts in their chest at the same time. The first donor heart was in the piggyback position and the second, that had replaced the patient's own heart, was in the normal (orthotopic) position. At the time of writing this book, the first of these two boys, whose original piggyback transplant was performed by Marius Barnard, remains alive and well more than thirty-five years after his first heart transplant. To my knowledge, he is currently the longest-surviving heart transplant recipient in the world. Now married with children, the efforts made by the Groote Schuur team in the early 1980s and subsequently have proved well worthwhile.

In the other boy, the second transplant also eventually failed from chronic rejection and he underwent a third graft, again in the orthotopic site, and thus became one of the few humans to have had four hearts in his lifetime: his own, a piggyback transplant, and two orthotopic transplants. Sadly, he proved a persistent 'rejector' and eventually died from graft failure.

## Cross-Species (Xeno) Piggyback Heart Transplantation

In the late 1970s, Barnard and Losman and their colleague, Alan Wolpowitz, used this piggyback technique to take yet another step into an area that was largely unknown. They transplanted, first, a baboon heart into a woman, and, second, a chimpanzee heart into a man in desperate attempts to keep them alive. Both patients had undergone conventional heart surgery, but, at the end of the operation, neither could be weaned off the heart-lung machine. This meant they would die unless they could receive a heart transplant. As no human donor heart, nor any form of mechanical heart, was available at that moment, both patients would have died had Chris and his colleagues not attempted to keep them alive by implanting an animal heart.

It was already known from experimental and clinical studies reported by other groups that xenografts—organs transplanted between one species and another, such as a chimpanzee heart into a human—elicited a more vigorous rejection response than when the organ is from the same species as the recipient (for example, human-to-human). Chris and his colleagues, therefore, realised that (even with intensive immunosuppressive treatment) they could not keep their patients alive for very long with an animal heart while they waited for a human donor heart to become available.

The animal heart was placed heterotopically, that is, as an auxiliary heart alongside the patient's own heart, so that both hearts could contribute towards keeping the patient alive. The hope was that the donor animal heart would help support the circulation until the patient's own heart recovered sufficiently to manage alone; if this occurred, the animal heart could then have been removed. Alternatively, if a heart from a deceased human became available, the animal heart could be removed and replaced by the human donor heart.

On the first occasion, a baboon heart was transplanted, but this was too small to support the circulation sufficiently, the patient dying some six hours after transplantation. In the second patient, the chimpanzee heart successfully maintained life until irreversible rejection occurred four days later, the recipient's native heart having failed to recover during this period and no human donor heart having become available.

Baboons were readily available in South Africa, being caught by farmers when they threatened to destroy their crops or by municipal authorities when they behaved aggressively and dangerously towards humans, usually when they were scavenging for food. Chimpanzees, however, are not native to South Africa. It is uncertain how Chris obtained the chimpanzees, as in various publications he mentions that he 'bought them', or they were 'a gift' from a Dutch breeding centre or from the South African Chamber of Mines, but Dene Friedmann clearly remembers them being a gift from a primate breeding colony in the Netherlands. According to Marius, 'the female chimpanzee went into total mourning for her mate, on which we had experimented. She cried for him and stopped eating. Her grief was intense, real and uncannily human-like. She was soon given away to a zoo.' Dene Friedmann confirmed that this experience upset the entire team, Chris included.

The chimpanzee heart transplant resulted in a fierce argument between Chris and Marius, who opposed it completely and refused to have anything to do with the procedure. Chris told me that he abandoned further attempts at xenotransplantation (cross-species transplantation) since, in his own words, 'I became too attached to the chimpanzees.' However, these two surgical experiments demonstrate both Chris's ingenuity and boldness in his attempts to save the lives of his patients.

Others on Chris's staff also did not much care for these transplants. Senior operating room nurse, Pittie Rautenbach, remembered:

When the sedated animal [a baboon on this occasion] was brought in, a strange feeling came over me—very hard to describe. Was this the beginning of a new era of animal sacrifice in order to save the lives of humans? It was a glimpse into a scientific future I did not think I was going to like. That same year I assisted when Professor Barnard transplanted a chimp heart.

Soon after, Chris received a letter from a former colleague who now lived in New Zealand. He informed Chris of a book, *Slaughter of the Innocents*, that had been published in New Zealand, and which gained considerable publicity both in that country and in the UK and the USA. In it, the author made dubious claims about Chris, including that he had removed the heart from a chimpanzee that had not been anaesthetised. Chimps are very strong and quite aggressive, even vicious, and so this would clearly not have been possible even if somebody was inhumane enough to consider doing this. On legal advice, Chris instituted legal proceedings against the media in New Zealand and the UK, and was awarded compensation by the courts. Chris's American lawyers advised him not to instigate proceedings against the author in the US on the grounds that Chris was a public figure and it was therefore very unlikely that any claim he made would be successful. Chris was not impressed that, in the 'land of the free', people could make untruthful claims about you with impunity.

Prescott Madlingozi, an extremely able laboratory technician who ran the heart-lung machine for the animal experiments in the laboratory, had another reason to complain about these transplants.

I was very upset with the professor at one stage after he had performed double heart transplants in two patients using baboon and chimpanzee hearts. The professor was being sued by someone for some reason and he needed support from his laboratory staff to say that all the research had been done appropriately ... I therefore drew up a letter that all the laboratory staff signed and handed it to Professor Barnard's attorney. The outcome of the case was in Professor Barnard's favour, but he never ever thanked anyone for this letter or the work that had been done. Later when we saw him again after the trial, there was nothing said and life just continued as normal.

Even before Barnard's attempts to support patients with baboon or chimpanzee hearts in 1977 (and excluding James Hardy's attempt in 1964), two dramatic attempts had been made to keep patients alive with animal hearts.

Whereas Donald Ross in London and Denton Cooley had carried out their first human heart transplants on the same day in 1968, they also both made rather rash attempts to keep patients alive by animal hearts. In Ross's case, he chose a heart from a pig, whereas Cooley selected a sheep. Although I spoke to both of them about these attempts, I failed to ask them their reasons for their choices of animal donor.

In 1968, Ross found himself in the unenviable position of having two patients in different operating rooms at the National Heart Hospital whom he could not wean from their heart-lung machines after routine heart surgery (just as Chris faced in 1977). Unfortunately, this was not that uncommon in those relatively early days of open heart surgery. Just as Chris later tried, Ross attempted to support the first patient by stitching in a pig heart as an auxiliary (heterotopic) heart—the first really true 'piggyback' heart transplant. He devised his own rather cumbersome technique. The pig heart was rejected within minutes (what we term hyperacute rejection).

In the second patient, therefore, Ross tested a second pig heart simply by attaching it to the heart-lung machine and perfusing it with the patient's blood. If it survived for more than a few minutes, he would suture it into the patient as an auxiliary heart. In the event, it was also hyperacutely rejected. Sadly, both patients died.

Like Ross, Cooley had become caught up in the frenzy to perform heart transplants in the late 1960s. On one occasion (also in 1968), when a human donor heart was unavailable, he transplanted a sheep heart that, like Ross's pig hearts, was rejected within minutes.

None of these three attempts was in any way 'scientific'. Particularly with what we know now from experimental cross-species organ transplantation (Appendix I), there was not even a glimmer of hope of success. Even from experimental studies carried out in the mid-1960s, it was clear that these attempts would be doomed to failure. Both Ross and Cooley later admitted to me that they felt some embarrassment over these efforts, even though they clearly had the patients' well-being in mind. Yet as Shakespeare wrote in *Hamlet*, 'Diseases desperate grown, by desperate appliance are relieved, or not at all.'

## Further Progress

The piggyback heart transplant—using human donor hearts—played a major role in the Cape Town programme for ten years. In total, excluding the two nonhuman primate transplants, forty-nine consecutive piggyback heart transplants were performed between 1974 and 1983 with moderately good results for that era. Nearly all were carried out with immunosuppressive therapy consisting of the basic drugs that had been introduced into kidney transplantation in the 1960s: azathioprine, corticosteroids, and anti-lymphocyte globulin.

The operation of piggyback heart transplantation was largely phased out in Cape Town following several advances that were introduced in the 1970s or early 1980s, which diminished its advantages. In particular, improvements in the diagnosis and prevention of rejection (thus reducing the need for the native heart to provide support during a rejection crisis) and in the management of deceased potential donors (thus reducing the risk of inadequate function of the heart immediately after the transplant) led to its demise. These advances are discussed in a subsequent chapter.

The use of a piggyback human or animal heart transplant in a patient whose own heart does not recover good function after open heart surgery, to allow a period of circulatory support while awaiting recovery of the heart, has now been supplanted in the current era of heart surgery by the use of mechanical devices, such as ventricular assist devices or total artificial hearts (discussed in Appendix I).

The operation of piggyback heart transplantation never caught on in a major way in most other heart transplant centres, possibly in part because the surgical technique is more complex than orthotopic heart transplantation. For some years, it continued to play an occasional role in some major cardiac transplant programs, as there are certain patients who, for various reasons, might not survive if their own heart is removed. Today, however, it is rarely carried out. Its small role in the development of heart transplantation has passed, but I believe it played a valuable role in Cape Town in those early years.

# 20

# Second Wife, Second Life

Not deterred by his recent matrimonial problems, Chris soon found a second wife, on this occasion choosing a beautiful nineteen-year-old, Barbara Zoellner (Figure 20.i) who, furthermore, was the daughter of a multimillionaire industrialist, one of the wealthiest men in South Africa. His marriage to an immensely wealthy girl, twenty-nine years his junior, only added fuel to the media fire. They became engaged only three months after his divorce from Louwtjie had become finalised.

Barbara's parents—father Fred, who initially was against the marriage, and mother Ursula (Ulli), who was greatly in favour of the marriage and encouraged it enthusiastically—were independently wealthy and cultured people. Their marriage, however, had been turbulent for years, in part due to Fred's infidelities. Barbara may have been looking for stability and even security in her marriage, but, if so, though she loved Chris very much, she certainly selected the wrong husband. His frequent travels and flirtations did not lend themselves to stability.

Denton Cooley, as always, saw the funny side of the situation. Chris announced to Cooley's wife, Louise, that he, then nearing the age of fifty, was going to marry Barbara, a nineteen-year-old girl, and would probably bring her to Houston on their wedding trip. Louise immediately answered that Chris and his wife would be very welcome and that she and Denton would invite some of their children's friends over to meet Barbara.

Barbara was a beautiful woman: tall, slim (perhaps too thin) and elegant, with dark hair and doe-eyes, always immaculately dressed, at least in public (Figure 20.ii). Deirdre Barnard remembers her first sight of Barbara. 'What I saw was a tall beautiful girl more or less my own age in a very plain dress, all pinks and purples, who looked as if she'd walked straight off the cover of *Vogue*. I don't think I fully realised until then that when my father left Zeekoevlei he didn't just move to another place;

he moved into an entirely different world.' Perhaps adding to Barbara's appeal was what Deirdre described as her 'slightly aloof manner and her lovely smile that lit up her face.'

In Deirdre's opinion, Barbara was to prove to be a good wife, a wonderful mother and one of the most modest people you could ever hope to meet. It is perhaps remarkable that Deirdre did not hold some bitterness towards Barbara because she had learnt of her father's engagement to Barbara from a newspaper placard, just as she had heard of her parents' divorce. She recollected that 'at that moment, being so peripheral seemed to make me count for very little indeed, and it hurt.'

Chris, like Ronald Reagan, was in many ways the 'great communicator' to the public and to the medical profession, but perhaps not to members of his own family.

At first, Deirdre was shocked and appalled that her father was planning to marry a girl born in the same year as she had been, but soon accepted the situation. She was then torn between wanting to participate in her father's new 'glamorous' life, but not wanting to upset her mother. Louwtjie understood this need and was generous in encouraging Deirdre to see Chris whenever she wished, even after his marriage to Barbara. Deirdre therefore entered this new world. She wrote:

> Everything was wonderful the day we first had lunch at the Zoellners. They had invited a small party of people and we all sat outside and had drinks before lunch. There was gin and tonic and ice and lemon and everyone very polite to everyone else and I thought to myself that if I had never seen 'elegant' in my life before, I was surely seeing it now. Barbara was there, of course, looking tanned and beautiful with her lovely long hair hanging loose. She was absolutely glowing with happiness. Lunch was beautifully prepared and everything set out just so. All we needed was a photographer to come and take a picture for a lifestyle magazine. It was just so perfect they wouldn't even have needed to bring a stylist with them.

Deirdre clearly admired and interacted well with her new stepmother. Both were later to open separate boutiques in Cape Town. Deirdre reports that 'in those days Barbara was at her most beautiful and she had a wonderful glow that seemed to float around her. My father was very proud of her and although the dynamics of my life had changed, in a very short time she fitted into the broad scheme of things so naturally that it seemed to me she'd always been there.'

Deirdre gave an example of Barbara's dignity and charity. When Chris and Barbara were to be married, Barbara ordered a wedding cake but, unknown to her, the caterers put it on public display, presumably because it would be of public interest, but perhaps also because it would be good publicity for them. This upset Barbara very much. It was an affront to her sense of privacy on such a special occasion. She therefore auctioned off the cake for charity, and had another cake prepared for her wedding.

Her generosity of spirit was also exemplified by other acts of charity. For example, for three years, in 1984, 1985, and 1988, Barbara was on the South African *Sunday Times* 'Best Dressed' list of women. On one of these occasions, she won a prize of a trip overseas. She gave it to a young woman battling cancer. Those close to her knew this was 'a gesture that was both natural to and typical of her.'

Deirdre also pointed out that Barbara chose to give birth to her two sons at the Mowbray Maternity Hospital, which was a state hospital, and not in a private clinic, which she could easily afford (Figure 20.iii). She had married Chris, who worked within the state system of health care. Her attitude was that, if a state hospital was good enough for her husband, it was surely good enough for her.

## Weathering the Storms

Deirdre seemed to weather these emotional storms remarkably well, though she did need professional counseling for some time. She wrote:

> I went to a psychiatrist. I talked a lot and yes, I talked about my parents, the divorce and all those things that were written in the newspapers. I talked about all our private family business being hung out for everyone to see. As if someone had come into our house, rifled through all our most private things, picked on what they thought was the juiciest stuff and gone off, gleefully and triumphantly, carrying their loot with them.
>
> It is good to talk and it made a very pleasant change to have someone who listened and understood as the psychiatrist did, but talking and listening—getting a nice cleansing brainwash, if you like to put it that way—is not going to do the trick all by itself. Being angry isn't going to get you anywhere. You can't stay still and wallow in anger, no matter how tempting that may sometimes appear to be. You have to let it go. Easy to write down, not so easy to do, and yet it can be done and it's important that it should be done.

The more introverted André did not weather these storms so well. Although we do not have André's recollections to read and gain insight into his state of mind during these turbulent years, it would seem that he did not handle them as well as his sister. Just as he may have felt abandoned when sent to boarding school in Pretoria, he may have felt equally isolated when his father entered the new world of celebrity, in which he perhaps did not feel comfortable.

Chris again proved insensitive to his former wife's feelings. He married Barbara on St. Valentine's Day, one minute (12.01 a.m.) after Louwtjie's forty-fifth birthday (Friday, 13 February 1970), having sent her a telegram wishing her 'a happy birthday'. Louwtjie recalled, 'Each year when I celebrate my birthday, I will be reminded of his remarriage.'

In his defense, Chris pointed out that he purposely delayed the wedding by a minute so it would not coincide with Louwtjie's birthday; he thought it would be 'insensitive' to arrange the wedding for the thirteenth itself, but perhaps a date more distantly removed from the birthday would have been preferable and possible.

Adding to Louwtjie's sorrows was the unbelievable behaviour of some people who wrote anonymous letters to her or made anonymous phone calls condemning or cursing her at a time when she was emotionally at rock-bottom. Having struggled for months to re-adjust to her new situation in life, these accusations gave her an inferiority complex and she often gave way to self-pity. 'I began to consider myself a complete failure,' she later wrote. 'I felt as if I had not only failed Chris, but the world as well. It took me a long time to overcome this. I only succeeded because I called upon the strength of God to help me fight this battle.' Fortunately, for every nasty anonymous letter, she received ten inspiring ones in which people previously unknown to her expressed their empathy.

Only a handful of guests were invited to Chris's lavish wedding to Barbara, which took place privately at her father's palatial mansion in Johannesburg. As Barbara was a Roman Catholic, they were married in a civil ceremony by a local judge who was a family friend. Deirdre chose to attend, but André did not. Bill Pepper took a photograph of the newlyweds kissing, and it sold for $2,500, which was a great deal of money in South Africa in 1970.

The morning after their midnight wedding, Chris and Barbara left for Europe on honeymoon, with Bill Pepper tagging along. They were again greeted by literally thousands of well-wishers and inquisitors when they arrived at Rome airport; Chris could again not believe his eyes. While in Rome, Chris put aside a significant amount of time to examine children in need of heart surgery, many of whom he arranged to operate on later at GSH. They also met the fashion editors of *Harper's Bazaar* and *Vogue* magazines, who persuaded Barbara to do some modelling for them. When Barbara put on the elegant clothes, Chris thought 'she looked absolutely stunning and I was the proudest husband in the world to see her beautiful face on the front covers at news-stands all over the world.' Not only had he suffered a massive mid-life crisis but he had now gained himself a 'trophy wife'. He liked to joke that 'a man who married a beautiful woman and a good cook was a bigamist.' I do not know how strong Barbara's cooking skills were.

Chris's marriage to Barbara appears to have been a happy one for several years, providing him with two sons, Frederick and Christiaan, Jnr. Fortunately, Barbara received a substantial monthly allowance from her father, and so the couple was able to move into a bigger apartment in La Corniche in Clifton, a beachside suburb of Cape Town (Figure 20.iv), which Barbara's mother helped them furnish. The novelty of living in rooms with wall-to-wall carpeting and antique pieces of furniture was not lost on Chris. Later, Barbara's father bought them a house in the upmarket suburb of Constantia. In their extensive grounds, they built an aviary and began a collection of exotic birds native to South Africa. Perhaps surprisingly, Chris claimed he enjoyed growing his own vegetables in their garden—not the sort of activity one associates with a jet set celebrity—but I wonder how much of the 'yard work' he actually did himself.

The poor boy from Beaufort West was now living in a style he could never have imagined as a barefoot child. When overseas on his numerous visits abroad, sometimes accompanied by Barbara, his lifestyle was even more upscale. He stayed in some of the most luxurious hotels in the world, for example, the Savoy in London (Figure 20.v), the Athenee Palace in Paris, the Oberoi in Delhi, and the Pierre in New York, and was entertained by the very wealthy in their homes.

Deirdre described a typical scene.

He and Barbara were in Italy. They were staying with the Mondadoris, Giorgio and his wife Nara, members of the famous publishing family which had published his first book (*One Life*). He asked me if I would come to spend some time with them there. The house, when I eventually reached it, wasn't a house at all. It was more like a palace surrounded by gardens with cherry trees, immaculate lawns and a swimming pool. The Mondadori house was pretty much how you would expect such a house to be. You walked into it and it kind of swallowed you up. Barbara was used to such places and comfortable in them, but I wasn't.

# The Accident

At a time when Chris had been an outspoken critic of the government's apartheid policy, he and Barbara were hit by a car while crossing the road after leaving a restaurant in Cape Town. Both sustained significant injuries. Several vertebrae in Barbara's neck were fractured, but fortunately without injury to the spinal cord. She required hospitalization for several weeks. As the car had been parked, but, as soon as Chris and Barbara appeared, it left the kerb at high speed and did not stop after hitting them, there was the possibility that it was a planned event. Whether it was intended and, if so, whether it was an extremist right-wing reprisal for his criticisms of the government, remains uncertain. Marius 'stepped up to the plate' and played a major role in their care in hospital.

# The Final Rift with Marius

Steadily, Chris became distracted by his travels and by his increasing social activities and other interests. One of his junior colleagues at that time commented to me that, after Barnard's second marriage, he did not keep up with advances in surgery anymore. Throughout the 1970s, when he was away from Cape Town at frequent intervals, Chris was greatly helped by his brother and surgical colleague, Marius (Figure 20.vi), who maintained the routine day-to-day running of the department of cardiac surgery in his absence, which was an enormous help to Chris. Nevertheless, whenever Chris was in Cape Town, he was the driving force and wanted to remain the leader of the team.

I asked Chris how well he and Marius had collaborated professionally.

As well as brothers can. We didn't get on that well, but we were very close. When I was away, he kept that unit together. He took my place. He was a competent, dedicated surgeon who looked after his patients well. But working with Marius was in some ways a big problem for me because I didn't want to favour him because he was my brother. So, in fact, I did the reverse. I kept him back more because I didn't want to show the people I was favouring him. At the end, we didn't get on too well together because he wanted to take over the unit, and I didn't want that. I was wrong. I should have let him take over so the unit would have been in good shape. I was very upset that he had made the suggestion, but he was absolutely right. That's what I should have done. If I had allowed him to take over the clinical side, and I had just remained in administration, I think things would have gone very well.

Chris's statement that 'we didn't get on well together' may be something of an understatement. Marius's initial decision to accept the appointment offered by his brother had been influenced by the fact that no other position was open to him at GSH at that time (April 1967), but later, he clearly regretted accepting Chris's offer. Marius felt continued tension, irritation, and frustration working under Chris, and eventually could stand it no longer.

In his memoirs, Marius wrote:

My one year of cardiac research in the mid-sixties under Chris's supervision had resulted in many clashes, some of which had been terribly acrimonious. This had convinced me of two things: firstly, that I never wanted to be a cardiac surgeon, and, secondly, that I never again wanted to work in the same department as Chris. Yet here I was, working in his department once more. I have to admit that I owed the appointment to him, despite the fact that his difficult relationship with the head of surgery had probably been the source of [Professor] Louw's attitude towards me. I often wonder how the rest of my life might have panned out had Chris not felt some compassion for me. I have to acknowledge that he must also have had doubts about appointing me, knowing in his heart of hearts that I would be trouble for him. Our youth together had not been rich in brotherly love and our two years together in one room as medical students were based on, to say the least, a hostile truce.

Most of my responsibilities [in the department] were a challenge and enjoyable. Why, then, was I so miserable and anxious to leave? Chris's moods were unpleasant and he had the unfortunate habit of venting his spleen on innocent staff. He was most unreasonable at times, but was unaware of the hurt he caused. His demands on the time of his residents were also unreasonable and resulted in a hard-working but unhappy team.

... [Marius realised] someone now had to take over the responsibility of the cardiac unit when Chris was abroad. This, of course, required that it be a surgeon on the permanent staff. Rodney Hewitson and Terry O'Donovan, both senior to me, were in private practice and had only part-time appointments at Groote Schuur Hospital. They assisted with operations but had no post-operative duties. This left only me, so Chris asked me to assume his duties at both Groote Schuur Hospital and the Red Cross Memorial Children's Hospital.

But as my relationship with Chris deteriorated, I became more of a hindrance than a help to him and the discord between us became counter-productive to the unit. One of us had to go. Since Chris was the leader of the team, it wasn't going to be him, so I was slowly moved out of the program. Chris and I now enjoyed a no-greet, no-speak relationship, and my only relief from this unpleasantness was when Chris was overseas.

Marius and one of the other faculty surgeons tried to resolve the problem with Chris.

We told him that he could get all the honour as head of the unit and that he could travel as much as he wanted to. Furthermore, we would guarantee him that we would not only maintain the standard of work, but also increase the volume of operations. This was all we wanted. We had another condition, however, and I was blunt about it. I told Chris that he was now a hindrance, not a help, and that he should remove himself from running the unit. He could still get all the credit, but he should just get out of our way.

Thinking back, I must have been very naïve or just plain crazy to think that Chris would meekly accept my proposal. To his credit, he didn't rant or rave although, in retrospect, I have to admit that he had every justification to do so. Not surprisingly, he rejected the proposal in no uncertain terms and showed us the door.

The day was the final nail in my coffin at Groote Schuur Hospital. My dream of taking over from Chris in the future was blown out, like Elton John's well-known song 'Candle in the Wind'. My vision of building a world-class unit, one that would provide the paediatric cardiac surgery that I loved, and sufficient facilities and staff to operate on hundreds of patients from all over the world, particularly those from poor countries with no cardiac surgery facilities, was now shattered.

Looking back, I think I was unfair to Chris and that I could have tried to achieve my aims and objectives in a more tactful way. But the opportunity was lost forever and my dream never realised. It is now too late for tears, but I still regret his decision. It could have been so different. Instead, Chris fought back in a cool and calculated way to destroy me.

Chris sent the following written message to Marius:

As to your statement late in the day that I am jealous of you, I find this difficult to understand as you have excelled in the field of cardiac surgery only in projects that I have initiated. A claim I believe you cannot make of me … I am deeply distressed to inform you that I find your behaviour unacceptable and have put up with it long enough. I have therefore decided that from now on you will be treated as any other member of the staff and I will judge you solely on your merit.

This equated with demoting Marius who Chris no longer considered his deputy. However, as Marius records:

> My demotion during Chris's absences also had a ridiculous side. Joe [Nobrega, another of the staff surgeons] was most uncomfortable and ill at ease with this situation and, in practical terms, he allowed me to run the unit. During our Saturday meetings at the cardiac clinic, where we'd discuss cases we had operated on and select cases for the following week's list, things went on as if nothing had happened. Professor Wally Beck and his team still regarded me as the most senior cardiac surgeon and I was, therefore, still obliged to make all the final decisions. This situation didn't last long. With no admission from Chris about his ill-directed actions, he restored me to my previous position at Groote Schuur Hospital, but continued to work me out of the Red Cross [Children's Hospital].

The above description of Marius's interaction with Chris demonstrates Marius's lack of tact and diplomacy (even though Chris could sometimes be accused of the same failing). I did not know Marius well as we hardly ever worked together in the few months I spent at GSH before he resigned, but he was not known by my colleagues and his juniors for his tact. In his memoirs, he provided a further example of his tactless and questionable manner.

> One such dinner I remember attending was at Groote Schuur, the prime minister's residence, and I had to hire a tuxedo for the occasion. We were met by our very charming hosts, John Vorster and his wife, Tienie. I recall very little about the evening except that we ate tahr meat. When we eventually stood up to leave, to the amazement of my colleagues I said to Mr Vorster, 'Mr Prime Minister, I found you quite pleasant, so the next time I vote against you, the mark will not be so deliberate as before, but I'll still vote against you.' Unsurprisingly, this elicited no response, he simply walked away. Chris was incensed and considered my remarks totally uncalled for. But I actually enjoyed making them.

Despite Chris's own failings with regard to his interpersonal relationships with the members of his team, I do not believe he can be held entirely responsible for his failure to work amicably with his brother. My opinion is strengthened by a comment made to me by a long-standing member of the heart surgery team which was that 'after the first heart transplant Marius would denigrate him [Chris] to the staff and tell them he was going to take over.'

Marius's frustrations in trying to work amicably with Chris are perhaps best summed up by the suggestion, quoted by author Donald McRae, that Marius had contemplated entitling his own memoirs as *The Chris I Have to Bear.*

## Marius's Resignation

In 1980, Marius resigned his position, leaving no obvious 'second-in-command'. Although his dysfunctional relationship with Chris was the prime reason for his resignation, he might also have felt the need for a break from the continual responsibilities of heart surgery—from the persistent pressure of helping to run a heart surgery unit, particularly without the ultimate authority to make the important decisions. Certainly, he would not have resigned if Chris had given him full control of the unit.

In his memoirs, Marius admitted that 'I had always dreamt of running the cardiac unit at Groote Schuur, but knew that, should Chris leave, the long knives of the provincial government and hospital authorities would be drawn and used against me. In any event, I felt that they wouldn't tolerate another Barnard.'

The 'long knives' may have been drawn because of Marius's penchant for outspoken criticism of the Nationalist government, but also sometimes for the Provincial Administration or the administration of the hospital.

> My main reasons for leaving Groote Schuur Hospital, were not only my enduring problems with the provincial and hospital authorities, but also my disappointment in Chris. This was not because of his lifestyle or his publicity addiction, but rather due to the restrictive, non-forward-moving and irrational ways in which he managed the cardiac unit. Another major reason for my disappointment was that he allowed the Nats [the ruling Nationalist Party] to use him, both at home and internationally, for their foul plans and policies.

In 1980, Marius was selected as the Progressive Federal Party's parliamentary candidate for Parktown (a suburb of Johannesburg) and therefore planned to resign from the staff of GSH. Officially, he had to give a month's notice, but he had irritated the administration so much by his political activities that, in his own words, 'they wanted to exercise one last bit of authority and unpleasantness, and this legal requirement was waived.' One day later, he received a call stating that he had been relieved of his duties and was to leave immediately. Predicting this would happen, he had already cleared most of his belongings from his office and the rest he packed in his car.

'After three years as a registrar [surgical trainee] and thirteen as a cardiac surgeon,' he wrote, 'during which time I had given my all in time, dedication and a high standard of patient care—I left without even saying goodbye. I was treated badly and was given no farewell—not even a cup of tea.'

Apart from a short note of thanks from Dr Sanders, the medical superintendent, he received no other form of recognition for his services. In the more than thirty years left in his life, he never once entered Groote Schuur Hospital again, and only once returned to the Red Cross War Memorial Children's Hospital.

Marius was very aggrieved at the way he had been treated. According to him, even Chris did not thank him for his services, although when asked to comment publicly, Chris stated, 'It's very difficult to get surgeons of his quality and therefore it will be very difficult to replace him.' Since that day in 1980, Marius and Chris met less than half a dozen times over the next twenty years before Chris died, although during the last few years of his life, Chris phoned Marius frequently—what a sad outcome.

In the event, Marius moved to the Johannesburg area where he continued to carry out heart surgery, though not heart transplantation, in private practice on a part-time basis, less stressful than running a busy academic unit, particularly when you are having to work with a brother with whom you are no longer interacting amicably. He stood for parliament for the Progressive Federal Party as a liberal 'anti-apartheid' candidate. He won a seat and was active in parliament for several years. I admired his open opposition to the government's policy. In this respect, he was markedly more open and outspoken than Chris.

Between 1980 and 1989, he served in the House of Assembly as a member of parliament. He represented his small party as its spokesman on health. He held onto his seat in his constituency in 1987. The Progressive Federal Party was disbanded during his last term in parliament.

Marius's resignation from GSH had a major effect on me personally in that Chris offered me the position on his staff that Marius had vacated, which was a great stroke of luck for me. I will always be immensely indebted to Chris as he allowed me the opportunity to expand my surgical experience and pursue my research goals.


## Chris as a Writer

It was during his second marriage that Chris began what can only be considered his 'second life', a life not dominated by surgery and the hospital. As his interests in surgery slowly waned, which began quite early after the initial transplants, so his other interests began to widen. During the 1970s and later, he wrote—at times with research assistance and collaboration by others—several books on matters of health for the layman, particularly relating to the heart, which were well-received. One on the South African political scene was also published during this period. He became interested in the potential role of euthanasia in patients whose lives had become unbearable, and put down his views on this controversial subject in another book. The books he wrote or contributed significantly towards are discussed in Chapters 27 and 28.

How much of the writing was actually penned by Chris, and how much was written for him by others, remains uncertain. Chris himself, however, was quite open in admitting that, although the ideas came from him, their translation into actual words was frequently provided by others.

With regard to his academic work, early in his career he was active in reporting his surgical data personally, and took the lead in this respect. So keen was he on publishing his excellent surgical results that I feel sure he then would have prepared the manuscript himself. However, by the 1980s, from my personal observations, he had been largely unwilling to put together more than a page or two of prose without substantial assistance. For example, during the several years I worked with him in Cape Town and Oklahoma City, I can never recollect him writing a medical paper himself; someone else always wrote the manuscript, and he would read and approve it, but rarely suggest any significant revisions.

For example, on one occasion when he returned from giving a lecture on heart transplantation at London's Royal Society of Medicine, he came to me and explained that the Society had requested him to submit a paper on the topic of his talk for publication in its journal. He asked if I would prepare the manuscript for him.

'But I don't know what you said,' I told him.

'Yes, you do. I reviewed all of our results.' I prepared the manuscript, and it was subsequently published. He readily agreed that I should be credited with co-authorship.

He also developed an interest in writing more creatively. When I visited him for the second time in Cape Town in 1973 (well before I joined his staff in 1980), he told me that he then only carried out two or three heart operations each week as he wanted to spend more time on his writing. He collaborated with the established South African writer, Siegfried Stander, on three novels that were generally well received, and wrote a fourth without significant help (Chapter 27). Although publication was certainly facilitated by his instant name recognition, they were certainly as good as many others that are found on the bookstands. Like many novelists, he drew heavily on his own experiences, for example, in medicine, to provide the background for his stories.

Without wishing to minimise Chris's achievements in this field, one is forced to ask the question of whether his novels would have been accepted for publication if he had not already been well-known. Although it was possibly slightly easier thirty to forty years ago, it is notoriously difficult for an unknown writer to get a first novel published today, and there must be some doubt as to whether Chris's novels would have seen the light of day if the name of Chris Barnard had not been under the title. The chances of publication were greatly helped, of course, by Chris's collaboration with a professional writer in the person of Siegfried Stander.

I was under the impression that Chris would not have had the patience to write an entire novel or book by himself. He had the ideas, but needed someone else to perform the laborious task of putting those ideas on to paper, at which time he would step back into the arena and rearrange, or at least suggest a rearrangement of, the words whenever they did not conform to his original ideas. His 'laziness' in this respect had, I suspected, steadily increased with the years.

Apart from allowing him to express his views on various topics, the books for the general public and the novels brought in extra income to augment his salary from the Provincial government, which was still only R1,200 per month. Writing for the South African newspapers formed another source of income.

## Chris as a Journalist

For many years, Chris contributed a weekly syndicated column to the leading local English language newspaper, the *Cape Times,* on any topic of his interest. These were edited by Bob Molloy, a Cape Town journalist, and were invariably both entertaining and thought-provoking. Chris had the gift of seemingly always finding an anecdote to illustrate the point he was making, and the knack of stating a fact or opinion in a way that caught the reader's attention. We will discuss his writing in a subsequent chapter, but a handful of examples of memorable statements from his publications relating to medicine follow here.

> The engineering and architectural departments of any university annually turn out more guarantors of the nation's health than any medical faculty.
>
> Basics such as good nutrition, clothing and housing are the foundations of a healthy nation. Any national health program, no matter how copiously funded, is simply pouring money into a bottomless pit unless these minimum essentials are taken care of.

A man called Thomas Crapper made what was probably the largest stride in terms of preventive health measures in London in the last century when he developed the flush toilet.

Whether these quotes from Chris were all original to him, or 'borrowed' from previous writers, I am unsure, but I have not seen them elsewhere. In any case, the ability to recall an appropriate phrase to illustrate a certain point is one of the skills of writing (although one should credit the source). Two selections of these articles were later collected and published by Bob Molloy, who had collaborated closely with Chris over a number of years (Chapter 27).

Many years later, I wondered, as I had on several previous occasions, whether or not Chris really wrote the weekly newspaper columns that appeared under his name in the *Cape Times*. I knew that Bob Molloy 'edited' these articles, and secretly suspected that he ghost-wrote them after being given a general idea by Chris as to what he wanted to say. It is clearly much easier to come up with a general theme for an article and let someone else do the research and put it all together for you than it is to sit down and put the words on paper yourself.

To clarify the degree of involvement that Chris had in these articles, and indeed to confirm my own suspicions that he probably contributed relatively little, I wrote to Bob Molloy, by that time the editor of a newspaper in New Zealand, and put this question to him, 'Did Chris really write the newspaper columns himself?' Or, put another way, 'How much "ghosting" did you do?'

I believed these questions to be of some importance, as the answers would confirm whether or not Chris Barnard was a skilled and entertaining writer, or whether he was merely allowing his name to be used to attract readers to a particular weekly column.

I here reproduce Bob Molloy's reply in full.

Dear Dr Cooper,

Your query concerning Chris Barnard's authorship of his various books and newspaper columns is a recurring theme in the media, almost as if the questioners believed that one day the real Chris Barnard might stand up and we could all go home secure in the knowledge that the greatest hoax of the twentieth century had been at last uncovered.

Alas, the truth is always too mundane for the Bessy Ballpoints and Noddy Notebooks who inflict 'tabloiditis' on us all. The short answer to your question is that insofar as my own involvement is concerned he was always the prime mover.

His columns, which appeared in the South African Morning Group papers for eight years without a break, were from beginning to end his own work. I, as the editor, spent too many weary hours drafting and redrafting the work not to be fully aware of who was calling the shots.

There were times when we disagreed so strongly in a phrase or theme that it seemed the column would never appear. Usually I compromised, most of my objecting being to infelicitous use of metaphor or phrasing, almost never to the main concepts. He was at once an exhausting and stimulating person to work with, with a quicksilver mind that threw off ideas as a catherine wheel does sparks.

I also edited three books, two of which were collections of his columns and one on the 'Moment of Death' controversy (*Good Life, Good Death*). The first two have been discussed above. The third was based on collaborative research by myself and an American writer, the whole being pulled together and largely reworked by Chris. He initiated all the issues, discussed the research findings and drew his own conclusions. My involvement was mainly T-crossing and I-dotting.

To sum up: Chris was (is) the consummate Renaissance man, master if not of all trades at least of those he turned his hand to. Editors, including myself, may have anglicised his more Afrikaans phraseology but that was about the extent of it.

Sincerely,

Bob Molloy

Mr Molloy's reply makes it quite clear that Chris's writings were predominantly his own, although Chris himself indicated to me that he thought Mr Molloy was being very modest and minimising his own contributions to their collaboration. Even more does he earn my respect in this regard as the articles, produced weekly for several years, were invariably stimulating and frequently amusing.

Chris continued to accept invitations to lecture abroad to doctors, speak to laymen, and participate in charitable events, such as telethons. As time progressed, his diminishing stature in the medical profession was illustrated by the fact that he was less often being invited to address a medical audience and increasingly being invited to speak to lay people: more as an 'entertainer' than a serious surgeon. To be a good lecturer, especially when addressing an audience of lay persons, it is helpful if the lecturer is something of a 'performer' or actor, and so Chris must have had something of the thespian in him. Chris's new lifestyle also distanced him from many of his surgical peers, who no longer considered him a major player. His participation in major surgical meetings declined dramatically.

He lectured on the British liner *QE2* on a number of occasions, joining the vessel as a celebrity guest in one part of the world, and disembarking a few days or even weeks later at another exotic location. He enjoyed these sojourns at sea not only because of the social aspects of the cruise, but also because they gave him time to think. 'There's nothing like having a deck rail to lean on and starlight on the sea for promoting long thoughts,' he wrote. 'I must have spent hours staring at the sea while feeling that we were all on a freeway, hell-bent on going somewhere and completely oblivious to the accident victims at the roadside.'

On one cruise, the ship docked in the Kenyan port of Mombasa, where, because of the apartheid policy still in place in South Africa at the time, the local authorities would not allow the South African passengers to disembark. Chris went to reason with them, pointing out that he had operated on several Kenyans with heart disease (usually children) at Groote Schuur Hospital. Indeed, while I was on the staff of the hospital, I remember very well a delightful and wealthy black gentleman from Mombasa who underwent heart transplantation. Chris pointed out that many of the Kenyan patients, particularly the children, had received all of the surgeons' and hospital services in South Africa free. As long as the patient could find funding to get to Cape Town, possibly provided by their home country's government or from family and friends, all other expenses had been covered by the hospital (ultimately by the Western Cape provincial administration—effectively, the South African government). We even had one or two American patients who could not afford a heart transplant in the USA who came to South Africa for the procedure. Chris would accept almost all of them if they could get to the country.

The Kenyan authorities, persuaded by the arguments of the well-known surgeon, eventually agreed that he could leave the ship, but not the other South African passengers. However, Chris pointed out that it was these very South Africans who, through their taxes, had paid for the care of some of the Kenyan child patients, and many others from other countries in southern and central Africa. Eventually, if I remember correctly, he managed to persuade the authorities to allow all of the South African passengers to disembark for a sight-seeing trip.

His high profile enabled him to participate in several business ventures. As his finances allowed, he invested in several restaurants in the Cape Town area, most notably La Vita, at which he frequently dined and with which he was closely associated for the remainder of his life. Some of the restaurants were successful, others less so. He acquired a cattle ranch along the south coast of South Africa, and later exchanged it for a couple of sheep farms in the Karoo, not very far from Beaufort

West, where he had been born and brought up as a boy. Was this, one may ask, a yearning to return to his roots, to the 'real' South Africa, as he knew it, the South Africa of the farmer and the '*dorps*' (small rural towns)?

For years after his fame had peaked, Chris continued to receive letters from all over the world. A short and amusing example is one from a young man in the Middle East who wrote to Chris in the early 1980s, approximately fifteen years after Chris first came to the public's notice. I reproduce it here in full.

> Venerable Doctor Christiaan Barnard
>> Dear Mr.
>> I hope you are well and in good health, and I send the best greetings from utmost of my heart to your Majesty. I was very hesitant before writing your Majesty because of my great shame, but my great inborn love to your Highness gave me a push and encouraged me to write to your Majesty, hoping to realise my wish and only dream in my life.
>> My utmost hope and full dream is to speak English fluently as an aboriginal.
>> I think that the best means of learning the mother tongue is to live among the American people.

When Chris's secretary gave me the letter to read, you can imagine my disappointment, as an Englishman, when I read that the writer thought he could best learn English by living among Americans. Chris hugely enjoyed the letter.

Although an extreme example of the regard and even awe in which many of the world's citizens viewed Chris (admittedly, not many gave him royal status), the letter does illustrate how he and heart transplantation had captured the public's attention even in countries thousands of miles from South Africa or the western world. The fact that it was mailed fifteen years after the 'great event' confirms the impact Chris had made worldwide.

## A Secretary's View

A secretary's perspective on their boss is always worth knowing. For several years of his career at GSH, Chris was supported by Celeste Blaettler-McCann, who had briefly worked for Chris's second wife, Barbara. After expressing an interest in the job, she had been 'warned off' by the personnel department of GSH, who told her that, because of his volatile temperament, he did not keep secretaries for very long. Her first impression of him was that 'he was pure dynamic energy.'

As she had no previous experience of medical secretarial work, her 'first month was pure hell.' He dictated far too fast, and made numerous deletions and changes. However, they eventually 'became great friends and communicated very well ever after.' She found him to be a perfectionist 'with the memory of an elephant.'

His worst fault, according to Celeste, was 'his bad temper. When things didn't go according to his plans, he would become enraged at the slightest provocation and, unless you were brave or stupid enough to confront him, the best defense was to try to keep calm and not say something dumb. He just didn't suffer fools.'

Celeste noticed that when he appeared at any gathering, he was 'one of those people with a distinct "bearing" and poise, and couldn't be inconspicuous even if he had wished.' Once engaged in conversation, he was charming, quick-witted, humourous, occasionally scathing, purposely shocking just to test reactions, and became bored easily. In fact, it was a feat to keep his attention for more than a few minutes.

His most attractive attribute, in her opinion, was 'his ever-youthful and lively interest in almost any subject.' Furthermore, he was a superb host and took pleasure in serving his guests personally. She admired him for always having the courage of his convictions. Despite his quick temper, she had 'very happy memories of that period of [her] life.'

Throughout these years, Chris's critics often accused him of being a publicity seeker, and the frequency with which his name appeared in the media might seem to provide some justification for this accusation. Initially, it was his medical achievements that put him in the public eye, but it was his charisma that ensured he would remain a subject of public interest. Thereafter, he suffered the fate of innumerable other celebrities; seemingly everything he did or said, good or bad, was deemed worthy of reporting. He complained to me that, over the years, many reporters and media people requested, even begged for, an interview with him, and, when granted, one of their first questions was 'why are you so much of a publicity seeker?' He patiently pointed out to them that it was they who had requested the interview, not he.

I asked Chris whether he regretted any aspects of his lifestyle during the period after the first few transplants.

The trouble was not of the lifestyle, but it stopped me from concentrating on the hospital and on research. I left it all to other people. When you leave things in other people's hands, eventually it gets out of your hands. Eventually, I started falling behind because I didn't know things and I was not up with all the monitoring. The cardiac surgical unit really suffered a tremendous amount from that. If I had it all over again, I would have limited the amount of traveling that I did. I travelled too much. The second regret is that I didn't retire earlier. I should have retired in maybe 1980 or 1981, but not stayed on until 1983. I stayed two years too long.

During these last two years, Chris played an ever-decreasing role in the running of his department. Although I frequently heard him say that he should have been far more selective in accepting invitations to lecture and to attend meetings, whether his 'addiction' to the celebrity lifestyle would have allowed him to decline more invitations is uncertain, but, I suspect, doubtful.

# 21

# Insight and Innovation: Subsequent Progress in Heart Transplantation

With increasing experience and several minor innovations, the results of heart transplantation slowly improved. As a consequence, towards the end of the 1970s and in the early 1980s, other cardiac surgical groups slowly came back into the field and resuscitated their transplant programs or initiated new ones. For example, I had the privilege of being closely involved in the initiation of the programme at Papworth Hospital in Cambridge in the UK, headed by Terence English, which carried out its first three transplants in 1979. These were the first heart transplants in the UK for about ten years. However, a quantum leap in the results awaited more major innovations, three of which we will discuss here.

## Endomyocardial Biopsy

The first important innovation related to the diagnosis of acute rejection of the heart and involved the development of the technique of endomyocardial biopsy. A long instrument with small 'jaws' at the end is passed along a vein (usually in the neck or arm) into the transplanted heart, where a small 'bite' (or biopsy) of the heart muscle is taken from one of the pumping chambers (ventricles) (Figure 21.i). The instrument is withdrawn, and the biopsy processed and examined under the microscope to detect whether the patient's white blood cells are invading the heart muscle—whether rejection of the heart is developing. If it is, then extra immunosuppressive therapy can be administered. However, if there is no evidence of rejection, then no extra therapy is given, thus reducing the risk of infectious complications.

The technique and the instrument (the bioptome) necessary to take the sample had been introduced in Japan some years earlier (in 1962), but the instrument and technique were modified by a member of Shumway's team in Stanford, a young Northern Irish surgeon named Philip Caves, and was introduced into heart transplantation in 1973. This proved a major advantage in the management of patients with heart transplants, whether they were orthotopic or heterotopic. When rejection was suspected by the clinical examination of the patient, such as developing features of early heart failure, or even when no features were obvious, a biopsy could provide strong evidence to confirm or deny that rejection was developing. Endomyocardial biopsy soon became the standard technique for diagnosing rejection of the heart.

If endomyocardial biopsy had been available when Chris had carried out his transplant on Mr Washkansky, the biopsy would have demonstrated an absence of rejection, strongly suggesting that the shadows seen in the lungs on chest X-rays were not associated with rejection of the heart (or the nebulous 'transplant lung'), but were more likely associated with pneumonia. As a result, extra immunosuppressive therapy would not have been administered, but antibiotics would have been given immediately, possibly saving the patient's life.

Sadly, Philip Caves was destined to enjoy only a short life himself. After returning to the UK, he was soon appointed as professor of cardiac surgery in Glasgow, but within a few years, died of a heart attack in 1978 while playing squash. He was only thirty-eight years old.

## Introduction of Improved Immunosuppressive Drugs

The second, and most important, advance came from Europe, largely through Roy Calne (Figure 8.iii) and his junior colleague, transplant immunologist David White. This was the testing and introduction of a new, much more potent, immunosuppressive drug: cyclosporine.

With the introduction of azathioprine, Roy Calne had become a leader in the concept of immunosuppressive drug therapy. Although azathioprine administered alone had a relatively weak immunosuppressive effect, when Tom Starzl and others combined it with high-dose steroids, the combination was able to prevent or reverse rejection in a good percentage of patients with kidney transplants. Nevertheless, this regimen was far from ideal, and the overall one-year survival of patients with kidney, heart, or liver grafts worldwide remained only about 50 per cent. A better drug was required if organ transplantation was to become a truly successful form of therapy.

## Cyclosporine

It fell to Calne again to take this next step forward by introducing a new drug called cyclosporine and, once again, it was Starzl who showed that its combination with steroids had a beneficial effect. The combination of cyclosporine, azathioprine, and corticosteroids, first suggested by Maurice 'Taffy' Slapak in the UK, proved even better. Within a few years, one-year graft and patient survival after kidney, heart, or liver transplantation rose to approximately 80 per cent.

The laboratory work of Jean Borel, a scientist at the Swiss pharmaceutical company, Sandoz (later to become part of Novartis) on cyclosporine (derived from a soil fungus) became known to David White, a young immunologist in Calne's department, who heard a basic science lecture by Borel and realised that cyclosporine had potential in transplantation. The senior executives at Sandoz were investigating cyclosporine as an antibiotic (in which role it was weak), and were not interested in it as an immunosuppressive agent because they felt the potential commercial market for it would be too small. In their opinion, the number of patients undergoing organ transplantation was very small (as it then was) compared with the number who needed treatment for conditions such as infection, high blood pressure, diabetes, and so on.

However, White and Calne managed to persuade them to provide a little cyclosporine for testing in animal models. They investigated cyclosporine in rats and dogs with kidney grafts, and in pigs with heart grafts, and found the drug to be far better than any other agent previously examined in any of these models. A pilot safety study was carried out in patients.

They finally obtained regulatory authority permission in the UK to treat severe rejection episodes in kidney transplant patients who were not responding to high-dose corticosteroid therapy, which was then the standard treatment for rejection. Cyclosporine proved effective in reversing rejection, at least in the short-term. At that point, Calne began treating all of his patients who were receiving organ transplants with the new drug. It soon became the mainstay of immunosuppressive therapy, usually in combination with corticosteroids with or without azathioprine.

The dose they initially gave to the patients was the same they had given to the laboratory animals, but this proved too high, and in humans this dose caused kidney failure. It was ironic that cyclosporine had not been documented to be toxic to the kidneys in any of the animals in which it had been tested, but it proved toxic in humans.

'Furthermore,' Professor Calne told me, 'there were two patients who developed fatal lymphoproliferative disease (a malignant disease associated with too intensive immunosuppressive therapy). It took us a long time to realise we were giving about three or four times the dose of cyclosporine that was required in patients.' When these problems had been resolved, cyclosporine proved to be arguably the greatest advance in organ transplantation to that date.

Although the Sandoz senior executives were originally of the opinion that their company would not make any money by developing cyclosporine for patients with organ transplants, White had heard that cyclosporine subsequently made approximately US$2 billion for Sandoz. I hope the executives were suitably grateful to Calne and White for persuading them to develop the drug.

If Dimitri Novitzky's memory is correct, and I have no reason to doubt it, it was in regard to cyclosporine that Chris Barnard missed a great opportunity. It appears that the distraction provided by a pretty young lady lost Chris the opportunity to be one of the first to test cyclosporine in patients with heart transplants. At a gala dinner in Europe, Dr Jean Borel approached Chris and offered the use of the drug in cardiac transplant patients. It had already been shown by Roy Calne's group to be effective in patients with kidney and liver transplants. Chris mentioned to Dimitri that he very much regretted that he had ignored that offer, but at the time, he had been distracted by the attentions of an attractive young girl. The kudos of being the first to use cyclosporine in heart transplant patients went to the Stanford group in the USA.

When we eventually began to utilise cyclosporine in the heart transplant programme in Cape Town in the mid-1980s, we briefly suffered the same problems that Professor Calne had experienced in that we gave too high a dose. This was because the Stanford group had reported that a high dose was needed to prevent rejection in animals with heart transplants, but this dose was unnecessarily high in humans.

Cyclosporine also enabled the first truly successful transplantation of the heart and both lungs in the world in 1981, carried out by Shumway and his junior colleague Bruce Reitz.

## Tacrolimus

Cyclosporine proved an immense step forward, but about ten years later, interest in another immunosuppressive drug, initially known as FK506 and subsequently as tacrolimus, developed. Tacrolimus (derived from a different soil fungus) worked in a similar way to cyclosporine, but was about 100 times more powerful. It had been identified as a potential immunosuppressive agent by another pharmaceutical company, Fujisawa (later Astellas) in Japan. It was Tom Starzl (Figure 8.iv) who tested it in numerous animal models and then was the first to administer it to patients in his transplant centre in Pittsburgh (to where he had moved from Denver).

The introduction of cyclosporine and, even more, tacrolimus opened the door to successful transplantation of organs that had hitherto proved difficult, such as the liver, lung, pancreas, and even the intestine and, ultimately, the hand and face.

## Newer Immunosuppressive Agents

Other drugs followed, which, when combined with either cyclosporine or tacrolimus, proved beneficial. By the turn of the twentieth century, therefore, severe rejection became largely a phenomenon of the past. The risk now was to be tempted to immunosuppress the patient too vigorously, opening the door to infectious or malignant complications.

Both Calne and Starzl went on to make further contributions to the development of organ transplantation, and deservedly received many honours for their work. There are many scientists in the field of organ transplantation (myself included) who believe they should have been awarded the Nobel Prize (Chapter 29).

## The Detrimental Effect of Brain Death on the Heart

In my opinion, a third significant innovation took place in Chris's own department at Groote Schuur Hospital. Towards the end of his active career in Cape Town, Chris was much less involved in the day-to-day care of patients than in his younger days, when his untiring attention to them was legendary, but he still maintained a considerable interest in the research being conducted in his department's experimental laboratory. He encouraged young men such as Winston Wicomb, a biochemist, and Dimitri Novitzky, a surgeon, and stimulated them to make important advances.

Largely through the work of Winston Wicomb (Figure 21.ii), a system for storing isolated hearts out of the body for up to forty-eight hours was developed. The system involved cooling the heart to about 4°C, reminiscent of the pioneering work in hypothermia for heart surgery (Chapter 4), and supplying it with oxygen and other nutrients by pumping a special solution through it continuously, a system known as 'hypothermic perfusion' (Figure 21.iii).

Winston's work was another example of how Chris had demonstrated his vision for the future. He had employed Winston with the specific aim of developing a system of storing hearts so that they could be transported (without detriment) from other centres in South Africa to Cape Town. However, in Chris's vision, this would just be the beginning. He wrote, 'How much better it would be if complex organs such as the heart could be stored for weeks or months so that we could establish organ banks on which the world could draw at well-planned leisure.' Others had similar aspirations, of course, but Chris took early steps towards this goal.

After much work in the experimental laboratory, we were eventually able to store a baboon heart by hypothermic perfusion for twenty-four or forty-eight hours, and then transplant it successfully into another baboon. Even when these laboratory studies were in their early stages, Chris encouraged us to use the storage system in the clinical transplant program. Winston and I were a little hesitant to use it in patients at this stage as we had only tested it successfully in a small number of experiments. 'Does it work or doesn't it?' Chris asked us. When we replied that it did work, he then urged us to use it when we were next informed of a suitable deceased human donor from outside Cape Town, which we did.

In some other countries, such as the US and in Europe, the transplant surgeons could fly by private jet to collect a donor heart, but the cost of private jets was beyond our means in South Africa at that time. At best, we could hire a single-propeller-engined plane to take us to another city. However, as the safe storage time of a cold (4°C) donor heart (stored in ice) was only four hours (which included the operating time it would take to implant the heart into the recipient), this meant effectively we were confined to Cape Town. The development of the hypothermic perfusion machine, initiated by Chris and perfected by Winston, was therefore a case of 'necessity being the mother of invention.'

For the first time in the world, in 1981, Winston Wicomb stored a human donor heart by means of a perfusion apparatus. Thereafter, he used the device successfully on several occasions. To attempt to store a human heart in clinical transplant practice was a very ambitious step at the time. Unfortunately, when Winston left Cape Town to take up an appointment in the USA in mid-1985, the storage system was no longer used, mainly because the solution he perfused through the heart was quite complex to prepare and needed his expertise. It has been only in recent years (more than thirty years later) that similar perfusion devices have been reintroduced elsewhere in the world.

On the first occasion of its use in 1981 (16 September), the donor heart was obtained in Port Elizabeth (a city in the Eastern Cape almost 500 miles from Cape Town), transported on the hypothermic perfusion machine by plane to Cape Town (Figure 21.iv), and implanted in the recipient patient almost thirteen hours after it had been excised from the donor. At that time, this was by far the longest period that a human heart had remained outside of the body between donor and recipient. Very fortunately, we transplanted the heart in the piggyback position because, for the first several hours, the heart, though it looked healthy and was beating regularly, was not generating enough force to expel any blood, the patient being maintained alive by his own heart heavily supported by intravenous drugs that stimulated it.

To say the least, this experience was disconcerting as it was in such contrast to our experimental results. We had never seen a situation like this in the laboratory where the stored heart had always functioned strongly immediately (and where the heart was orthotopically transplanted when it would, of course, be dependent on itself, as there was no native heart to help it). After some hours, however, the pulse trace indicated that the donor heart was improving dramatically, and the patient recovered quickly from the operation.

This phenomenon of delayed function suggested to us and to Chris that temporary depletion of the heart muscle's energy stores had occurred. Whereas in the baboon experiments, the heart had been removed from a healthy anaesthetised animal, in the clinical situation, the heart had been excised from a human donor who had undergone brain death. This alerted us to the fact that brain death must have a detrimental effect on the heart, and led to extensive investigations into the changes that take place in the body, and particularly in the heart, during and after brain death, and the implications of these changes. This work, led by Dimitri Novitzky (Figure 21.ii), was the first comprehensive study investigating the effects of brain death ever carried out. I presume this was because what happens during and after brain death was not of great interest to physicians before organ transplantation became a form of therapy.

The results were surprising to us. We documented that hitherto unrecognised major endocrine changes, particularly a reduction in thyroid hormone, contributed to the reduction in heart function. Remarkably, after brain death, the body can no longer use oxygen to replace its energy stores (even if oxygen is supplied). Without being able to utilize oxygen, the energy stores in the heart muscle, for instance, rapidly become depleted and the heartbeat gradually fails. It is these changes that result in failure of the heart even if all conventional support of the brain-dead potential donor, including artificial respiration, is maintained. Prolonged storage of the heart (such as by Winston Wicomb's perfusion machine) exacerbated the loss of heart function after brain death.

Dimitri Novitzky developed a concept of hormonal replacement therapy, particularly with regard to thyroid hormone replacement, which experimentally was documented to allow the body to use oxygen again, and therefore replace and maintain the energy stores in the heart and improve heart function. Today, thyroid (and other) hormone therapy of potential organ donors is increasingly widely practiced worldwide. Thanks in considerable part to the early persistence of Dimitri, more than 70 per cent of potential organ donors in the US benefit from thyroid hormone therapy today. This has contributed to a significant increase in the number of organs that are retrieved from deceased donors each year, and thus in the number of transplants that can be performed.

With more assurance that the donor heart was likely to function well immediately after transplantation (through treatment of the donor with thyroid and other hormones), the reduced incidence of severe life-threatening rejection episodes (through the administration of cyclosporine), and the ability to confirm rejection (provided by taking a biopsy of the heart muscle), we in Cape Town resumed orthotopic (rather than piggyback) heart transplantation. The advantages of the piggyback transplant were no longer so obvious.

The impact of endomyocardial biopsy, cyclosporine, and hormone therapy to the donor can be illustrated by the fact that only about 50 per cent of the patients my colleagues and I treated in Cape Town in the early 1980s survived for one year, whereas by the mid-1990s (by which time I was working in Oklahoma City), more than 90 per cent or our patients lived for longer than one year.

## Vision and Curiosity

Even when the results of heart transplantation began to improve in the early 1980s, not all leading medical centres had the vision or enthusiasm to accept the challenge. For example, in the mid-1970s, Ben Cosimi, a Harvard kidney and liver transplant surgeon, visited Shumway's group to assess whether Boston's famed Massachusetts General Hospital (MGH) should begin a heart transplant program. The hospital authorities decided that the complexities were too great at the time and the benefits insufficient. Even in February 1980, the MGH Board of Trustees decided that 'the resources that would be required outweighed the potential patient benefits.' It was only five years later (in 1985), with the proven value of cyclosporine, that MGH (a hospital that likes to believe it is in the forefront of medical advances) began a heart transplant programme, almost twenty years after Barnard's pioneering effort.

The lesson from this is that it frequently takes a single-minded enthusiast or zealot with a great sense of his or her 'mission' to push ahead with new technologies in their early stages. The great pioneer of kidney and liver transplantation, Tom Starzl, told me once that he never worried about a 'career' in the usual sense of the word, such as obtaining steady promotion with gradually increasing responsibilities, prestige, and financial reward; he was only interested in what he saw as his mission in life, namely establishing organ transplantation as an effective means of surgical therapy. Without these visionaries (surgeons like Lillehei, Barnard, Shumway, Hume, Calne, and Starzl), progress in medicine would be much slower. Pioneers like these men are prepared to proceed often in the face of intense active opposition or at least obstructive lethargy from the more cautious or reactionary members of the profession.

In my own experience, those in opposition to such an advance often become almost as single-minded and zealous in their efforts to prevent its success as do those trying to accomplish the mission. They will resort to spurious arguments against the aims of the pioneers and distort facts to suit their goals. Despite the fact that the underlying aim of the new therapy is to save patients' lives or at least improve the quality of their lives, the reactionaries find many reasons, some of which superficially appear quite reasonable, to oppose progress.

Transplant surgeon Tom Starzl aptly summed up his attitude to surgical research, and how a form of treatment evolves with time: 'History tells us that procedures that were inconceivable yesterday, and barely achievable today, often become routine tomorrow.'

Roy Calne once told me that he believes an important quality of a true researcher is that he or she should have immense 'curiosity', continually asking questions and seeking answers. Why does that happen? What would be the outcome if we did this? In his autobiography, *The Ultimate Gift*, he quotes an article from the *British Medical Journal* in 1978.

> The greatest discoveries, the ones which change the direction of world-established disciplines, often occurred because of utterly irrational persistence, following up of seemingly trivial observation, or sacrilegious crossing of disciplinary lines. Virtually never has a specialised researcher, well trained in a particular discipline, discovered anything of importance by pursuing a project thought reasonable by an expert committee.

Professor Calne also wrote, 'the most important advances have been achieved by obsessively driven and curious individuals. Their motives are often mixed but usually involve the challenge, excitement and intense personal satisfaction of surmounting obstacles in order to achieve an objective.' He went on to state that 'although virtually all science starts with an educated guess, or hypothesis, it is only the repeated successful testing of such a theory that qualifies it to join a body of knowledge that is accepted by most sane people.'

Hungarian 1937 Nobel Prize winner Albert Szent-Gyorgyi, wrote, 'Discovery is seeing what everybody else has seen, and thinking what nobody else has thought.'

George Bernard Shaw may have been correct when, in *Man and Superman*, he wrote, 'The reasonable man adapts himself to the world; the unreasonable one persists in trying to adapt the world to himself. Therefore, all progress depends on the unreasonable man.' In this regard, Chris was to some extent an 'unreasonable man'.

Chris had his own opinions on research and researchers.

> In truth, research is neither glamorous nor dull. It has, like any job, its routine side and from time to time its monotony. And it has its moments of sheer joy, when results come out according to expectations or, even more exciting, when the data unexpectedly yield an insight that then leads perhaps to a major accomplishment. As someone who has done a share of research, I reckon that to do it successfully you need a dogged sort of curiosity, a tireless approach to problems, however tiny, that drives you to worry at them until they either yield to a solution or reveal themselves as issues that are simply not worth pursuing. Good researchers, of course, need good brains. But they also need a streak of stubbornness in their makeup that makes them hang on, limpet-like, to their objectives in the face of fatigue, boredom, and sometimes acute despair.

## Impressions of the Researchers

Winston Wicomb worked under Chris's supervision for several years, and so his opinion of Chris is worth recording. Chris 'had an excellent sense of humour, could dominate any debate, charm any woman, and take any chance in life if he believed in it. Taking that chance in life—for example, using my heart storage system in a patient for the first time—excited me most about him, and that is what I admire about Christiaan Barnard.'

However, Winston added that Chris 'was very aggressive and frequently threatened to fire members of the staff, me included, which he did on one occasion … [But] the next day, as far as he was concerned, all would be forgotten, though I would still be boiling inside. It was sometimes very difficult to communicate with Barnard at this stage of his career.'

Chris sometimes asked Winston to investigate other topics he found interesting. For example, he persuaded Winston to treat some rats with tablets that it was hoped would prevent the injury to the lungs that smokers normally experience. Winston remembered that 'getting rats to "smoke" [by placing them in a smoke-filled bell jar] was not fun, nor was giving them the tablets morning and evening.'

For reasons I could never fully understand, and nor could Winston, Chris took Winston (who was thirty years his junior) into his confidence more than anybody else. Winston recollected that, 'during part of my time with him, he went through a period of intense interest in things sexual. He would say he had an interesting story to tell me. We would sit down in my office and he would reveal some romantic fantasy. These fantasies had me excited as well. Any attractive female might be the proposed object of his desire.'

Winston, Dimitri, and I worked with a small team of excellent research technicians, as I have commented on earlier. A selection of their memories of Chris is also of interest.

Prescott Madlingozi, the excellent heart-lung pump technician for the animal experiments, recorded his opinion:

Professor Barnard was very hard-working and 'pushy'. No one ever messed around with him. He was very 'neutral' with the staff members—neither especially friendly nor unfriendly. If he were showing visitors or friends around the laboratory, however, he would always be joking and having fun, but never communicating directly with the laboratory staff members. It was very seldom that he would ever have anything to say directly to us. He could make derogatory statements that reduced one to nothing. He would just tell you outright that you were 'stupid' and leave it at that. You could have no backtalk at all as he held the main strings. He always seemed to want everything for himself and nothing for others.

Ferdinand Barends, a young man who, like Hamilton Naki, helped in the laboratory and became an excellent, largely self-taught surgeon, remembered:

One unusual observation about him was that although he claimed he never smoked, he would often come running around the laboratory asking for a cigarette. Sometimes he would ask me to go out and wash his new car, standing outside the medical school building, but that was about all the personal contact we had. Sometimes the professor would ask us to work on weekends, and he would promise extra payment to us as well as a day off. We got the payment and also a present of some wine, but we never got the promised day off, which was rather upsetting.

John Roussouw, who meticulously cared for all of the experimental animals, told me:

[Chris's] character was very unpredictable. One day he was very nice to you and the next day he would fight violently with you. After such a confrontation, he would always totally forget everything as if nothing had happened. Whenever Professor Barnard came to my house to pick me up to take me to his home to do a job for him he was always extremely pleasant and nice to me—I sometimes wondered whether this was partly because I was going to help him out, but, in truth, whenever he saw me on the road or anywhere he would always greet me.

These are all mixed memories, reflecting Chris's complex personality. These brief comments reflect his mercurial nature: his charm, yet his abruptness, and self-centredness. His tendency to use his technicians to help him with personal chores on occasions would be frowned on today, but was not uncommon in the past, even outside of South Africa. The innovative American surgeon, Alfred Blalock, would on occasions employ his equally innovative black technician, Vivien Thomas, in his Baltimore home as a barman or waiter when entertaining friends. In such situations, the technician was not treated with the dignity and respect due to him. In Chris's case, however, although they undoubtedly felt they had little choice in the matter, the technicians may have been grateful to earn some extra money, although that was not always the case.

## Heart Transplantation in Babies and Children: Leonard Bailey and Baby Fae

There was one more step forward in heart transplantation that is worthy of mention, and that is the initiation of heart transplantation in babies and young children. As Adrian Kantrowitz first noted, paediatric heart surgeons were frustrated by the almost total lack of donor hearts of a suitable size to transplant into babies born with otherwise untreatable heart defects—conditions such as hypoplastic left heart syndrome in which the main pumping chamber of the heart (the left ventricle) is almost nonexistent (a condition for which Chris had devised an earlier operation, but which was only partially successful). Despite all efforts, the newborn infant often suffered a very early death, often within days. One surgeon, Leonard Bailey, working in Loma Linda University Medical Center in California, became so frustrated that he took the very bold step of transplanting a small baboon heart into his patient.

Encouraged by the fact that cyclosporine had greatly improved the results of the transplantation of human organs, in 1984, Bailey and his colleagues transplanted a baboon heart into an infant who became known throughout the world as 'Baby Fae'. As there was no benefit in retaining the patient's own, very abnormal heart (as Chris had done in his early cross-species transplants), Bailey replaced it with a small baboon heart.

The baby survived for twenty days after the transplant, at which time the heart was rejected. The initial plan was to use the baboon heart only as a temporary support or 'bridging device', and to replace it with a human donor heart as soon as possible, but no suitable human heart could be found before the baby died.

This attempt at cross-species transplantation mobilised extremists from various animal groups. For days, there were demonstrations outside the hospital. There were threats on Bailey's life, and for several months, he was advised to wear a bulletproof vest. The strength of feeling about the use of animals for medical purposes is illustrated by the fact that the hospital where Baby Fae was treated received seventy-five letters from the public that expressed concern with the perceived misuse of the baby, but 13,000 letters protesting perceived misuse of the baboon.

The case prompted more questions about the ethics of research in human subjects. In particular, there were concerns about how adequate informed consent could be obtained under life-and-death circumstances, especially when a child is involved. For example, the permission form signed by the parents of Baby Fae stated that 'this research is an effort to provide your baby with some hope of immediate and long-term survival.' Although this truthfully reflected the surgical team's hope, long-term survival might be considered perhaps unduly optimistic for the science of the time unless a human donor heart could be found very quickly. However, although heavily criticised by some, Bailey's efforts were more accepted than those of James Hardy some twenty years earlier.

Len Bailey's experience with Baby Fae did not contribute much to our knowledge about transplanting animal organs into patients (a topic discussed in Appendix I), except to show that, even with cyclosporine, it was likely to be unsuccessful at that time, but the massive publicity it received drew the attention of the public and medical profession to the need for small donor hearts for infants and children dying of heart disease (usually related to a structural birth defect). Until Baby Fae, the dearth of donor hearts from brain-dead babies and children had been even worse than that in adults. After Baby Fae, Bailey was able to develop an extremely successful heart transplant programme (using human hearts from deceased babies and children) in infants and young children. Possibly because the infant's immune system is 'immature', and therefore more easily suppressed; the results have proved rather better than heart transplantation in adults.

Chris Barnard, who had always had a special interest in heart surgery in children, was very excited by Bailey's work, which he greatly admired.

At the time of writing this book (2017), heart transplantation is carried out in approximately 4,500 (adult and paediatric) patients worldwide each year (with approximately 2,750 of these being in North America). One and five-year survival of the patients worldwide is between 85 to 90 per cent and approximately 80 per cent, respectively. Today, heart transplant patients have more than a 60 per cent chance of living longer than ten years.

The major limiting factor remains the number of suitable donor organs that become available. Transplant teams are forever expanding the criteria to allow less ideal hearts to be used, such as hearts from elderly donors that would not have been considered acceptable a few years ago, and even occasional hearts that have stopped beating in the donor and require resuscitation (as in Chris's first case).

The early pioneers in heart transplantation, particularly Christiaan Barnard and Norman Shumway, who initiated and persisted with their programs, would be delighted to learn how it has developed into a successful and fairly routine form of therapy, admittedly in a relatively small number of patients (thousands rather than millions) for terminal heart disease.

# 22

# A Price Too High:
# Personal Tragedies

During the early 1980s, two traumatic events occurred that took their psychological and emotional toll on Chris Barnard, one occurring before and one after his retirement from Groote Schuur Hospital.

## Second Divorce

Chris's second marriage became strained, again in part due to his frequent absences abroad and his continued jet-setting lifestyle, as well as his wife's grave suspicions of his infidelity. Barbara was concerned when she saw that he was 'dancing with young women on his travels.' She would ask his secretary for his itinerary for the next few months, and Chris would tell the secretary not to give it to her because he knew she would be upset if she saw how often he was planning to travel. In 1981, after eleven years, their marriage failed rather abruptly. According to Marius, Barbara 'became extremely jealous of Chris, who persisted with his wandering eye until there was a final explosion between them.' This 'explosion' revolved around their housemaids' reports to Barbara that Chris had entertained two young women in their home when she had been away. Although he denied any impropriety, Barbara could not be persuaded, and initiated divorce proceedings.

If his first wife, Louwtjie, had shocked Chris by sending a car to meet him at the airport filled with his personal belongings, his second wife, Barbara, was equally decisive. The final break again came unexpectedly (for him) when he was on a visit to the USA; a phone call from his wife's lawyer informed him that he was not to return to the family home. Chris believed that, with some compromises on his side—curtailing his travelling, spending more time with his wife and family, and so on—this marriage might well have been saved, though personally I think there were more serious problems his wife was too discreet to make public. He had clearly not taken his wife's warnings seriously enough, and when the crunch arrived, he was shaken by her firmness and resolve to push through with the divorce.

Chris took temporary shelter with his two 'wonderful friends' Fritz and Maureen Brink, who collected him from the airport and gave him board and lodging in their Blouberg Strand Guesthouse (Rockhaven), beautifully situated on the rocks adjacent to the beach.

In his 1983 book, *Christiaan Barnard's Program for Living with Arthritis*, Chris gave his personal account of his relationship with Barbara and the events leading to his divorce, but I suggest they provide only a very slanted interpretation of these events. My understanding is that his wife, Barbara, did not agree and took legal action.

> She was young and beautiful, and we fell in love. The affair culminated in divorce from my first wife and marriage to Barbara. The effect on my arthritis, among other things, was dramatic … Certainly for several years after the wedding I virtually ceased to be an RA [rheumatoid arthritis] sufferer … Then came the bombshell. Barbara came to me one day saying she wanted a divorce. She had met a younger, more active man who, she said, could give her the sort of life that I could not … And then it came out that arthritis had played a major part in the breakdown of the marriage. Barbara was very active, and although she tolerated the fact that sometimes I was inactive as a result of arthritis, after we divorced she told friends and newspaper reporters that I used to sleep on Saturday afternoons and that I never used to play with the children or go out to the beach with her … I slept often during the weekends because I was exhausted by the inflammatory process that was burning in my body all the time—the constant pain … I had an extreme emotional reaction to the divorce. I felt that life was ended for me. I was terribly jealous because Barbara was going out with someone thirty years younger than I. [In fact, he is even much younger than she.] … The result was that I eventually felt that I was hopeless, physically, emotionally, sexually.
>
> I had never been jealous before in my life. If my wife doesn't love me, I thought, then she must do what she wants to do … I had no confidence, I had no desire to live, I contemplated suicide many times. And at those times I frequently blamed arthritis for my predicament.
>
> I honestly feel that I could have won Barbara back if it was not for my arthritis. I just couldn't do what she wanted me to do. If I had performed physically and sexually as well as this younger guy, she would have come back to me—or so I believed at the time … She was not prepared to

display the patience and understanding that I needed at that particular moment …

So there I was, an arthritic who blamed the loss of his wife on his disease and then found, to add injury to insult, that the marital breakdown was actually aggravating the arthritis. A truly vicious circle.

This account, obviously directed towards the readers of his book on arthritis, is of interest for several reasons. First, it is a good example of how, by providing anecdotal personal experience of the writer's own life experience, he or she (in this case, Chris) can capture the reader's attention in regard to a specific topic, in this case, the problems associated with suffering from rheumatoid arthritis. Second, it can be considered a good example of what I can only describe as 'propaganda' or at least a highly biased account (what the political pundits would now term 'spin') of the reasons underlying the divorce. As much as I admired and respected Chris, I do not believe for one moment that Barbara was so shallow to want to divorce him for the reasons he states. He totally ignored his own indiscretions and failings that might have contributed to the break-up of the marriage.

The account clearly suggested that Barbara had an affair with Chris that led to his divorce from Louwtjie, and also had an affair with the new man in her life before the break-up of her marriage to Chris. My understanding is that neither claim was true.

Indeed, while the divorce was proceeding, Chris wrote to a local newspaper claiming that Barbara was attracted to this other man because of his youth, and was 'ditching' Chris simply because he was getting old. This was clearly written to engender sympathy and support for his position. It reflected badly on Barbara. If my memory serves me correctly, when Barbara read Chris's comments (which were not very different from those which I have quoted from his book on arthritis), she immediately took legal action and Chris was forced to write a retraction of his claims. Chris does not come out of this episode with any 'Brownie' points, let alone covered in glory.

It is obvious that Chris, like many other husbands (and some wives), did not appreciate what he had in his spouse—a beautiful and elegant woman and, by all accounts, a very nice person who even visited his elderly mother each week—until it was too late. 'One of my mother's few pleasures,' he wrote, 'was the weekly visit made by Barbara. She took her cream doughnuts, which my mother loved, and stayed talking with her longer than any of her sons ever did. During my short monthly visits, she would often clasp her hand over her mouth in disbelief and say, "Chris, you are so lucky—she's such a good woman!"'

Chris either did not realise how fortunate he was, or like many of us, began to take his situation for granted, or his need for travel, high society, and extramarital liaisons was too strong for him to control.

## Visiting his Mother

The subject of him visiting his aged mother, Maria, had arisen on several occasions previously. After several years during which she was cared for by Louwtjie (and Chris) or Marius and his wife, she had to be admitted to a nursing home just before the first heart transplant. She had suffered a massive brain haemorrhage (stroke) some years previously and, after a period of coma, had survived, but the quality of her life was very poor. She remained largely paralyzed on one side, living (or, as Chris put it, 'existing') between her bed and wheelchair.

He did not believe his mother fully realised the changes that had taken place in his life. She was unaware that her son had become the most famous doctor in the world, nor did she have any memories for past events in her life. Barney, her eldest son, who lived in Cape Town, saw her perhaps once a year. Dodsley, who lived several hundred miles away in the northern Cape, had visited her only once during the six years that had passed since her stroke. Marius and Chris saw her more frequently, but Chris admitted 'certainly not as often as she would have visited us had the circumstances been reversed.'

While Louwtjie and Chris were still married, Louwtjie would frequently remind him to visit his mother who was resident in an old-people's home in the Cape Town area. She would ask him, sarcastically, 'Do you think, in your busy schedule, you can find time to go and see your mother again? You haven't been to see her since you've become famous.' Chris would not visit his mother, now aged eighty-five, for weeks or even months at a time, and to be reminded of this was painful to him.

Chris used this experience in one of his newspaper columns, which he titled 'Disposable People', from which I quote here.

> The room had all the soullessness of the institution, but the old woman had tried to make it her own, placing treasured possessions of a lifetime here and there like signals of her need to be somebody. 'Look! Look! I'm me!' they seemed to scream at the visitor, as if trying to blot out the effect of the too-polished floor, the sounds of people in the corridor and the official look of well-kept lawns beyond the window.
>
> A hand embroidered bedspread witnessed a life of loving and striving, of happiness in some great double bed of matrimony, of birth, illness and

inevitable death. A faded wedding photograph, the bride standing with her hand on the shoulder of her seated groom, as was the fashion of those days, and there had been youth and a joy in living. Other possessions added their chorus, a tale of a rich and full lifespan. Now she sat in that impersonal room, seeming almost shrunken in an overlarge chair, her head turned away from me, staring out of the window at the well-regulated garden.

Those eyes had seen more than seventy Karoo summers. At that moment it was doubtful if she could see anything through her tears. The hands, gnarled now and clasped in an attitude of uselessness on her lap, had been the hands of a lover, then later a mother, rearing a brood of strong sons under a Karoo sky.

The sons, grown to adulthood, had brought her here when the hands had become too fragile to cope with even her own simple needs. They were busy men, no doubt kindly, but each hard pressed with his own affairs and themselves fathers of families. They had brought her here in good faith, seeking the best that the bonds of family could wish, unaware that they were killing a loved one with strangers … Need we wonder, then, at a society which grants its senior citizens, after a lifetime of labor for the state, a pension just sufficient to kill them off in a genteel fashion from long-term malnutrition … These are the new Nothing People, no past and no future, for the past is safely isolated in some old-age cell and the future is left to the planners … Somebody like the old lady I told you about, sitting in her tidy, comfortable, well-serviced and lonely room. I still miss her. She was my mother.

The passage provides a poignant example of the sad circumstances that many elderly women (and a few men) find themselves in as they await death. Although it in no way excuses Chris (or his brothers) for not visiting her more frequently, at least he was honest in his appraisal of the situation. In my opinion, it is a well-written article that both paints a moving picture of the plight of many aged and infirm people, and also draws their plight to the readers' attention.

Chris's desire to hold onto Barbara had some unusual effects on him, and temporarily affected his judgment in odd ways. Perhaps the oddest was that he came to believe that an African 'witch doctor' (a *sangoma*) could cause the two women servants (who had 'spilled the beans' on him to Barbara) to suffer some form of punishment. He arranged to meet with this individual in a rather remote place on the Cape Flats (just outside of Cape Town), where the 'doctor' would bring evil spirits to bear on the women. Chris gave him a bottle of gin and R500 to speed up the process.

This story shocked me more than most other stories in my life. I could not understand how an intelligent and mature, scientifically trained surgeon could become involved with what can only be considered 'hocus pocus' and 'mumbo jumbo'. Later, I believe Chris could not understand how he had been so influenced himself. The incident illustrates how, under circumstances of severe emotional stress, even seemingly 'sane' people can make weird decisions.

Despite efforts on Chris's part to reunite them (even after the divorce), on 13 January 1982, a month before what would have been their twelfth wedding anniversary, the divorce was finalised in court (in Chris's absence). Their two sons were aged ten and seven, respectively, at the time, ages at which the major changes in their lives could well have impacted them emotionally. According to Chris, on this occasion, he was left with only his clothes, three pieces of furniture, and 'the bed and mattress on which I was supposed to have screwed this girl and screwed up my marriage.'

Deirdre pointed out:

It may seem a strange thing to say in the light of what happened to my father in his life, but he was old-fashioned in many ways. He believed in the institution of marriage and he believed in the family. My father, if you can believe it, wrote that he'd envisaged Barbara sitting alone at home after the divorce fretting over the loss of her 'wonderful husband', which just goes to show that his ideas about women were pretty outdated. It was something that was very hard for him to face up to. He couldn't bear the idea that there would ever be anyone else in Barbara's life, but of course she was a beautiful woman and a very nice person and it was inevitable that in time she would meet someone else. So it was not really surprising when she met and married Joe Silva.

I don't know how long it took before my father realised that the life he and Barbara had together was truly over. I think it may have been the evening he went back to Waiohai, the house in Constantia they'd once shared, and Joe—who was a frequent visitor there—offered him a drink. My father was the trespasser in what had once been his home, and Joe was the host. When Barbara, who had left the room to get ready for dinner, came back and asked him please to excuse them as they were about to eat, I think he finally realised that it truly was over.

Whereas Chris had bounced back from his first divorce quickly, and I believe with few regrets, the break-up of his second marriage plunged him into deep depression for several months. He would come to our research laboratory and tell us how upset and depressed he was. I am sure he bitterly regretted that his marriage had failed as it had been clear to all who knew him that Barbara was possibly 'the great love of his life'. Deirdre's view was that in Barbara my father found a particular mixture of attributes that was exactly right for him.'

During this period of depression, he sought help and counseling from his close friend, the Roman Catholic priest, Tom Nicholson. He told Tom that if he could get Barbara (a Roman Catholic) to return to him, he would become a Roman Catholic himself (which would have had his father turning in his grave). Tom told me that Chris would sit in his office and cry over the breakup of his marriage. 'He was a very emotional person and would cry quite frequently.' Remembering this time, Tom wrote, 'the great healer needed healing. He came to me. The mending of this heart took much more time than a bypass. It took hours and hours, days and nights, of sweat and tears and talking. If ever I came across a broken reed, this was it. But he was and is a man of rare courage, and time, coupled with the acceptance of the things we cannot change, proved once again to be a great healer.'

According to Dene Friedmann, 'Chris often told me that divorce was worse than death as death was so final, but with divorce the partners were still living, which made it much more painful.' Dene once said to Chris that, even if he got Barbara back, he would have continued his 'itinerant' lifestyle. He grinned at her while he was saying 'no, he would change.' She knew he would never have changed. In her opinion, 'he was a huge "ladies man", and couldn't resist a conquest.' The urge was to be with him forever.

Chris later wrote, 'There can be no more saddening experience than to sit in a divorce court and watch the legal process dissolve years of commitment in a few minutes.' However, ignoring the fact that he did not attend the divorce court, whether personally he had made a sufficient 'commitment' can certainly be questioned.

He also wrote, 'Quickie divorce has been likened to a street accident, the sudden disaster which hurls you instantly from the warmth and safety of familiar surroundings to a strange country of physical pain and mental anguish.' He certainly suffered months of anguish but, after a prolonged period of very considerable depression, he adapted to his changed circumstances, and bounced back to his usual self. He found himself again, at the age of fifty-nine, the eligible bachelor.

Nevertheless, Chris always retained a great affection for Barbara. When several years later, after both of them had remarried, she told him she had been diagnosed with cancer, he spent a great deal of time and an immense amount of energy to try to find a treatment that might help her. Sadly, his efforts proved futile and Barbara died in 1998 at the early age of forty-eight.

Deirdre recorded:

> My father was devastated at Barbara's funeral ... he wept inconsolably,
> like a child. His great friend Emiliano, of the La Vita restaurant days
> [when he and Chris shared ownership of the restaurant], the scene of so
> many good times and parties including my own wedding, put his arms
> around him to comfort him. I know that because of all that had passed
> between Barbara and him, because of all the happy memories he must
> have had of her, in that moment of final parting my father was beyond
> comfort.

I wonder whether there was an element of guilt in Chris's grief—not
because of his behaviour that contributed to their divorce, but for the
following reason. When Barbara was dying and he went to see her, she
asked him not to travel but to stay with her while she was dying. However,
he had already made some commitments abroad and so he still continued
travelling, perhaps again illustrating his addiction to the 'high life' or his
need to be the centre of attention, as he frequently was when abroad.
Many would consider his decision on this occasion—to put his own wishes
ahead of those of his dying ex-wife—to be inexcusable. When he returned
to Cape Town, Barbara, who was very disappointed by his decision not
to stay with her when she clearly needed his support, refused to see him,
again demonstrating her firmness and resolve, which greatly upset him.
Chris's behaviour on this occasion must surely be very unusual.

One can only admire the immensely dignified and courageous manner
in which Barbara faced her death. Before she became too debilitated, she
called on all her friends to say 'goodbye'. Thereafter, in the final weeks of
her life, she asked them not to visit her, but relied on the support of her
close family and Father Tom, who had been her trusted confidante and
counsellor for many years. Her last days were spent at home, cared for by
her second husband and her children. At her request, her funeral service
was conducted by Father Tom in his modest parish church in Plumstead, a
suberb of Cape Town, where she had always attended Mass.

Barbara's death from breast cancer followed only three years after her
mother's death from the same disease. After his wife's death, Fred Zoellner
donated a large sum (£1.5 million) to the University of Cambridge in the
UK to establish funds for research into cancer treatment. Chris acted as a
conduit between Barbara's father and the university. It surprised me that
the donation should have been directed to the University of Cambridge
and not to the University of Cape Town. As a young man, however, Fred
Zoellner had spent a year as a student in Cambridge and this may have
influenced his thinking, or he may have felt that the future of advanced

medical research was going to be limited in South Africa, as indeed it has now become.

My understanding (from a source at Cambridge who was involved in the transactions) is that Mr Zoellner first intended to make his donation to the Max Planck Institute in his native Germany, but Chris suggested Cambridge to him, and proceeded to make contact with members of the University. The Cambridge authorities were, of course, delighted to receive such a generous donation, and the Zoellner Chair in cancer research was duly established. However, Chris then requested 'a big present' from the University to recognise his role as a facilitator, a request that shocked and dismayed the senior University officers. Eventually, it was agreed that Chris would be paid a retainer (or salary) for the next few years to work as a 'fundraiser' to augment Mr Zoellner's initial donation. To say the least, he did not prove very active in this role. The episode left a 'bad taste in the mouths' of the University hierarchy who had been involved in the transaction, and does not reflect well on Chris.

## André's Death

The second traumatic event was the death of Chris's oldest son, André (on 29 February 1984). By this time, André was a young doctor in Cape Town, married with a young family. During a period of severe depression, for which he was taking prescription medication (and, I have heard from a reliable source, certain illegal drugs), André was found dead at his home one morning, having fallen asleep and drowned in his bath while under the influence of some drugs. Whether his death was accidental or not remained uncertain, although it seems most likely it was accidental. The death of his oldest son was a shattering blow to Chris. He later wrote, 'Grief is pain beyond belief,' and I suspect this related to the loss of André.

On reflection of André's short life, Chris felt ashamed that 'I remembered very little of where André had been on various important occasions' in his life. 'Where had my son been when I was given the Freedom of the City of Cape Town, where was he when Frederick and Christiaan were born?' It is interesting that Chris picks out events that were important to him, but not necessarily to André. Where was Chris when André got married? Where was he when André's children were born?

Chris had known of André's drug problems for some time. Some months prior to André's death, he had been called urgently by the professor of medical jurisprudence, who informed him that narcotic inspectors were aware André frequently bought prescription drugs, such as Wellconal and pethidine, which he had prescribed for himself. When Chris confronted

André with what he had learned, his son expressed relief that his father now knew. Chris later wrote that André professed that 'it started so innocently but now I can't control it. It was a stupid thing to do and I have to stop.' Tom Nicholson was sure that André was taking hard drugs intravenously during his last few years.

Chris made arrangements for André to see a psychologist, but by his own admission, 'I never bothered to check on his progress afterwards—my parental concern ended there.' Again, Chris is damned by his own (honest) words. Presumably, Chris was too wrapped up in his own life to devote sufficient time to the rehabilitation of his troubled son. At a time when André really needed some fatherly love and attention, Chris undoubtedly failed him.

Later, André was admitted to Groote Schuur Hospital, where Chris had to obtain special permission to visit him (presumably because the psychiatrist caring for André saw Chris as part of the problem). André had clearly deteriorated further, his personal life falling apart around him. Chris wrote, 'It broke my heart to see my son in this neglected state—dressed in jeans, unshaven and with no pride.' Chris's opinion was that 'my poor son—probably because of lack of support from me—had grown up being unable to cope with the cruel world around him. So he'd chosen the easiest way.'

However, André's condition temporarily improved, and he was able to leave hospital and return to his family and job at the Red Cross Children's Hospital and to what Chris called 'the harsh realities of life.' Chris admitted that André had not been a sufficient part of his (Chris's) life and that he had not played a sufficient part in André's life. He vowed to give André more attention. He convinced himself it was 'never too late'. However, Chris was again distracted from his good intentions as he had other commitments, such as being a celebrity speaker on a luxury cruise liner. He delayed contacting André.

Chris was again abroad when he received a telephone call from Fritz Brink, giving him the tragic news of his son's death. 'I have very bad news for you,' Fritz said. 'André committed suicide last night.' There remains considerable doubt that his death was a suicide. Death from drowning while drugged seems much more likely. Father Tom Nicholson reported that the psychiatrists caring for André did not believe he was suicidal.

Chris later wrote, 'While I was wining and dining on a luxury cruise in a fantasy world, my poor son was struggling to get to grips with real life. I was going to show how much I loved him when I got back! I sobbed into the empty room ... My words sounded hollow and my hands began to shake uncontrollably.' Chris deeply regretted he had not phoned André, 'or at least sent him a card', but now it was too late.

Chris returned home at once, embarking on the 'saddest journey' he had ever made. He was met at Cape Town airport by the inevitable photographers and journalists. There were dozens of them to 'welcome' him home. According to Chris, they had 'come to see whether they could capture my grief on film.' Chris's only comfort was that André, whose 'quality of life had deteriorated to the extent where there was no joy in living', had gone 'to a far better place than that from which he'd come.'

Some days later, when André's funeral service (held at the crematorium, and conducted by Father Tom, specifically at Louwtjie's request) ended, and the mourners had left the chapel, Chris turned back and 'could see black smoke coming from the chimney of the crematorium. All that remained of my son was a handful of ashes.'

With hindsight, Chris doubted whether during his last few months André could have been cured. 'The opportunity for treatment had been lost. I should have given him the love and affection he needed when he was still a little boy. It was my fault,' he concluded with honesty and without attempting to excuse himself.

What impact the divorce of his parents had on André when he was just a teenager will now never be known, but it was obvious to his family and friends that it was an emotionally stressful event for him. Leaving school one afternoon, André had read about his parents' separation on the newspaper posters. In retrospect, Chris realised the impact that 'such shocking news' could have on a boy of that age. He was also to learn of his father's engagement to Barbara and their wedding through the press, rather than directly from Chris. Communication between parents—Chris, in particular—and their children left something to be desired when it came to these personal matters.

Deirdre, with her great ability to 'weather the storms' that she faced in life, wrote:

My brother and I in our separate ways had learnt of our parents' divorce and [later] of my father's remarriage when we read the news on newspaper placards. As desirable ways of being told of a final and painful decision go, on a scale of one to ten, I would rate this pretty low down. My brother, who was doing his national service in the navy when news of my father's engagement to Barbara broke, was deeply distressed. The matter was so public that Admiral Biermann, then chief of the Navy, gave him a week's compassionate leave and sent him home to my mother for her to help him through it.

Deirdre remembered André as 'a nice, normal boy, pleasant to look at, with a good sense of humour, extremely gifted in some areas, just about average in others. Which is to say he was just the same as the rest of us. The trouble is that I am not quite sure how easy it is to be "normal" and stay that way when you happen to find yourself in a family like ours.' She realised:

> While I was taking up so much of his [Chris's] time and allowing him to fill my life the way he did, my brother, who was different from me and whose interests were different from mine, was losing out … I had always felt as if my father had somehow singled me out. I had thought that what made us special was that we were such a good team. I really had moments when I was on a high, when there was the 'rush' of having won and the slightly euphoric feeling that goes with it. It was only later that I realised that, as with everything else in life, this came with a price tag. It can be very hard when half the world seems to own a bit of your father. It was hard for my brother and it was hard for me.

André, who had always taken a 'back seat', began to move further and further away from the family despite the efforts of his mother and sister to engage him. However, Deirdre noted that 'André had also been sent away to school, probably as this was thought to be best for him during a period of turmoil at home, but he may have interpreted this as being unwanted.'

In her memoirs, Louwtjie Barnard, who was deeply upset by André's death, had described him as 'an attractive, sensitive young man and a deep thinker. He takes life very seriously, accepting nothing, questioning everything. He has already found courage, faith and strength. Deirdre and I love and respect him. He has taken his place as the man in the house.'

It may be that, inadvertently, this added to the stress of André's young life—to take on the role of the 'man of the house' when in his mid-teens. With his father now largely absent from his life and home, the burden of responsibility felt by André may have taken its psychological toll. Deirdre also mentions this point.

> André and I were very different in temperament. I realise now that because of the direction in which his own life had borne him, he had in a sense missed out on a crucial phase of his growing-up. He had, by his own choice, assumed a man's role when he was really no more than a boy … My brother, I knew, had been deeply unhappy, plagued by the kind of despair none of us seemed able to find any cure for.

Furthermore, after his divorce from their mother, Chris's glamorous new world did not hold the same attractions for André as it did for Deirdre. She wanted to be a part of it, 'even though to do so meant undergoing a kind of sea change as you moved from one world into another that was so very different', but André did not.

André never recovered from the divorce, and was always considered to be a 'sad' person by Father Tom, who played golf with him every week when he was a student at UCT and therefore got to know him well. André missed his graduation ceremony because he knew it would not be possible for both his parents to be there at the same time. His mother was probably more bitter than Chris, but he wanted them either to be there, or to have no ceremony. Tom told me that Chris's first wife was always a difficult person throughout life, even into old age.

There were occasions when Chris tried to bridge the gap between him and his son. For example, after his marriage to Barbara, knowing André's love of the British radio comedy, *The Goon Show* (a ground-breaking 1950s programme of very offbeat humour) Chris introduced André to the British actor Peter Sellers, who had been a prominent member of the 'Goons'. When Sellers came to South Africa (to learn from Chris what could be done about his coronary artery disease), Chris and Barbara gave a party so that André and his friends could meet the famous comedian, who entertained them informally throughout the evening.

## The Peter Sellers Connection

As an aside, the story of the interaction between Chris and the comedian varied slightly whenever Chris put it into print, but essentially it was as follows. Chris had first met Peter Sellers at a cocktail party in England to launch his book, *Heart Attack: You Don't Have to Die,* which he had written with considerable help from a medical colleague at UCT, Eugene Dowdle. Sellers was invited to the party as he had suffered a massive heart attack a few years earlier. Chris advised Sellers to undergo coronary artery surgery. As he thought it would be helpful to the actor to watch a coronary artery bypass graft operation, Sellers flew to Cape Town to observe Chris perform one but, as soon as he left GSH, he fled the country without even waiting to say goodbye. Presumably, watching the operation had not had the intended effect, but had proved too stressful for him.

Sellers subsequently consulted a faith healer or mystic in Manila in the Philippines. When Chris next bumped into Sellers, at the palace of King Hussein of Jordan, the actor told him 'Chris, I'm completely cured!' He claimed that the 'healer' had performed eleven operations on him in his hotel room without anaesthetic. Chris again urged his friend to see a cardiologist, if only to confirm the cure, but within a few months, Sellers was dead.

The fact that Chris met a friend who was a world-famous actor when they were both guests at a king's palace illustrates Chris's life during these years—quite different from his life before the first transplant and quite different from the average surgeon.

Chris was pleased when André decided to study medicine as this gave them a common interest, and he was pleased and proud when André joined him at the Red Cross Children's Hospital when he was presented with a gift to mark his retirement. However, father and son were never anywhere near as close as father and daughter.

There had been occasions when they felt close. In one of his newspaper columns, Chris wrote of one such occasion. When André was a final year medical student at UCT, not long before graduating as a doctor, he asked Chris to be his guest at the final-year dinner.

It was the kind of celebration every student knows, food and wine with good friends and happy conversation. He was obviously well-liked in his group. Afterwards we walked under the trees in the dark while he told me of his hopes for the future. They were high hopes. They took in the whole world. I realised then I was talking to a dedicated doctor. There are times in one's life when gratitude overflows. That was one of those moments. I felt very privileged and grateful for just being there.

Perhaps the family felt that André was gaining some stability when he met an English nurse, Gail, who was working in Cape Town, and they planned to marry. Gail was older than André and, for obscure reasons, Chris did not approve of her. Barbara and Chris held an engagement party for them at their home in Constantia, but Chris did not want to give a speech, though Father Tom persuaded him to do so. During the speech, Chris either could not remember Gail's name, or chose to make out that he could not remember it, which was embarrassing to everybody. Their wedding took place in the UK in 1978, but Chris did not attend it, though Louwtjie did. Even after the birth of his two children, however, André remained depressed and in need of the support that certain drugs could give him.

For years, Deirdre had watched André 'carrying a terrible sadness inside himself. He had reminded me of Atlas, the man with the world on his shoulders, but with his death that too had ended ... it was almost as if I could see that great heavy burden simply being lifted from him and André being free, walking upright again.'

André certainly received less attention from Chris than he should during the period when Chris was so heavily committed to his hospital work and when his spare time was taken up with training Deirdre as a water skier. This and the later turbulence in their family life, culminating in his parents' unhappy divorce, may well have contributed towards his depressive illness, and drug-taking, at an early age. Anyone, however, who saw the newspaper photograph of an overwhelmingly distraught and tearful Chris at his son's funeral can be in no doubt of the agony which the bereaved father suffered at this time, nor could anyone doubt the father's love for his son (Figure 22.i).

As might be expected, the press treated André's funeral not merely as a sad ending to a tragic episode, but as an opportunity to question Chris's relationship with his son. Chris was hurt and upset by one journalist, and wrote:

> Most destructive was the unlovely soul who dug around in a newspaper file to find a fifteen-year-old point of dissension between me and my dead son and then wrote it into an account of the funeral. All of us at times add to the sum of human unhappiness. Some out of love, some from hate—which is simply the other side of the same coin—and some for profit. The last category is the least forgivable.

Cape Town journalist, Bob Molloy, recalled this same tragic period of Chris's life.

> At the funeral service, photographers poked long lenses into private grief. Some reporters told their readers who sat where, who wept and who didn't. Long before the inquest, the media had flown every speculative kite a grubby mind could concoct, completely insensitive to the pain of the grieving family. One female reporter struck bone with quotes from a letter written to Barnard by his son as a young boy. In the letter the youngster, in anguish at the family breakup after divorce, harshly criticised his father. The breach, long since healed, had faded into family history until dragged anew into public gaze by the eager digging of a media harpie. While a father grieved for his son, the press lashed him for sins long forgiven.

Subsequently, when Chris was being interviewed by Tim Sebastian on American television, he was asked how he felt when his son died. Deirdre reported:

> My father replied very calmly. He spoke of his sadness at putting off a talk he'd been wanting to have with my brother. He had known he was troubled and had wanted to help him. His response was so calm and measured that you would almost have thought the moment had passed

and yet, after the question was answered, my father began to weep. It was a terrible thing to see. I couldn't bear to watch. I couldn't look at it without weeping myself for the sadness of it, because I am a part of my father just as my brother was. In front of millions of viewers my father wept for my brother, a man unable to contain his grief, his breaking for all to see. If you asked me what it was like to be Christiaan Barnard, then I would tell you that is how it was. You might consider this and then ask yourself if, given all the fame, the accolades and the good times, you really would choose to change places.

Nazih Zuhdi, the heart surgeon who later invited Chris to join him in establishing a heart transplant programme in Oklahoma City, also noted Chris's emotion whenever he spoke of his late son. Dr Zuhdi wrote, 'His eyes well up with tears at the thought of his son who passed away years ago, and trickle slowly down his cheeks.'

Chris addressed the subject of parenting in one of his later newspaper columns. He wrote, 'The problem with human parents is that many invest only money in the rearing of their children. Money is a poor substitute for time. If you haven't got the time, your money will only buy you grief.' Sadly, he must have been writing from personal experience.

Chris would appear to have had a better relationship with his two sons by his second wife: Frederick and Christiaan, Jnr (Figure 22.ii). For some years, Chris and Barbara were enjoying a generally happy marriage, providing a more stable environment for Frederick and Christiaan, Jnr, whereas André was surrounded by considerable tension and occasional bitterness by both his mother and father throughout much of his childhood. When married to Barbara, Chris joined in all the family's religious activities at the Catholic church, even though he was never a Catholic himself. If Barbara was away, he made sure the boys attended the church and followed all the religious rules. Although Barbara did not feel Chris spent enough time with his sons, he probably spent more time with them as they grew up than he had with his eldest son, who grew up during the period of Chris's maximum work commitment and activity (and, of course, his early celebrity traveling). Those of us in medicine, and particularly those in such a physically, mentally, and emotionally demanding specialty as heart surgery, will know just how difficult it is to ensure time for family activities, especially early in one's career. Competition between work and family has led to many divorces and many unhappy and disturbed children.

In one of his newspaper articles, Chris recounts a touching moment.

My seven-year-old son, Frederick, met me at the door as I arrived home. It had been a long day and a tough one and I was feeling every year of my age. As I bent down to his hello he threw his arms around my neck and asked: 'Daddy, are you famous?' The question caught me unawares. I must have mumbled something because he added: 'The other boys at school say you are.' Suddenly I knew that my son was proud of me. I'm sure it's been a helluva long time since a knight in full armor came riding home after killing the dragon. There can't be many people around who can remember the last occasion. But at that moment I knew exactly how it felt.

Chris had been given honours 'in glittering ceremonies attended by nobles and national leaders. I have known adulation you wouldn't believe. An exhibition of these honours and medals some years ago in Cape Town was described by a journalist as "an Aladdin's cave of treasures".' However, the knowledge that his little son was proud of him meant more to Chris than all of these other accolades.

## Thoughts Turn to Retirement

No longer with his brother's support, Chris found the chores of running a big and busy department increasingly onerous and irksome, and his thoughts turned to early retirement, although he had begun to contemplate this as early as 1978. This was the period in which, in retrospect, he believed he should have retired earlier. The medical school authorities persuaded him to remain in the post while they gave consideration to a successor. This he agreed to do, though later he came to regret this decision as he felt his reputation suffered during this period when he took little active interest in the activities of his department. He spent less and less time in the operating room and ward, and although the transplant programme and research laboratory maintained his interest longest, he eventually became little more than a spectator in his own department. In his final year on the staff, we saw him only on a handful of occasions.

Chris's approach to surgery had always been 'all or nothing'; he had to be involved in everything or nothing. It was not in his nature to delegate, as Marius had discovered. He had to be in charge and know exactly what was going on in his department. To give up the reins was clearly against his nature and was not the way he wanted to live life. However, sadly, during his final one or two years at GSH, he knew little of what was taking place in his department.

He readily admitted that he had begun to lose interest in surgery. 'On many mornings, I'd look for excuses not to go to the hospital,' he wrote.

Fortunately, he had surrounded himself with a small group of gifted young surgeons—Joe de Nobrega, Jannie Hassoulas, and Hector Sanchez—who, in my opinion, continued the high surgical standards the department was known for. The reliable Rodney Hewitson had taken responsibility for all of the non-cardiac thoracic surgery (mainly lung surgery) as early as 1972.

When Chris did come into the hospital or visited Red Cross Children's Hospital, he found he no longer knew the names of any of the patients, and frequently, he could not identify a single one he had operated on. He wondered how he had turned his back on what had been such an important part of his life for twenty-five years, a career that had given him 'so much joy and recognition. Was it because I no longer saw a challenge in heart surgery?' he asked himself. The younger surgeons had taken over and, although in his younger days he had clearly been jealous of his junior surgical colleagues, such as Bob Frater, he now found that he 'wasn't jealous in the least. I was quite willing to bow out gracefully and without a single regret.'

By this time (the early 1980s), Chris's phenomenal energy and zest for surgery had clearly waned. His overt reason for requesting early retirement (and, importantly, receiving his full, well-deserved pension) was that the rheumatoid arthritis—from which he had suffered for many years and which affected his hands as well as the joints in his legs—was steadily getting worse, making it increasingly difficult for him to operate. Several times, he told me that he was never without pain in his hands and several other joints. Even those of us who experience pain rarely can appreciate the relentless burden of never being free of pain. Thus, the effect of his battle with arthritis should not be ignored.

However, there is no doubt that the major reason for his request for retirement was that, by this time, he had lost interest in the day-to-day problems of heart surgery and, particularly, in running his department. 'When I retired in 1983,' he later wrote, 'they said it was because I had arthritis but that was just an excuse. Actually, it was because I wasn't hungry for the work anymore. I'd lost my enthusiasm.' Fortunately, his junior colleagues could carry out the various operations required of them. Hector Sanchez (originally from Argentina) and Jannie Hassoulas (a Greek South African) were excellent paediatric heart surgeons, the very experienced Joe Nobrega, Dimitri Novitzky, and I could cope with the routine adult heart surgery, and Dimitri and I ran the transplant program. The research lab was organised by Winston Wicomb, and, whenever essential, Chris asked me or one of my colleagues to attend important hospital meetings in his place. Even when he had been fully active, I do not believe he ever enjoyed administrative meetings and did his best to avoid them.

In one of his weekly newspaper articles, in which Chris described his situation at that time, he explained, 'I've never been a good spectator. Either I'm playing the game or I'm not interested ... There is no life situation that a spectator can look at from outside without missing part of the action. Anyone who has anything to do with advising others in their life problems should have that phrase mounted in bronze on their desks.'

At the end of 1983, he could wait no longer and, at the age of sixty-one, he took early retirement from his post at the University of Cape Town and its associated hospitals. On 31 December 1983, he left his office at the medical school for the last time (Figure 22.iii). With his retirement, this effectively ended his productive contributions to heart surgery and transplantation.

The 'burn out' that Chris (and possibly also Marius) had experienced from the continual stresses and strains of the highly demanding career of a heart (or organ transplant) surgeon is not uncommon. I know of many surgeons who felt the need to change career direction after several years in heart surgery. Many move into medical administration (for example, as a dean or sub-dean of a medical school or similar academic institution) or into healthcare administration, and others move into full-time research (as I did) or teaching. Still others take early retirement, as did Chris, some of whom follow a latent interest that has been on their minds for years, such as painting, cabinet-making, the study of history, or travel, or, in Marius's case, politics. For example, I know one former heart surgeon who retired very early and trained for the much less stressful position of a pathologist and, still later, trained as a chef, an option that had been fermenting in his mind for years.

I am sure Chris could have arranged to remain at UCT in a research capacity but, with his many other interests, I think by this time he wanted to make a complete break. However, looking back at his adolescence in Beaufort West when he had had to run home from 'illicit' dances with girls, he wrote, 'Heart surgery isn't standing still. Research is always exciting, and the undiscovered the most exciting of all. I will no longer be part of it. How does it feel? Just the same as that teenage kid felt—it's hard to leave while the music is still playing.' Nevertheless, the need to leave was overpowering for him.

Elsewhere, as he stepped out 'of a lifetime's concern with medicine and heart surgery,' he wrote, 'I feel as if I am deserting a child, though a child grown bigger and more sophisticated than I could ever have dreamed the day I assembled the first heart-lung machine at Groote Schuur Hospital.'

However, he had no regrets over his decision. His opinion was that 'If you wake up in the morning and you no longer look forward to your job, drop it and do something else.' He believed you should do a job 'with all one's heart or not at all.' Indeed, he believed that was good advice for life, not just a job.

GSH organised a formal farewell event to mark Chris's retirement, but his description of it in *The Second Life* does not sound as if it was a raucous occasion.

> After tea and sandwiches and the obligatory speech by the [medical] superintendent I received my gift 'for twenty-five years of faithful service', which was wrapped in a long box. A Rolex watch, I thought as I impatiently ripped off the wrapping paper. It was a hospital tie, the back label of which proclaimed it to be washable. There was also a party at the Red Cross Hospital which André, who was now a paediatrician, also attended and I was very proud to have him standing next to me. I didn't receive any gift at all there—perhaps they'd decided that one tie between the two hospitals was enough.

With his characteristic honesty (and lack of tact), Chris used the opportunity of his retirement party at GSH to criticise what he perceived as the falling standards of the clinical care being provided by the hospital. As a member of the faculty at that time, although there are always limitations to the care a national health service can provide, I must say I thought the standards remained pretty high at GSH. As Chris had not participated in any meaningful way in the care of patients in his department during the previous year, if not rather longer, I am not sure on what he based his opinion.

Chris's colleagues and juniors in his department arranged a more informal retirement party for him at his own restaurant, La Vita. The feelings of several long-standing members of his team were summarised by Pittie Rautenbach. When she looked back on the 'wonderful party at his own restaurant, La Vita, at Newlands, it was exactly twenty years after I had started training as one of his team, and I was sad, so sad that I hardly touched the delicious food served to us. To have worked for twenty years with a person of such drive, professionalism and perfectionism as Professor Barnard cannot leave anybody untouched.' In contrast to his GSH present, as a farewell gift, we gave him something we knew he would certainly appreciate (Figures 22.iv and 22.v).

Chris was made an Emeritus Professor of the University of Cape Town, which Professor Jannie Louw noted 'holds him in the greatest esteem, despite his own obstinate opinion to the contrary.' Early in 1984 the university established the Chris Barnard Chair of Cardiothoracic Surgery, to which Bruno Reichart from Munich, Germany, was appointed from 1 September 1984.

# Museums

At about the time of Chris's retirement, the citizens of his home town of Beaufort West showed their respect and affection by opening a museum in his honour, the 'Dr Chris Barnard Museum'. By this time, Chris's relationship with the citizens of the town had been assuaged by their efforts to renovate his father's church. The museum outlines his achievements and contains mementos of his career, including the many awards and honours bestowed upon him by states and institutions around the world (Figure 22.vi). Several of his colleagues in Cape Town, including myself, attended the opening ceremony and the reception that followed. One prominent absentee was Marius, who had never forgiven the citizens of the town for the way they had demeaned his father, who was treated by some with contempt for ministering to the coloured community.

Later, after the new GSH was opened, a museum was established in the old hospital; the Heart of Cape Town Museum opened on 3 December 2007, the fortieth anniversary of the first heart transplant. It preserved the actual operating theatre in which the first heart transplant was performed as well as many other memorabilia of Barnard and his team. There is also an excellent video interview with Chris in which he reminiscences about the historic operation. In my opinion, the museum is well worth a visit.

The museum had a collection of children's paintings sent to Chris after the first transplant, and also letters in various languages from children from around the world. One child wrote that 'heart transplantation is the greatest advance since false teeth.' Another asked how you would do a transplant, as she had two birds and wanted to do a heart transplant between them. Chris replied to most of them and wrote this little girl that she should visit his laboratory to see how to do it as it was not possible to explain it in detail. He was also sent a letter stating that he now had honorary membership of the London Playboy Club.

There were letters or telegrams of congratulations from many surgeons, including Drs Wangenstein, Lillihei, Shumway, DeBakey, Kantrowitz, and Cooley. There was a telegram from his former colleague, Walter Phillips, from New York City dated 5 December 1967. I was also interested to see another from the Royal College of Surgeons of England, signed by Sir Hedley Atkins, who was at that time the President of the College and had been a mentor of mine as a medical student at Guy's.

The lack of knowledge about South Africa by many in the world was illustrated by a letter from a UCT graduate living in the US, who said he was often asked why he wasn't black, and did lions roam through his backyard. The graduate was pleased that the transplant had been carried out as it put UCT and South Africa on the map.

There were, however, some critical letters. One mailed from Virginia in the USA stated that 'It is my profound conviction you are unmoral. A bunch of ghouls, all of you.' From Sussex in the UK came a 'memo to the great heartless transplanter. Well done, Messer-abouter. Transplanting pays you, does it not? If not, by good results, it does pay you from the money viewpoint?' A letter from Hong Kong called him a 'prime monster', and a writer from Melbourne, Australia, informed Chris that he had written to the chief of police in Cape Town advising him that Barnard should be arrested for murder.

No matter what a person does with his or her life later, retirement from one's major career activity is a big step in anyone's life. A retiree may look back on their contributions to society. A year or two before his retirement, Chris presented some of his thoughts on this topic in a newspaper article, 'Medicine Means Standing Up To Be Counted'. Contrary to what one might expect, it made depressing reading because he returned to the problem of malnutrition, which clearly concerned him.

What do you do when you take a look back at your whole career and realise with a jolt that you may have been barking up the wrong tree? In the almost fourteen years of heart transplants in South Africa we have operated on fifty-seven patients, of whom seventeen are alive. Of the remainder, a number had been granted good quality life long past the prognosis given before the transplant. Two have lived more than twelve years. It wasn't the transplant statistics that were worrying me, it was a report by the World Health Organization ... In a brief glance at the contents one fact stood out as if embossed on the paper—a statement that made nonsense of all our efforts. It said that in the previous fourteen-year period—the time it took us to rescue seventeen people from imminent death using the world's most expensive medical technology—some 400-million children worldwide had died of malnutrition. Looking at the world as a whole, our efforts vanished in the sea of misery in which mankind appears to spend most of its existence.

Although these data do question the wisdom of investing time, effort, and money in treating a relative handful of patients by heart transplantation, Chris underestimated the impact his work has had in medicine. Heart transplantation has by now proved life-saving to thousands of patients who would otherwise have died from terminal heart failure, and has stimulated the development of mechanical devices that can support a failing heart (ventricular assist devices) or replace it (total artificial hearts), which are now implanted into thousands more each year. The major limitation to heart transplantation is the limited number of suitable donor organs that become available each year, but this problem is likely to be solved by the use of genetically engineered pig hearts. Chris's contributions were therefore important and essential predecessors to innovations that will advance medicine considerably further.

Chris's enthusiasm for heart surgery had waned, but he had not lost his enthusiasm for life. He was keen to explore other opportunities and interests. From 1984, therefore, he directed his energy to other endeavours and expanded on those that he had already developed.

# 23

# Money Matters:
# Business Opportunities

'Many things drove my father,' wrote Deirdre, 'sometimes at great cost to those closest to him. He knew this and said so, but one thing he was never driven by was money.'

Although Deirdre was generally very perceptive about her father's actions and motivations, I am not sure this particular statement was entirely correct. Although Chris was never driven to make money from his surgical skills, after he became a celebrity, he took the opportunities provided to increase his income from several business ventures, some of which proved controversial. He was also paid handsomely for many of his speaking engagements. In these activities, I suggest his major motivation was to increase income so that he could, first, support his family, which was steadily enlarging, and, second, continue to live in the lifestyle to which he had become accustomed, partly through his marriage to the wealthy Barbara, and partly though his travels as a VIP.

His income as a surgeon from the Western Cape authorities had been sufficient for his needs in South Africa, but had been 'derisory' in comparison with what he might have earned in the US, for example, or even in the UK, if he had participated in private practice as well as in the National Health Service, as most of the London cardiac surgeons were doing. Once he began to experience the lifestyle of the glitterati, his needs naturally increased, very considerably, if he were not to be totally outshone. Particularly after his retirement, he was always pleased to accept an invitation that paid him well. Eventually, it is my understanding that, when he was in his seventies, he obtained the services of an agent who requested a substantial fee for Chris to lecture abroad, although the fees he requested nowhere matched the speakers' fees charged by most modern former politicians and other notables.

As a surgeon employed full-time by the Cape Provincial Administration, and thus one who had chosen not to be entitled to charge patients a fee for his services, Chris's income had never been high and it was, of course, substantially reduced after his retirement. On occasions, he had turned down lucrative offers of surgical work abroad, choosing to remain in his beloved South Africa, though he had, of course, accepted other invitations that provided income. Furthermore, when occasionally asked to see a wealthy patient, sometimes when he was traveling overseas, as far as I am aware, he never charged a fee for his professional opinion. When foreign patients were flown into Cape Town for a heart operation, he again never charged a personal fee.

When, in 1992, I requested Gloria Craig, a friend of Chris's family, to provide me with her reminiscences of him, she commented on his willingness to advise patients wherever he was without considering any financial remuneration. When once on vacation in Greece, she remembered:

> Chris visited the hospital on Rhodes, and 'worked' almost every day, even though he was on holiday and at the time his arthritis was troubling him quite a lot. At the same time people were approaching me at the hotel because I was part of the Barnard party—visitors, staff, etc.—begging to be allowed to be examined by the good Professor. He eventually examined every one of them, free of charge, as well as all the patients at the hospital.

His relative lack of 'greed' is perhaps illustrated by an occasion of which I had knowledge through someone who was present at the time. After his retirement, he was approached by a foreign businessman who wanted to explore a business venture in one of the 'homelands', set up by the South African government to create the impression that the black populations were being given equal opportunities for development as the white population. As the homelands were situated in rural parts of the country where resources were generally poor or non-existent, there was no reality that they provided equal opportunities. However, the homelands had their own governments—some would claim them to be 'puppets' of the South African government—that could make some decisions about their 'state'.

The businessman wanted Chris to accompany him to meet the president of one of the homelands, and Chris finally agreed. The 'carrot' was that, if the deal were made, Chris would receive a large sum of money for his role as the facilitator. After the businessman's proposal had been presented to the president and his cabinet, the president asked to speak with Chris (and my informant) in private. The three men left the room, and the president asked for Chris's advice. Was the proposed deal in the best interests of his people? Chris answered honestly, 'No, it's a crap deal,' and the discussion ended there. The businessman went away disappointed, pondering why his proposal had been declined, and Chris departed without improving his financial position. A less principled man would have persuaded the president to accept the deal.

However, at about the time of his retirement, Chris accepted several financially attractive opportunities. Indeed, he said himself that it was only after his retirement that he began to make real money. He continued to accept invitations as a guest lecturer around the world and, particularly, on cruise liners, which proved both a way of taking a pleasant vacation and of improving his financial status. He participated in advertisements, including some for Kellogg's in Australia and Ford in South Africa (Figure 23.i). This was certainly not something one would have expected of a distinguished member of the medical profession but I believe that, by this time in his life, he no longer cared so much for his reputation; he was more concerned with his bank balance. This may have been a more practical approach to life, but it saddened some of his friends to see him demean himself in this way.

Of interest to us in this respect was Chris's attitude to modeling. Chris's son, Christiaan, Jnr, and his granddaughter, Karen (Deirdre's daughter) both did some professional modeling for fashion events and magazines. According to Deirdre, Chris's view was that, 'while it is very nice to be beautiful enough to be a model, being beautiful is simply a bonus in life. It's lovely, if you have it, it's there for us all to enjoy, but it isn't enough all by itself. When you are put on this planet a little bit more is expected of you than that.' He felt that it was 'a nice sideline, perhaps, but not the way one should earn one's living.' Evidently, advertising cereals and cars was an acceptable way of earning a living, but not modeling.

Chris also benefitted through unofficial sponsorship, for example by driving cars provided for him by various car manufacturers (that at different times were said to include Datsun and Mercedes).

## Business Opportunities

Several business opportunities were presented to Chris. He lent his support to Aris Argyriou, a Greek businessman who wanted to open a health spa and an institute of preventive medicine on the island of Kos, the birthplace of Hippocrates (the 'father' of medicine), with Chris as his advisor and figurehead. Although this involved Chris in several visits to Greece, a country and whose people he came to love, to my knowledge, this project never came to full fruition.

# Clinique La Prairie

Of more importance to Chris from a financial perspective, he developed a financially profitable, but controversial, link with Armin Mattli, owner of the Clinique La Prairie in Switzerland, where he acted as research advisor. The Clinique's main interest and source of income was in the contentious field of 'rejuvenation' therapy, whereby cell extracts from fetuses of sheep were injected into people who felt they needed to renew their zest for life. Those seeking treatment in the clinic were housed in luxurious accommodation that impressed Chris 'much more than the knowledge of the medical staff.'

Armin Mattli appointed Chris as his scientific adviser, at a salary that Chris described as 'substantial' and the two of them became close friends for several years, although ultimately, they became estranged. For reasons unknown even to Chris, it was decided that he should undergo rejuvenation treatment himself, and he received injections of cells from eleven different sheep organs. I presume this was considered advisable from a public relations perspective.

Hearing of the activities of this controversial clinic, an American writer, Dan Greenburg, wrote a tongue-in-cheek, entertaining article for *Playboy* magazine about a visit he made to it to 'test the waters' or, more accurately, 'take the shots.' I include a few passages from it here.

> I began to hear a lot about a place in Switzerland called Clinique La Prairie, which has been around for fifty-seven years. Its specialty is giving people injections of live cells from sheep embryos, a process that is alleged to revitalise the system. Charlie Chaplin, a satisfied customer of Clinique La Prairie, was reportedly seventy-four when he impregnated Oona O'Neill ... Clinique La Prairie is a lovely white Swiss dollhouse with a brown peaked roof, yellow awnings and balconies spilling over with flowers (Figure 23.ii). It sits on a hill facing the lake and is right next door to a girls' finishing school.

In the clinic, Greenburg met Chris.

> Barnard took the injections himself for his arthritis. He's a handsome man with an infectious smile and vast personal charm. 'The idea here is not to conquer death,' says Barnard wryly, 'but to make people die as young as possible.' [Armin] Mattli [the owner of the Clinique] too, has had the injections. I ask both if the therapy has improved their sex lives. Mattli winks. Barnard says that area has never been a problem for him.
>
> Barnard explains Clinique La Prairie's success in regeneration of organs and tissue in patients who've been injected with live fetal cells as

follows. After injection, the fetal cells release cellular substances, which are absorbed into the blood stream of the patient and transported to the various organs, where they stimulate rejuvenation and regeneration. 'Some people think cellular therapy is a joke. It's not a joke,' says Barnard, passionately. 'I think it's stupid for the scientific establishment to ignore cellular therapy just because the scientific evidence has yet to be established—we take aspirin, and we don't know how that works either. Within a year, we will have definite scientific evidence to prove to the scientific community forever that it's not a hoax.'

Whether Chris really believed that the treatment was a joke or not is uncertain. Under the circumstances of his interview with Greenburg—in the presence of Mattli, the owner of the place, who signed Chris's salary checks—he may have felt bound to support the work going on there. After all, he was receiving regular fees from Mattli for his advice or public relations contributions to the Clinique. Furthermore, there was no proof either to support or condemn the therapy. Indeed, today, there is rapidly increasing evidence of beneficial effects of several types of cells, for example, mesenchymal stromal cells, when introduced into the body. These effects may be a direct result of the presence of the cells or an indirect activity resulting from substances they produce, for example, cytokines or chemokines.

Although many of us in the medical profession might look on the Clinique's form of therapy with great scepticism, many believing it to be nothing but a form of charlatanism, Chris kept an open mind about it, undoubtedly influenced by meeting patients who claimed how beneficial it had been to them, but possibly also influenced by the financial benefits that would accrue to him personally from his participation in the activities of the Clinique. In his book on rheumatoid arthritis, Chris commented on this and other forms of alternative therapy:

When I first began to look seriously into the claims of the so-called alternative therapists, I was heavily skeptical. My training had seen to that. For me they represented a kind of updated medical mumbo-jumbo, a mixture of superstition, folklore, misplaced faith, and downright ignorance ... At the time, the late 1960s, I was beginning to notice how often alternative treatments such as acupuncture, biofeedback, and homeopathy were creeping into medical discussions. More and more doctors seemed to be opening their minds to the possibility that what had so often hitherto been dismissed as suspect quackery could contain more than an element of genuine usefulness. Intrigued by this thought I began to read, discuss, and try to make up my own mind on the matter. I also ... tried one or two alternative therapies for myself.

Chris was not alone in believing that some alternative therapies should be critically examined. Several major medical schools worldwide have established such research programmes, some of which have been supported by national fund-awarding organizations, such as the US National Institutes of Health (NIH).

Chris took considerable scientific interest in the claims of the Clinique, and although aware of the scepticism of many members of the medical profession, he continued to feel that, on balance, one should keep an open mind until proof one way or the other was forthcoming. He did, in fact, make some effort to research whether the claims of the Clinique and some of the patients were justified, though perhaps never in a comprehensive, fully scientific fashion. For example, he persuaded Winston Wicomb to begin some studies in his laboratory at the UCT medical school, though no significant results came out of them.

Chris was particularly interested in some studies carried out by an Austrian scientist, Frans Schafer. Chris was first shown microscopic slides that indicated that the cell therapy offered by the Clinique might be beneficial. When fetal and adult cells were cultured together, the fetal cells survived with the aging cells, but this would not happen in the living body because earlier studies had demonstrated that the sheep cells were destroyed by the patient's own immune system, as would be expected from studies on xenotransplantation (cross-species transplantation). Perhaps, while they remained alive, the fetal sheep cells produced a substance that rejuvenated the patient—a substance that increased genetic repair so that aging was slowed, or possibly the fetal cells stimulated the recipient's own cells to make such a substance.

Dr Schafer thought that it was the glycosphingolipids that might do this. These are fat structures [lipids] that can be found in the outer membrane of most cells and which have many varying biological functions. Dr Schafer carried out experiments in his laboratory that suggested that glycosphingolipids, by stimulating repair by increasing the synthesis of proteins, to some extent protected tissues from the damaging effects of irradiation. Glycosphingolipids might therefore also protect from the effects of aging. Chris's love of research and his life-long desire to remain young were genuinely stimulated, and he became excited about the possibility of determining whether glycosphingolipids had this potential. 'Maybe there were still exciting days ahead for me', he wrote.

## The Glycel Episode

Nevertheless, valuable as this research might prove, Chris's association with the Clinique harmed his reputation in the medical profession, particularly when it led him into the realms of the marketing of cosmetics.

The single incident that did his image and reputation most harm was a development that came out of the new research on glycosphingolipids. This was his involvement in the marketing of the rejuvenating skin cream Glycel, that it was claimed had 'anti-wrinkle' capabilities. He had been associated with the production company as an advisor on research.

Armin Mattli had developed a new product that contained glycosphingolipids, which Dr Schafer had demonstrated in the laboratory could help repair damage to cells caused by ultraviolet light. Excessive ultraviolet light damages certain tissues in the skin. It was, therefore, suggested that the new cosmetic could help delay, or even reverse, a part of the aging process of the skin.

In *The Second Life,* Chris claims that he pointed out to Mattli that just because glycosphingolipids worked in culture (when grown in a flask or dish in the laboratory), they would not necessarily have the same effect on cells in the intact skin. Mattli responded by telling him that Dr Schafer had developed what he called a 'transdermal factor' that allowed the glycosphingolipids to penetrate the outer layer of the skin and become incorporated in its deeper layers.

As Chris had not been involved in the production or the testing of the cosmetic, he initially refused to promote it. However, after persuasion, he did agree to speak about the experimental work he had been associated with at Dr Schafer's laboratory. According to Chris, he received a written agreement which stated that his sole involvement would be to talk about the research he had done with Dr Schafer, and that his name could only be used in the promotion of Glycel after the text had been approved by the American Medical Association. Chris still felt uncomfortable, but thought all the loopholes had been closed. The Christiaan Barnard Research Institute had been established by Mr Mattli, and Chris had agreed that it could use his name in the sale and promotion of products, as long as it did not interfere with his practice as a physician. For this, he would receive 10 per cent of its earnings. This was another agreement he later regretted.

When Chris arrived in New York for the cosmetic promotion, he was given a large suite at the very expensive Pierre Hotel where he was 'wined and dined like a king'. At the time of the marketing of the cream, Chris gave a talk on the research he had been involved with, and demonstrated how some of the constituents of the cream (the glycosphingolipids) could slow the aging process in collagen, which is an important constituent of the skin. He did not say that the cream itself, applied externally, could prevent skin aging, but, as it contained glycosphingolipids, his remarks were interpreted as such. Theoretically, at this stage, he had in no way been involved in making any claims for the cream, although his comments, whether intended or not, were excellent publicity for the cosmetic.

When Chris spoke to members of the press, they kept referring to Glycel (Figure 23.iii) as 'your cosmetic'. He repeatedly explained he had not developed the product, nor ever tested it, and that he was only qualified to talk about the research on glycosphingolipids. Yet Glycel became known as 'Barnard's cream'. His name then started appearing on the boxes and jars, but 'instead of putting my foot down ... there and then and telling both Alfin [a business colleague of Mr Mattli] and Mattli that I was withdrawing from the contract because they hadn't kept to its conditions, I let it ride'. He admitted he had been 'seduced' by the Pierre Hotel suite, the French champagne, and all the five-star wining and dining (and possibly, I might add, the thought of the 10 per cent commission).

To some of the public, claims such as 'anti-wrinkle', 'anti-aging', and 'rejuvenation' were not considered merely to be cosmetic claims, but were medical claims, particularly as they appeared to be backed by a well-known doctor. Some members of the medical profession were outraged by what appeared to be blatant advertising. Whether the indignation was justified or not remains a moot point. Indeed, certain medical organizations and individuals, mainly American, behaved so precipitously in criticising Chris and in 'requesting an explanation' that one suspects they had been seeking an excuse to 'cut him down to size' for some time.

Well-known dermatologists, some of whom were employed by competing cosmetic companies, appeared on television programmes saying that Chris's claims were false, but rarely gave any scientific reason to support this conclusion. Chris was not invited to appear with them to defend himself or the glycosphingolipids. Indeed, in Chris's opinion, some of the competitive cosmetic products made more outrageous claims than Glycel, but no one questioned this, whereas Glycel received criticism from every quarter. The Federal Trade Commission began an investigation that largely accepted Dr Schafer's experimental evidence. A reputable academic research group in Oklahoma City subsequently confirmed that glycosphingolpids provide protection from ultraviolet light injury in living cells.

The worst, however, was still to come. The American College of Surgeons informed Chris that, as a Fellow of the College (which had been an honour he had received), he had to appear before a disciplinary committee for 'unprofessional behaviour'. Their claims were based on stories in newspapers and lay magazines, not from scientific reports. As all of the promotional material for Glycel was supposed to have been passed by the American Medical Association (AMA), Chris thought this might resolve the problem, but was then told by his business colleagues that only 'a doctor belonging to the AMA' had approved the text, a quite different state of affairs.

Chris wrote a letter to the College of Surgeons, telling them that he was 'surprised such a prestigious institution could charge a highly respected fellow with 'unprofessional behaviour' based solely on newspaper reports.' He sent a report on Dr Schafer's research and ended by stating that he 'didn't have the time or the inclination to continue this ridiculous argument and that if they felt it should be dragged on they should accept my resignation.' A few weeks later, he received a brief reply stating that they had accepted his resignation.

A jar of Glycel sold for about $200. In the event, it has been estimated that Chris made approximately $200,000 from the sales of the product, with Armin Mattli and his business colleagues, Chris claimed, making millions.

These forays into the world of commerce, although they may have been financially worthwhile, exposed Chris to considerable criticism and, added to the image he had gained as something of a playboy, certainly damaged his professional reputation. If his publicised private life brought him detractors, then his perceived forays into the world of business and advertising brought him even stronger criticism.

Chris considered his decision to speak about the experimental work on glycosphingolipids at what was clearly an event for the promotion of a cosmetic cream to be 'one of the greatest mistakes of my life—and I've regretted it a million times since.'

What is certain is that many of his friends and heretofore admirers were disappointed and saddened to see him involved in this controversy. The impression gained, rightly or wrongly, was of trading a hard-earned medical reputation for promotional or advertising fees. I have presented a gross over-simplification of the whole affair but it certainly appears that he may have been less than wise in putting himself in a position where his name could be linked so openly with a cosmetic product. Whether he was merely a pawn in the commercial jungle or not, he can be criticised for not insuring that his reputation was not damaged, as it undoubtedly was. Again, although he primarily blamed himself, he had a tendency to present himself as the innocent who had been used unwittingly, but this image was clearly untenable in someone so intelligent and, in later years at least, so experienced in the ways of the world.

It may be, of course, that he went into it openly, to ensure some financial security in his retirement years, and only later regretted the course the events had taken. His pension from the University of Cape Town could certainly not keep him in the style to which he had become accustomed. It is likely that his frequent and increasing contacts with the wealthy, the famous, the 'glitterati' of the world instilled in him the desire, even the need, to increase his income later in his life. He still had financial commitments to several members of his family. Perhaps, therefore, he went into it with eyes open, believing it was worth risking some of his reputation for a substantial financial return. Yet those of us who respected and admired him hope that this was not the case, preferring to believe him a victim of poor judgment rather than a contemporary Faust.

One could reasonably ask what he really had to lose—perhaps his reputation, but this was already somewhat tarnished by his various social activities, and his place in medical history was already assured. Financial security for himself and his family may have appeared more important to him during these years than any possible further damage to his reputation.

Should we criticise him for making what was surely an attractive business decision? At the time, the medical profession—and perhaps even the public—was not yet fully attuned or mentally prepared to see its leaders appear on the billboards or in the commercial breaks. With time, however, this attitude is changing. It was not many years ago that the elite members of the acting profession and former top politicians declined being seen in adverts. This is no longer the case: the lure of the 'almighty dollar' has proved too strong. Similarly, in the USA, it is now common practice for hospitals and doctors to openly advertise for business, and for prescription drugs to be advertised directly to the public, which was not the case that many years ago.

For example, certain doctors and surgeons feature openly under titles such as *Best Surgeons* in airline and several other magazines, and apparently do not get censured for this. These members of the medical profession have reputedly been selected by an independent organization for their expertise and highlighted because of this, but, in practice, it could be seen by some to be a form of advertising. I am not saying this is in any way wrong, but is it in any way different from when Chris Barnard endorsed a product? It may not be long before prominent physicians are seen promoting prescription drugs, and then it is only one small step for them to begin promoting other health products. Indeed, this is already happening; Chris Barnard may have been only a few years ahead of his time. Nevertheless, Chris greatly regretted being involved in the Glycel controversy, which undoubtedly, he should have had the good sense to avoid.

His playboy image and his involvement with both the activities of Clinique La Prairie and the marketing of Glycel were probably major factors in why Chris was not honoured or formally recognised by many of the world's leading universities. For example, although he received honorary doctorates and fellowships from many academic and professional institutions, he was not recognised by the Oxfords and Harvards of the world. Although he rarely mentioned this, he was aware that some institutions with which he would have enjoyed being associated, had quietly ignored him.

For example, while in London on one occasion, Chris was invited for lunch at the Royal College of Surgeons of England. He later recalled, clearly with some disappointment, that 'that was the only recognition this prestigious college ever gave me for my achievements. In fact, I've received awards and honours from most Western countries, the only exception being Great Britain.' It does seem a little surprising that, during the early euphoria after the first few transplants, and with South Africa's historical association with Great Britain, he should not have received any honour from the College or other major British medical organization. In contrast, Norman Shumway was awarded the Lister Medal, one of the College's most prestigious awards. I suspect, however, that his subsequent behaviour alienated some of the senior members of the College who felt he demeaned the standing of a proud profession.

As a caveat to the work at Clinique La Prairie, as the potential of cross-species transplantation began to be discussed, the Swiss government became concerned that the injection of sheep cells into patients might result in an animal infection being transferred to the human recipients, and then possibly to those in close contact with them. The Swiss put a ban on the injection of animal cells. This should have put the Clinique out of business; after all, the claim was that the cells directly or indirectly stimulated the patient's immune system. I inquired from a Swiss colleague what was the present status of the Clinique, and was told that it was still in business, but now the sheep cells were administered by mouth, not by injection, keeping the therapy within the law. Eating or drinking sheep cells should have no greater therapeutic effect than having a good lamb chop. To my mind, this casts grave doubts on the Clinque's claims that the cells have a rejuvenating effect.

# 24

# New Horizons: Oklahoma City

In 1984, soon after Chris took early retirement from his professional post at the University of Cape Town, he accepted an invitation to go to Oklahoma City in the USA to advise the surgeons at Baptist Medical Center (Figure 24.i)—now Integris Baptist Medical Center—on initiating a heart transplant program. The drive to establish a transplantation centre was led by one of Oklahoma's leading heart surgeons, Nazih Zuhdi (Figure 24.ii), who had known Chris briefly when they had been surgical fellows together in Minneapolis in the 1950s. Chris was appointed scientist-in-residence and spent six months each year in Oklahoma for a couple of years, advising on the establishment of this program. My understanding is that the salary he received each month would have taken him two years to earn as a professor at the University of Cape Town.

Chris did not perform the operations or care directly for the patients in Oklahoma City, but as scientist-in-residence, his experience and expertise, as well as his support, were helpful to the group. Merely by lending his name to their endeavours, he eased progress and stimulated referral of patients. This excellent private hospital, which had ambitions to become a significant transplant centre and raise its public profile locally, also used him as a public relations man (Figure 24.iii). He did Baptist Medical Center much good by his public relations activities, speaking wherever and whenever he was invited, whether on *Good Morning America* to millions of television viewers or in small Oklahoma towns to a handful of doctors or lay people. His efforts proved valuable, as there was soon not only an active transplantation programme at Baptist Medical Center, but also a productive research group working on related problems. Apart from the frequent and tiring traveling, his life there was relatively undemanding and financially rewarding.

His rheumatoid arthritis, however, continued to hinder what would have proved a very pleasant way of life. It had become so troublesome that he had been prescribed treatment with injections of gold, a rather old-fashioned remedy that was only employed in severe cases. This treatment could prove damaging to the kidneys and bone marrow, and thus required frequent monitoring. Oddly, I do not remember his other health problem (his asthma) being problematic while he was in Oklahoma City.

There was already an active kidney transplantation programme in the hospital. To help with the establishment and running of the heart transplant program, at Chris's suggestion, the hospital invited Dimitri Novitzky and me to move from Cape Town to join its team, which we did in early 1987. With the active involvement of many of the local physicians and surgeons (some of whom were outstandingly good), the programme rapidly developed, and achieved a minimal hospital mortality and excellent medium-term survival following heart transplantation. It was in Oklahoma that I perhaps came to know Chris best. We frequently lunched together and, free of the burdens of active surgical practice, he had more time to talk and reminisce.

## Nazih Zuhdi

During his time in Oklahoma City, Chris and Nazih Zuhdi became good friends, and so a few comments here about Nazih Zuhdi are apposite. Dr Zuhdi was originally from the Middle East, having been born in Beirut, Lebanon (in 1925), and came to the USA as a young doctor to train in surgery. He spent several years working with some of the major pioneers of open heart surgery, including Walt Lillehei in Minneapolis, which is where he first came into contact with Chris. He then took up an appointment as a heart surgeon in Oklahoma City, where he built a very successful clinical practice. For several years, he combined this with some innovative and important research, which resulted in simplifying open heart surgery very significantly.

In the early days, the heart-lung machine needed to be primed (filled) with fresh blood before it could be connected to the patient and used to support the circulation while the heart was stopped. Several units of fresh blood were needed, which necessitated drawing blood from numerous donors on the morning of the operation. Each donor's blood needed to be compatible with the blood type of the patient. The need for such large quantities of blood for each operation limited the number of operations that could be carried out each day, and clearly increased the costs and complexities of such procedures. It was particularly problematic when an operation needed to be carried out as an emergency.

First, Dr Zuhdi demonstrated that it was not necessary to use fresh blood drawn from donors on the day of the operation as stored blood would do just as well. This greatly simplified the entire procedure. Second, and much more importantly, Dr Zuhdi demonstrated that it was not necessary to prime the heart-lung machine with blood at all, and that a simple sugar solution (dextrose) was all that was required. Indeed, he showed that there were significant advantages to the patient if dextrose were used rather than blood. By diluting the patient's own blood with dextrose, during the operation the blood flowed more readily through the small blood vessels in the patient's organs and tissues. At the end of the operation, the high content of sugar in the blood resulted in the patient passing a great deal of urine, which was good for the kidneys and also had the effect of 'concentrating' the blood again—the red blood cells returned to their original concentration. It is perhaps even more remarkable that this research was carried out while Dr Zuhdi was in practice in a relatively small private hospital in Oklahoma City (not Baptist Medical Center) and not in one of the mega academic medical centres where most such research is undertaken.

This contribution to heart surgery, though it may appear rather minor, was, in fact, a major advance. Without the need to obtain large quantities of blood, open heart surgery could be carried out in a much larger number of patients on a daily basis and in emergencies. Denton Cooley was quick to catch on to Dr Zuhdi's idea—indeed, many surgeons were under the misconception that 'hemodilution' (diluting the blood with dextrose) was Cooley's invention, which was not the case—and began to carry out open heart surgery on a scale not previously envisaged. I have seen one operating schedule from Dr Cooley's operating rooms at the Texas Heart Institute where no fewer than sixty cardiovascular operations were planned for a single day, many of them being open heart procedures. This escalation in operations involving the heart-lung machine would not have been possible without Dr Zuhdi's research.

As I worked with Dr Zuhdi on a daily basis in Oklahoma City for several years, I came to know him well. Like Chris, he clearly enjoyed the publicity that heart transplantation brought to a surgeon and to his institution. For example, he did not miss an opportunity to appear on local television programmes to announce an advance in the transplant programme at Baptist Medical Center. His association with Chris obviously increased the attention that he and his institution received.

Dr Zuhdi was a very good technical surgeon, and had made a great deal of money from his skills. He was also a man of vision in that he proposed to develop an excellent organ transplant centre in the city where, at the time, only kidney transplants were being carried out. In this, he was successful since, apart from heart transplants, he also introduced lung and heart-lung transplantation, and attracted young surgeons and physicians who established liver, pancreas, and intestine transplantation programmes there. Sadly, his good relationships with several of these excellent surgeons were not maintained, and the programme suffered when, as a result of their deteriorating interaction with him, they moved on to positions at other transplant centres. Nevertheless, others replaced them and the hospital remains an active transplant centre today.

## Oklahomans' Impressions of Chris

As part of his public relations duties at Baptist Medical Center, Chris was sometimes asked to address medical or lay groups in the surrounding towns, usually in Oklahoma, but sometimes further afield. He had not lost his abilities as an entertaining speaker. On one occasion, Stanley Hupfeld, the CEO of Baptist Medical Center at that time, accompanied Chris, Dr Zuhdi, and me on a visit to the small Oklahoma town of Beaver, where Chris addressed several groups. When I asked Mr Hupfeld to put his memories of his association with Chris on paper, he centred his attention on the proceedings of that particular day.

> During that trip, Dr Barnard had the opportunity to speak to a group of physicians, a community group of lay citizens, and a group of children of all ages at the local middle school. His performance was extraordinary. In each instance, he was able to touch the exact chord necessary to entertain, delight, enthrall and stimulate his audience. I was significantly impressed that he knew just at what level to pitch his message, depending upon the sophistication and the age of the audience. With the physicians, he was appropriately sophisticated while recognising their desires as rural physicians for an overview of the programme without a great deal of detail. He was able to inspire confidence and to make them feel comfortable despite his obvious celebrity status. The local community group remarks were funny and his engaging personality warmed everyone in the room. With a great deal of finesse, he told his story with poignancy—both triumphs and failures. He completely won their affection and received a standing ovation.
>
> Most remarkable of all was his ability at the local school. Here he managed to entertain children with a wide diversity of ages, most of whom had never heard of Christiaan Barnard except what they were told by the school officials. They had no real appreciation for the sophistication of a heart transplant, but they recognised that they were in the presence of true greatness. His ability to reach out and communicate with these children, to not talk down to them, but to stimulate their imaginations and give them something to remember was truly remarkable.

I came away from that day in Beaver with amazement at a man who, for all his 'notoriety', possessed real grace. His personality was unaffected by his visibility. His sincere, genuine love for people showed through in every instance. All in all, it was a remarkable day.

Kenneth Bonds, Chair of the Board of Baptist Medical Center, was similarly impressed by Chris as a speaker. Although he recognised Chris's medical achievements and his ability to address physicians and surgeons, he was even more impressed by Chris's success when addressing laypeople.

I've found him to be even more convincing, however, when he speaks to groups on his views about life, religion, politics, and the greater importance of quality of life over quantity. Talking to a group of bankers on a particular occasion, most were choking back tears as he concluded a moving address saying, 'Death is not man's worst enemy; man's inhumanity to man is the real enemy.'

Chris recycled many of his presentations over many years, as many speakers do.

By the time he was living in Oklahoma, Chris was, of course, in the later years of his life—the early and mid-sixties represented an older stage of life then than they do today—and so the impressions of some of the people with whom he interacted there are interesting to compare with those of people who knew him in earlier years.

Sue Edwards, Chris's secretary at Baptist Medical Center (whom he shared with Dr Zuhdi), noted:

The experience of being Dr Barnard's 'Ole Secretary' is one that I will never forget. It was exciting, frustrating, rewarding, and nerve-racking all wrapped into one extraordinary event in my life ... Dr Barnard, as I am sure is true of most famous people, was used to getting his own way and being 'pampered'—he could therefore be very demanding, impatient and critical. On occasion, I remember leaving work wondering what terrible deed I had done to deserve putting up with his temperament and demands, excusing a portion of his disagreeable attitude to the pain he was in on any given day due to his arthritis. However, for the most part working for Dr Barnard gave me a special feeling of worth and pride, knowing that I was contributing what I could to make his work day and daily life easier and more efficient. I generally knew by the comments he would make that my efforts were appreciated.

In 1992, her assessment of him was as follows:

> Dr Barnard has a special sense of humour and is always ready to have
> a good time. He loved country and western dancing and on several
> occasions during his visits he would have me arrange for everyone he
> was closely associated with at Baptist to enjoy an evening of dinner
> and country and western dancing at one of the local establishments. He
> would be out on the floor every dance, laughing and obviously enjoying
> the 'cotton-eyed Joe' and other such dances [Figure 24.iv]. The next
> day he might come into the office obviously in pain, his hands and feet
> swollen as a result of the activities from the night before, but he never
> regretted having the fun.

Philip Newbold, a senior executive at Baptist Medical Center at the
time, was grateful for the positive role Chris played 'in all of the endless
negotiations it took to establish our [transplant] programme, as well as
have an enormously positive impact on our Board of Trustees and our
community leadership.'

Philip and his wife, Mary, also commented on the wonderful relationship
Chris developed with their little daughter.

> Recently, our six-year-old daughter, Anne, had a big 'thrill'. Upon
> arriving home from school, she was delighted to have received a very
> special letter in the mail. It was a wedding photograph and letter from
> Chris and Karin [his third wife]. As we read it together and talked about
> the beautiful wedding gown and flowers, she began thinking back to
> her special relationship with Chris and Karin. Her eyes danced as she
> talked about climbing up on his knee [on several occasions] at dinner
> and the special little gifts they would always bring when they came for
> an evening. It warmed our hearts to see such a wonderful closeness and
> understanding between a small child and a famous heart surgeon. We all
> treasure those memories and know that this represents another way that
> Chris has shown [to us personally] his care for all human beings.

## Twentieth Anniversary of the First Heart Transplant

It was during Chris's stay in 1987 in Oklahoma City that Baptist Medical
Center generously sponsored a celebration of the twentieth anniversary of
the first heart transplant (Figure 24.v). Chris remembered that the hospital
'didn't skimp on making this a very glamorous and memorable occasion'.
At the end of a splendid evening, at which Dr Lillehei, Dr Cooley, and

several other eminent guests participated, Chris concluded his speech by proposing a toast to Dr Norman Shumway, who had carried out much of the experimental work that prepared the way for human cardiac transplantation. This was perhaps a rather belated, but nevertheless I believe sincere, recognition of the pioneering role Dr Shumway had played.

To mark the event, which received wide media coverage, Chris was flown to New York to appear on the popular television program, *Good Morning America*. He greatly appreciated that President Ronald Reagan wrote him 'a beautiful letter of congratulations', and disappointed that the South African government, many of whom he had alienated because of his political views, did not mark the occasion by contacting him in any way.

Chris used his greatly improved financial situation, both from his Oklahoma salary and his income from Clinique La Prairie, to invest further in South Africa. He relinquished a cattle farm he had purchased in Sedgefield, but took an interest in two large sheep farms in the Karoo (Ratelfontein and Bloemhof), not many miles from his origins in Beaufort West. He replaced the sheep with African game, including rhinoceros, and set up the reserve to attract tourists. This had been a dream of his for some years. He selected some animals, such as certain breeds of zebra and antelope that he felt were in danger of extinction, which he hoped to 'save for my grandchildren'. He later wrote that he found 'just looking at these wonderful animals gives me a sense of serenity'.

The reserve extended over 13,000 hectares (30,000 acres or 132 square kilometers) and eventually contained seventeen different species of game. However, although he profited financially from the tourist hunters, he developed 'utter contempt' for some of them who 'cowered from the safety of their trucks, but who could now boast that they'd shot a lion.'

My personal view is that the few years before and following his retirement were perhaps not used as productively as they might have been, though I would be the first to admit that he had contributed more than his fair share of work to society during the earlier years of his career, and undoubtedly deserved a rest. Perhaps, too, I am influenced by the fact that I did not know him well at an earlier stage of his career when he was tireless in his activity and immensely productive. Very few of us do not eventually run out of steam, and I should not begrudge Chris his desire for a less demanding life. The heavy responsibilities that he bore for many years, and the immense demands placed upon him as a surgeon had clearly taken their toll. Yet I believe that he personally retained some feelings of frustration and regret over those later years.

His early retirement years were therefore taken up with his responsibilities in Oklahoma City, his various other business interests, occasional lecture tours on cruise ships, and promoting books he had written. These were all time-consuming activities, yet I still feel he could possibly have used his time more profitably. He was still only in his early sixties, and, apart from his arthritis, he remained in fairly good health. His duties at Baptist Medical Center were not overly demanding, and he was provided with good secretarial help.

However, he did eventually—after his return to Cape Town—write a sequel to his original autobiography (again with professional help in the person of Chris Brewer), this time entitled *The Second Life,* which documented his varied life in the near thirty years since the first heart transplant. Equal attention was paid in the book to his personal and social life as to his professional life, reflecting his changing priorities during these years.

Before publication, he sent the manuscript to me for my comments. In his effort to make the book a spicy 'tell-all', he had included two passages that recounted events that would have been highly embarrassing to certain others, and so I strongly recommended he omit these sections, which I am pleased to say he did.

As I have mentioned in previous chapters, in many ways his life—with its extreme highs but also its deep lows—reads like a movie script and, indeed, there was some interest by Hollywood in making a film of his life. According to Chris, a film producer and a script writer visited Cape Town and bought the rights to his life story. Although movies have been made about him, I do not believe any have really captured the essence of his charismatic personality and dramatic, rollercoaster life.

In 1992, at the time of the twenty-fifth anniversary of the first heart transplant, I invited sixty people who knew Chris or had known him at some stage of his life to contribute towards a collection of reminiscences about him (*Chris Barnard: By Those Who Know Him*). These various contributions provided a word picture of him that illustrates the many facets of his personality and character as well as his achievements. Most 'pictures' of him were reasoned and balanced, some were adulatory, several were generally benign but had a 'sting in the tail', and one or two were outright critical of him. I should also add that one or two who declined to contribute clearly retained a touch of bitterness about their relationship with him or expressed concern that what they might write would be the basis of a lawsuit against them. Notably, neither of his two former wives responded to my request, though his third (and at that time his current) wife did.

My own impression of these contributions was that, in general, those who had known him longest, particularly those who worked with him during his most productive years in Cape Town, gave rather more balanced opinions of him than those who had known him for a shorter period, particularly if that was in his later years, for example, those who worked with him in Oklahoma City. His Cape Town associates tended to comment on the irritations and frustrations of working with him, whereas my impression was that his Oklahoma colleagues were less aware of any such problems. This is perhaps to be expected as Chris was certainly a more difficult person to interact with during the period when he was trying to establish himself and make his name as a world-class surgeon than when he had semi-retired.

I sometimes wondered whether it was fair to him to publish this collection. Few of us have to suffer such a public scrutiny of our character and achievements. I ask you, the reader, to stop for a moment and consider what your own 'friends' and senior and junior professional colleagues would say about you if given the opportunity—that is after accepting the premise that your life's achievements are such that you would warrant such a book.

# 25

# 'Three Strikes and You're Out': Third Marriage

Before his retirement, Chris's second marriage had been dissolved, and so he was free to begin friendships with other young women. When the press speculated about whether he would marry again, he responded jokingly that the more important question was whether any future wife would be more than twenty-nine years his junior, as Barbara had been. This proved to be the case.

By this time, Chris was in his early sixties. The new woman in his life was a blonde, whereas both Louwjtie and Barbara had been brunettes. Karin Setzkorn, an attractive part-time fashion model forty-one years his junior, became his constant companion. Karin had been born and raised in Cape Town and, after leaving school, she worked full-time as a fashion model for a year, before beginning a course at the Cape Town Technikon, studying food and clothing technology. When she met Chris, she gave up the course, and began accompanying him on his travels to many parts of the world, including Oklahoma City. When it looked as if they would marry, a reporter asked Chris whether there was a health risk because of the difference in their ages. Chris replied by saying that, if there were a health risk, his young girlfriend would just have to accept it.

Chris enjoyed joking about his preference for much younger women. Nick and Olwyn Enslin, his friends in the water skiing days, had a daughter, and years later, Chris once remarked that he was thinking of marrying her. The daughter was quick to point out that surely she was too old for him. Chris asked, 'How old are you?' She was thirty-one. Chris thought for a moment and finally decided, 'Yes, you are too darn old.'

John Chaffin, an excellent surgeon at Baptist Medical Center who carried out many of the heart transplants there in those early days, had a daughter at high school. He arranged for her to meet with Chris to discuss a school project on euthanasia on which she had to write a paper (for which, by the way, Chris was extremely helpful). Some months later, when she was dressed in sophisticated clothing, wearing high heels and make-up (and no longer looking the school girl), she bumped into Chris in a shopping mall. She approached him with a smile, but he did not recognise her as his colleague's daughter and misunderstood her friendly approach and asked her out for dinner. When she told him who she was, the high school daughter of his colleague, he was very embarrassed.

Karin Setzkorn recollected 'the only obstacle we met in our relationship was that people kept reminding us about the difference in our ages, although this was something that never bothered either of us personally. Of course we discussed it, but to us it was never a major problem. We were criticised a great deal, but luckily the criticism didn't affect our relationship.'

Chris's appeal to, and success with, the fairer sex perhaps swelled the number of his detractors, both male and female. Some men may have been jealous of his ability, even in his sixties, to attract beautiful young women. Surely, it was enough for him to be acclaimed for his work. Surely, God was being unreasonably generous when he also made him attractive to women. However, some older women may not have been able to forgive the fact that he overlooked their generation, his chronological rightful partners, in favour of younger competitors.

Certainly, part of Chris's charisma, and, in particular, his appeal to women, was his youthful image. At the time of the first transplant, he was forty-five, yet looked almost twenty years younger, almost boyish, with his unsophisticated fashion sense, rural directness, and disarming charm. It was amazing that such an incredibly young man—surely hardly out of medical school—could perform such brilliant work. Later in life, he retained what youth he could by attention to his appearance and dress, and by judicious cosmetic surgery (I know of at least two facelifts) and, until the last few years of his life when he was plagued by facial skin cancer, still looked maybe ten years younger than he was (Figure 22.iii).

One interesting aspect of his relationship with Karin is that, as a much younger man, but after the first transplant by which time he was well-known, he had, by chance, met a married couple who had asked if they could photograph him with their young daughter, a little girl aged six. He readily agreed (Figure 25.i), not imagining that this pretty little girl would one day grow up into a beautiful big girl and become his wife (Figure 25.ii).

After they had been dating for a couple of years, Chris gave Karin a twenty-first birthday party at his restaurant, La Vita. As he had done at Deirdre's wedding, the entire Dean Street Arcade in which the restaurant was just one establishment was taken over for the festivities. To entertain the guests, he gave a slide show that recounted various stages of Karin's life until then. The first slide of Karin as a baby was accompanied by a recording of Louis Armstrong singing 'Hello Dolly', which was evidently Karin's father's favourite song. The photograph of her as a six-year-old sitting on Chris's lap was another of the slides shown, and was accompanied by Maurice Chevalier singing 'Thank Heaven for Little Girls.' After several other slides, the photograph of the grown-up Karin, once again sitting on his lap, was accompanied by the Beatles number 'When I'm Sixty-Four'. By this time, Chris was almost sixty-four.

To entertain their guests further, Chris and Karin then mimed the words to the song by Sophia Loren and Peter Sellers, 'Goodness Gracious Me', which they had rehearsed. This was a song that Chris had sung or mimed on several occasions with other celebrities, usually for charity. The party was a huge success.

Perhaps guilty because in his past he had not informed, let alone consulted, Deirdre on the steps he was about to take in his private life (such as his plan to marry Barbara), on this occasion, he asked Deirdre if she would be happy if he married Karin. Deirdre, who was by now, of course, several years older than her father's intended wife, was pleased he would have companionship and love again.

After two years of helping Dr Zuhdi establish the heart transplant programme in Oklahoma City, in December 1987, Chris resigned his position with Baptist Medical Center, wishing to spend more of his time in his beloved South Africa.

Just as my own career benefited when Marius resigned from the staff of GSH, so it did again when Chris resigned his appointment at Baptist Medical Center. Although my role in the activities of the hospital did not change, I was eventually appointed by Dr Zuhdi to fulfill Chris's role as scientist-in-residence, which I appreciated very much. It was an honour for me to follow Chris in this capacity.

In 1988, immediately on his return to South Africa, at the age of sixty-five, he married for the third time. Father Tom Nicholson performed the marriage ceremony in the La Vita restaurant (Figure 25.iii), the entire arcade again being used for the celebrations. The couple had actually been married very quietly and secretly on the evening before the wedding by a friend, who was a magistrate, in Tom's apartment. Nazih and Annette Zuhdi acted as witnesses at the wedding. The ceremony itself was therefore really only a blessing of the marriage. In the La Vita ceremony, Chris was close to tears on several occasions, as was Karin. Chris gave the only speech that evening, putting out that this was his third and last marriage. He congratulated Karin on becoming a wife, a mother, and a grandmother overnight, and he promised that her parents would soon become grandparents (even though Karin was not pregnant yet).

Believing that the media had made enough money out of the Barnards, Chris sold the exclusive rights to photograph and report on the wedding to a South African magazine, *Rapport*, and 'was pleasantly surprised at how much they were prepared to pay.' Several of Chris's close friends, including Armin Mattli, Nazih and Annette Zuhdi, Aris Argyriou, and biotechnology entrepreneur Manny Villafana and his wife Elizabeth, attended the wedding and even accompanied the married couple on their honeymoon in the game parks of South Africa, beginning with a memorable rail journey to Johannesburg on the famous Blue Train. The press followed the activities of bride, groom, and guests closely. Dr Zuhdi was impressed by the public interest in the wedding and the honeymoon.

> The people of Cape Town outside La Vita (the restaurant where the reception took place) were held back by mounted police, as they all wanted to see Christiaan and get a glimpse of Karin ... The honeymoon started with a trip of endless pleasures on the Blue Train from Cape Town to Johannesburg ... At Beaufort West, where the train was to stop for a few moments, we were delayed about thirty minutes by the crowd of people wanting to see Chris and Karin [Figure 25.iv]. It was one of the most moving scenes of my life as there were hundreds of people, all black, chanting and serenading Chris and Karin with their haunting soul music and songs. Chris was their hero because he always was for the oppressed and the non-privileged. Chris jokingly pointed out to me that here in his place of birth there was no white man to greet him when the train stopped ... In Johannesburg, the train's final destination, there were hundreds of reporters and photographers to meet the newlyweds.

The absence of many white well-wishers is perhaps surprising as, by this time, Chris had resolved his differences with the town's officials, even though many of them still objected to his expressing his liberal views on apartheid.

After the honeymoon, the newlyweds returned to their townhouse in Welgemoed, a suburb of Cape Town. Karin and Chris settled down to domestic life, interspersed with his speaking engagements abroad and visits to the Beaufort West game reserve. This third marriage provided him with two further children, Armin (Figure 25.v) and Lara, the younger born in 1997 when Chris was aged seventy-four—forty-seven years after the birth of his first-born, Deirdre (Figure 25.vi).

In view of his advancing age, Chris was particularly proud of fathering these two children. He once told me that he was keeping a record of the exact days on which his wife would be 'most fertile'. He was in Beaufort West and Karin was in Cape Town when he realised that this was such a day. He immediately drove to Cape Town. Nine months later, Armin was born.

When, in 1992, I put together the collection of reminiscences by people who had known Chris, Karin kindly contributed her personal thoughts. At the time she wrote the article, she and Chris had had one young son, Armin Adam, clearly named for Chris's good friend, Armin Mattli, and his own father, Adam Barnard. Karin's comments on Chris are of interest (particularly because neither of his two former wives accepted my invitation to write about him).

Chris is a very intense person with a big heart. He always recognises and appreciates the small things in life. In addition, he has a very good sense of humour and always tends to see the funny side of any situation. One of his very good characteristics is that he holds no grudges and never breaks off relationships for reasons of bitterness or unhappiness with past associations. I think all of these characteristics attracted me to him, and most of all because he is such a down-to-earth person.

I am very proud of my husband. He is an absolute perfectionist. He has great determination and a very strong will, and a big sense of achievement. There is nothing or nobody that will stop him from doing something he really wants to do. He does have some bad characteristics, of course—after all, he is only human. He has absolutely no patience, and, indeed, the word doesn't even exist in his vocabulary. He is also very impulsive and sometimes gets himself into trouble by acting on the spur of the moment. He loses his temper too quickly, sometimes about very minor things. Tact is also a quality he does not have in any great abundance, and he tends to say things irrespective of the consequences.

Little Armin was born to us in February 1989. Chris was very worried about whether our baby was going to be normal, although he was reassured by several doctors that the age of the father was of no significance in this respect. I had the baby by Cesarean section under epidural anaesthesia and Chris watched every move of the anaesthetist and surgeon with his 'perfectionist eyes'. The baby was born completely normal and we were very grateful and Chris, in particular, was over the moon.

I must say that he has proved to be a wonderful father. He got up at night, winded the baby, and did everything—except change the nappies.

He spends a great deal of time with little Armin, playing with him, taking him for walks, driving him to the beach, and appears to enjoy every moment with him. Of course, Armin's first word was 'Dada', not 'Mummy'.

One of the hazards of being married more than once is that there is a risk of forgetting who you are married to at any particular time. Deirdre provided an example of this in Chris's case. 'Once in Greece when he was married to Karin, in a speech to an entire village, he thanked his wife 'Barbara' for her love and support.' However, Deirdre added, 'No matter how many other things he had on his mind, at no time in his life did he ever get my mother [Louwtjie] confused with anyone else. If you knew my mother, you'd understand why.'

Deirdre, who admitted that her father was not 'Top of the Pops' with absolutely everyone, agreed with all of Karin's comments, and believed that, with regard to his bad characteristics, her father was fully aware that all three of his wives felt the same way about him. In response, she reports that Chris claimed 'I am a moody, selfish, irritable perfectionist. I am never wrong and modesty isn't my strong point. But apart from that I'm really quite a nice guy.'

Sadly, Chris's marriage to Karin broke up in 1999, again with some suggestions that he had been womanising. If true, some of us now in our seventies have to admire his stamina. However, it seems that a major underlying problem was the differences that had evolved in their lifestyles. Karin placed emphasis on their home life, whereas Chris was still attracted to foreign travel and his Beaufort West game reserve. Their divorce was not finalised until 15 March 2001, less than six months before he died. He found the acrimonious divorce negotiations particularly stressful, as we shall see later, and suffered another long period of depression, similar to that he had suffered after the break-up of his marriage to Barbara. My understanding is that Karin received a generous settlement. She has since married again.

By this time, through his various business interests, particularly Clinique La Prairie and Glycel, Chris was a relatively wealthy man, though he never publicly admitted it. It is said that he maintained a significant bank account in Switzerland.

Chris could be quite philosophical about subjects such as relationships. Perhaps writing from personal experience, in one of his *Cape Times* columns, he wrote:

There is a sociological theory that human relations are based on debits and credits. The theory states that while there are enough credits on both sides the relationship will last ... a few of the credits [are] youth, power, influence, fame, wealth. I would add love, warmth, understanding, co-operation. Together, they form a complex of feelings that make a relationship durable. Should the balance sheet go into the red—for example with the loss of youth, health, fame or influence—there may still be enough credit in wealth to keep the relationship going. But often even that is not enough. If the loving, the understanding, the warmth and the ability to work together is not there, the relationship is based on a false premise. You can add all the other credits you like to the balance sheet but they weigh little against these basics.

In *50 Ways to a Healthy Heart*, he provided more of his thoughts on marriage and divorce.

As I write this book I am going through another divorce. I would like to say only one thing about this. It is—once more—my fault that I did not try harder in our relationship to make things better. I don't want to say any more about my private life. One thing, however, is certain: I am going through very difficult times and I am in a very different state of mind from normal. You may find what I'm about to say a bit strange coming from me of all people. But marriage is for me the most important business in the world. And it is a business that must never be neglected; it needs constant attention.

The fact is that partnerships—and I mean well-balanced relationships between two people—can promote one's general feeling of well-being and positively influence one's health. One of the most serious threats to such a relationship is boredom. I know what I'm talking about here. Even in your 'Good morning' and your 'Good night', in the interest you show in clothing or the planning of a holiday, every spoken and unspoken communication with your partner should contain a little spark of creativity which gives new drive to that partnership. It's all contained in that not-so-old adage: Variety is the spice of life.

Every relationship has its crises. Money, education, sex—anything can be the subject of a dispute. Statistically speaking, marriages are most threatened after two, seven and twenty years. Why? Because people develop differently; because the couple may not have developed a system for coping with arguments or they may have nothing to say to each other anymore; because a new person has entered the scene, or because one of the partners feels that they are being taken for a ride and constantly treated as the dumb one in the relationship. Finally, it might be because one partner wants to experience the fascination of a new relationship once more. Almost every relationship can be saved if a couple begins early enough. Practice prevention before all the crockery has been smashed.

Michael Lukas Moeller, a German psychologist at the medical faculty in Frankfurt, mentions one factor in relationships that can lead to illness: an inability to face conflict. I agree with this completely. My three marriages probably failed because I belong to this type. I don't like arguing. The better couples are able to communicate, the better and healthier their relationship.

In this same book, Chris commented on his pending divorce from Karin.

A few months ago I was in Europe and perchance I glanced over a copy of the Bild am Sonntag newspaper. There I came across a story about me. After reading a few lines it was as if I had been struck by thunder. It said my wife had asked for a divorce because she had found condoms and Viagra in my travel bag. The next day the telephone went wild. The whole world was apparently obsessed with finding out about my sex habits. How potent did I think a seventy-six-year-old man should be? What was I like in bed? And last but not least, what was my true opinion of Viagra?

I have remained silent about these things because I am of the opinion that my private life should be respected and is nobody's business but my own. However, the wild rumours flying about from time to time have convinced me that it's time to clear a few things up.

It's true that Viagra was in my travel bag, but I have never taken it. I don't know why my wife made such a big deal about it. We had separated some time previously. I had in the meantime moved from my home in Cape Town to another house. At the time she found the Viagra, we had already made the decision to go our separate ways. Perhaps my wife only wanted some degree of finality. I know that some people find it easier to detach themselves from a former loved one if they look for and exaggerate his or her mistakes. It helps them to distance themselves.

… I have no qualms about people using any means they can to help with sexual problems. I tell you this because I think we should rethink our approach to sex. If we have problems with our circulation, then we consult a doctor. When we are ill we take medication. However, if we suffer from impotency we take nothing for it, and suffer in silence. We are ashamed to admit that we need help.

I know of no other method which relieves stress as effectively as sex. You can sleep as much as you want, go to a health farm or indulge in relaxation exercises—nothing frees your mind or reinvigorates your soul like a satisfying love-making experience.

This does not apply to everyone. For some people sex does not play a dominant role and they do not suffer because of it. In contrast, my whole life has been filled with passion—something I still have today. I have often experienced, both as a doctor and as a friend, how men take impotency to heart. The loss of virility is not comparable to any other kind of stress. Men are proud, they lose their dignity when they can no longer perform adequately.

Chris was to write about sex further in some of his newspaper columns (Chapter 28). It was clearly an important part of his life (as it is for many men).

# 26

# The Media:
# Make and Break

In various parts of this book, we have mentioned Chris's interactions with members of the media. Early in his career at GSH, he was keen for his achievements and those of his team in the field of heart surgery to reach the public, and so he used his contacts with journalists adroitly. There were those who thought that perhaps he was too conscious of the value of publicity, but his opinion was that 'ultimately it is the public who pay for medical research and they are therefore entitled to know what is going on.' Many would agree that it is sensible to keep the public interested in medical developments, but there is a fine line between attempting to do this and self-publicity. Occasionally, his desire for publicity might backfire on him, as was the case with the two-headed dog. He had misjudged the public response.

After the first transplant, he showed natural skill in dealing with the media. He was personable and articulate, seemingly candid and honest, and enjoyed being the centre of attention. He was comfortable in giving interviews and participating in television programmes. Later, at times, he resented the intrusion of the paparazzi, who infiltrated his life to a degree that was irritating to him, particularly when it aggravated the marital problems he faced at the time. From the time he returned to Cape Town from Minneapolis in 1958, therefore, he interacted with the media in one way or another.

Chris's own thoughts on his interaction with the media are of interest. Immediately after the first heart transplant, Chris felt that he and his colleagues were simply overwhelmed by the unprecedented media attention. In his book, *South Africa: Sharp Dissection*, he wrote:

> All the 'no comments' we could have mustered would have done nothing to diminish the story; they might, however, have diminished its accuracy.

Perhaps in naiveté and inexperience, perhaps even through a readiness to receive recognition for an achievement we felt was as, if not more, important than many that are feted in the daily press, or perhaps by a reluctance to offend by failing to respond, we co-operated with press conferences, radio talks and television interviews.

When the media interest continued while further transplants were carried out, Chris wrote:

Admitting the good and accepting some measure of the blame, it is nonetheless important to note that there were many negative aspects to the publicity we received. Firstly, it created dissension among members of our profession ... As a result of this, many firm professional and academic friendships were damaged—some of them irreparably ... Secondly, the publicity sparked off a spate of band-wagon transplantations by teams ill-equipped to perform them, but constrained to try by motives that were far from ethical ... When patients died, as we as scientists recognised would happen in some cases after heart transplantation, the public became disillusioned. People felt cheated and this contributed significantly to the unpopularity of heart transplantation in the mind of the layman ... Because of the tremendous publicity, however, many surgeons became scared of the operation and stopped doing it.

The publication of irrelevant and often sordid details of the circumstances surrounding the death of the donor, left doubt in the minds of many regarding the ability of the hospital to respect confidentiality. Sanctimonious newspaper leaders calling for enquiries into the definition of death and fatuous articles under such headlines as 'Was the donor really dead?' caused concern in the minds of the patients that the doctors at Groote Schuur Hospital were more concerned with snatching hearts than healing ailments.

One patient who Chris used as an example was Dorothy Fisher (the fifth patient at GSH), who at the time of his comments was 'our longest heart transplantation survivor, about whom long articles were written to the effect that she was without food and money to buy bread and that the hospital authorities had turned a blind eye to her plight. The impression was created that Miss Fisher was treated in this way because she was coloured. In actual fact, she was paid to write these anti-white articles and make these anti-white statements; it is interesting to note that when they had been written, the newspapers forgot all about her and her poverty.'

I had the personal privilege of caring for Dorothy, who attended the transplant clinic regularly during my first two years at GSH. She was a delightful, gentle lady who I am sure would have said nothing detrimental about anybody unless she had been pressed, bribed, or even coerced into doing so.

Chris drew attention to another case in which he had used the heart of a thirteen-year-old coloured girl. The press claimed:

> The hospital authorities refused to provide the money to cover the cost of her burial [though for a hospital to do this is illegal in many countries]. I spoke to a reporter afterwards and asked why he had not come to me before he published this report, as I would willingly have given the burial money, which was only R100, from my own pocket. He could not really answer that question because he would then not have had a sensational story. I asked him why, if he had felt so bad about the matter, he had not arranged for his newspaper to pay for the burial, as newspapers are quite wealthy, and he just kept quiet.

In regard to the media's attitude to South Africa, Chris soon developed a jaundiced view. In *South Africa: Sharp Dissection*, he wrote:

> You do not get headlines if you say anything good about South Africa— but say something unfavourable and you will be 'splashed' on the front page ... Likewise, our radio and television news commentators pontificate every day on crucial national and international events, often expressing views that do not accord with those of thousands of their listeners. Those who control these views are never required, as would be a politician, to be exposed to in-depth and impartial cross-examination in their own media on the stand they take daily ... Today the motto of the news barons is no longer 'the news as it is'. Rather it is: 'Indoctrinate the world and the world can be made to go in your direction.'

On occasion, Chris consulted lawyers to discuss various reports that had appeared about him in newspapers, but the legal advice he received was always 'to let the matter lie, because the newspapers would just make more stories out of the lawsuit and get more publicity and sell more newspapers.'

His opinion was that 'the so-called free Western press is not totally free because it is shackled by economic interests and responsibilities ... [it] has to make money and sell its advertising space. I believe that because newspapers are always geared to commercial gain, powerful interests will always hold sway over "freedom of the press".'

In a newspaper article entitled 'The Press', Chris wrote:

More exposure to the media made me realise that many journalists are involved not so much in the information business as in selling an image. If the image isn't intriguing or saleable enough, then it has to be revamped, and what better way of doing it than through the subject's own mouth. There's also the 'new angle' aspect. The reporter can't simply repeat what the opposition newspaper has already published. There has to be a new angle even if it means raking out details of the subject's private life.

On some social occasions, I have found myself steered almost willy-nilly into the immediate presence of some beautiful woman while the rest of the group were almost entirely male. A camera flashes and, next day, a blow-up picture appears, cut to show a couple seemingly alone and obviously in some intimate situation.

But it is almost inevitable that the public spotlight will find the unguarded yawn at the important dinner, the spinach-in-your-teeth smile and any surreptitious scratch, blink or scowl. Not only will it be recorded but also interpreted and not always with the kind of accuracy that the subject would like. You learn to live with it or you think you do, until the next purple revamp comes your way.

Some of those who have written about him had commented on this aspect of his life. Deirdre wrote:

For all of his 'famous' life my father's comings and goings were of great interest to the press and in the nature of things, sometimes that interest was generous and genuine. More often, though, it was simply probing and prurient. Once he became a public figure there was no 'no-go' zone, no private place in my father's life. A great many things were said about him. Some were probably true, a great many were totally untrue and some of them were deeply personal and hurtful to our family and to me. I read somewhere something that stays with me. 'We tolerate a level of intrusion into people's private lives which makes journalists barely distinguishable from the stalkers.' I have had some experience of this and it makes me sad.

One day everybody loves you. You make them feel good and they can't do enough for you. Then something goes wrong. Nobody loves you anymore except when you die. Then it's all right to say that maybe there was a time once when you weren't so bad after all.

Deirdre's own personal activities were followed and reported closely in the press for several years. She quoted examples of how readers or commentators would tire of them. She would receive comments such as 'When are we going to see the end of these Barnards?' and 'What's her claim to fame after all? She was only Chris Barnard's daughter.'

Marius commented on his brother's relationship with the press. 'His personal life was manna to a remorseless press, who first built him up with endless praise and adoration and then gleefully set out to destroy him. Unfortunately, he played to their tune and became aware of the dangers of man-made fame only during the last few years of his life.'

Was Marius correct? Did the press 'set out to destroy him?' Who better to address this point than a member of the press, Bob Molloy.

At my invitation in 1992, Mr Molloy, the journalist who edited Chris's weekly column in the *Cape Times* for several years, wrote about this aspect of Chris's relationship with the media. There follows a summary of an article by Mr Molloy that he entitled 'I Went to the Crucifixion', in which he provided a good deal of insight into Chris's relationship with the media.

## 'I Went to the Crucifixion'

Barnard hunters tracked down every Barnard appearance on the social scene, wrung the last drop of innuendo out of every Barnard utterance, and kept a ready lens to record every likely female who came within focus of the charismatic doctor. The hunters themselves were a fascinating breed, ranging from the ordinary muckraking gossip writer to top journalists on leading newspapers around the world. At one time or another they all put in an appearance at the press club—chasing 'a good Barnard story and to hell with the facts' as one reporter put it.

It didn't take long to discover why. The overseas slush magazines and gutter press were clamoring for any hint of a Barnard item, and would often outbid each other in the race to publish. The retailer of a 'good'— i.e. sensational—Barnard story could practically name his price for it.

'The guy doesn't get paid enough to have a haircut,' was the angle adopted by a Canadian journalist. With a prediction—'One smell of the gravy train and it's goodbye Cape Town.' That sparked a nicely scurrilous run of stories speculating on when the professor would be bought by an overseas research institute. It was my first experience of check book journalism, having cut my reporting teeth on a very straight, short-back-and-sides provincial daily. The cash offers, in terms of my income, were mind-boggling. Apparently, all I had to do was supply the 'background' and they would write the story.

There was one slight snag. It seemed my stories were too 'tame'. I was writing about the Barnard team's medical Camelot where surgical miracles were almost daily fare. A place of hope for heart sufferers who would otherwise die. But the check-toters didn't want stories on Barnard at work. It was Barnard at play they were interested in. Exasperated, one West German journalist finally asked, 'Where's the dirt?' His American-accented English was good enough to allow him the luxury of sarcasm. 'Dirt sells,' he explained in a pretend-kindly voice. And added, 'Everybody's got some dirt somewhere and the professor is a natural. All you gotta do is dig for it and [again the now familiar phrase] the hell with the facts.'

It seems hard to credit, but otherwise ethical journalists appeared to delight in giving every Barnard item a gloss. The media even had a name for it: faction—the basing of fiction on fact, with a little twist of the fiction to make it more factual. The 'creative' photograph, in which judicious cutting brought the professor closer to some attractive female in the group, was par for the course. Other pictures and stories were simply setups with unknown models and stray good-lookers willing to have their names linked with the famous surgeon.

For his part, the professor didn't try too hard to stay out of the limelight. He worked long and he played strong, and rather obstinately didn't see what the hell it had to do with the world's press. He also couldn't see he was on a one-way street. Barnard-knocking had become a media sport which extended even to television where he was seen as fair game to the chat show hatchet men. He wasn't an easy mark. An entertaining after-dinner speaker and a devastating debater, he generally gave more than he received.

Here Barnard trod on more toes, this time political. An anti-apartheid battler from his student days, he broke every rule in the book by refusing to segregate his wards according to race, bluntly advising the alarmed hospital bureaucracy to 'like it or lump it.'

Authority wasn't slow to react. His loss of favour became most noticeable at South African airports where he enjoyed red carpet treatment as South Africa's most famous son. VIP privileges, such as use of private lounges and fast-tracking through the formalities were withdrawn. Airport officials, recognising him in the crowds, would often apologise and blame it on 'orders.' He never deigned to query the official change of policy and preferred to take it on the chin without comment.

Perhaps that was the factor which triggered the academic backlash. Perhaps it was inevitable that jealousies would surface. When they did, the Barnard-baiters were there, angling for the story. Suddenly we were reading sour comments from medical colleagues who hated to see such largesse flowing into heart research while they had to battle for paperclips.

One respected medical authority lashed the surgeon for 'turning his department into a media circus,' Barnard shrugged it off with another of his one-liners—'It takes a clown to know one.' And, pressed for more comment—'Some people see dung where others see horses.'

The barbs went deep in the medical establishment and won him no friends. But the Barnard charisma—beamed out at countless after-dinner speaking engagements and in tireless speaking tours of America and Europe, plus media coverage of every transplant—was bringing in the cash. Whatever he touched turned to gold.

## The David Frost 'Vendetta'

The relationship between Chris and the media perhaps reached its denouement in the television interviews he gave to the well-known British media personality, David Frost. Bob Molloy summarised the relationship between the surgeon and the TV personality.

'The anti-Barnard faction was growing,' observed Molloy, 'and looking for any opportunity to bring him down. A case in point was the David Frost vendetta. Frost, a top TV interviewer [in both the UK and the USA] who specialised in verbally dismembering his victims on screen, waited a long time for his moment.'

This was, in fact, Chris's third encounter with Frost. In the first two, Chris had come out of them very well, but Frost was itching for one more try to bring down his quarry. Molloy continued:

> Frost needed a *coup de grâce*. It came in a last-minute challenge to Barnard to appear live on screen during a four-day speaking tour of United States medical research centres. Frost had correctly guessed that the surgeon's mile-wide ego would be unable to resist it. And so it proved. Barnard crammed an extra few hours into a busy schedule and arrived for the fray totally unprepared and dog-tired. Leading, as usual, with his chin.
>
> A surprise guest on the show was an anti-apartheid activist, a courtroom-hardened lawyer, who attacked Barnard personally for his country's racial policies. Slow-thinking and jet-lagged, Barnard launched into a historical explanation of his country's predicament when all he had to do was agree and point out reasonably that he was on the same side. His slightly rambling dissertation came out as a defense of apartheid. Frost couldn't believe his luck. Easily orchestrating his studio audience into a shout-down, the inevitable happened. Barnard lost his cool and it was all over bar the credits.
>
> Overnight, the smear stories bloomed like fungi. Those newspapers which always had space for anti-South African copy immediately

damned Barnard as an apologist for the regime—and the tag stuck. Doors which once stood wide open for the golden boy began to close. People who fell over themselves to be seen with Barnard the surgeon were at pains to distance themselves from Barnard the racist.

I watched a tape of the show with disbelief. It was the finest hatchet job I had ever seen. I had to hand it to Frost. If character assassination is a learned skill, he was a master of the craft.

Barnard, a country boy from an unsophisticated background, had come up the hard way and believed in being bluntly honest. As a public figure, he survived for a surprisingly long time on plain speaking but in the end he was no match for the media manipulators. It was years before he learned to fight them on their own ground, with a hard-hitting syndicated newspaper column which targeted everything from the government to the church, and left a few bloody noses in the world of journalism.

Of the Frost debacle, he wrote, 'The kick-in-the-teeth feeling has eased enough to allow me to get closer to reality, which is that a top lawyer and a leading TV entertainer have much in common—they both work from a prepared script. They never perform without knowing the score, drawing on a team of advisers, director, gag writers, make-up artists and professional hand-holders to ensure the show not only goes on, it goes on successfully.'

Barnard later offered Frost a return bout on primetime in South Africa. Too wily to be caught off base, Frost 'regretted' that a busy schedule prevented him meeting Barnard on his home turf. 'Perhaps I should have said that when he first called me in New York,' a rueful Barnard told me.

Ironically, six months after the death of Peter Sellers, his widow, Lynne Fredericks, married David Frost. Chris wondered whether Frost had maybe got the better of both of them.

In one of his newspaper articles, 'Frostbite', Chris also reviewed his interactions with Frost.

I'd never heard of David Frost until he asked me to appear on his programme some years ago. His approach, a very successful one, is to interview well-known or controversial people in a live broadcast show. He may switch roles from that of friend and host to adversary or interrogator and the success of the show depends on how quickly he can rattle his guest. As the experienced quizmaster, he succeeds often; so much so that many politicians and celebrities have refused to appear on his show.

It is a matter of record that his first bout with me was a top-rated show but a personal disaster for him. I had been worked over by tougher inquisitors and hadn't faced a generation of UCT medical students without learning how to protect myself in debate. I'm told that he vowed to even up the score and, some time later, he had his scouts fly into the Republic on a Barnard dirt-digging tour. What they found was a lot of fodder about my first marriage, my personal life and an accusation that I'd once failed to get consent for the removal of donor organs. This duly went on screen. I'm told it was a qualified success, qualified by the fact that I wasn't there, a case of bowling at the wicket while the batsman's away.

He followed this up with an invitation to a return bout, a show in which he engaged some outside help, a top medical writer who was supposed to fire the ammunition supplied. The result was a duck for the Frost team as I kept the interview on strictly medical lines and soon found that the medical expert was a bit undergraduate when it came to a topic such as heart disease.

By this time, you're probably wondering why he kept coming back for more and why I should bother to go before a camera to play Judy for somebody else's Punch. In David Frost's case, I'd guess that, as a thorough-going professional and a world-rated television personality, he knows the value of controversy and is tough enough to take a tumble as part of the game.

For my part, there was an audience of several millions out there, practically all of whom saw me as representative of South Africa. Few had ever seen the Republic at first hand and their knowledge was based mainly on what they read, much of it unsympathetic. In view of the world-wide-no-holds-barred propaganda war being waged against us, I believed it would be criminal to ignore such an opportunity. And that was my downfall.

On my last visit to the United States I had another invitation to act as David's Aunt Sally, 'to give you an opportunity to put your country's case.' With hindsight, I can see that he had sussed out my psychology as much as I'd taken note of his. The rest is history. I couldn't resist the chance to take on Frost again, even though I was on a punishing rat race of speaking engagements that left me physically exhausted and hardly the scintillating guest personality the show required.

Frost made no mistakes this time. He sprung an ex-South African on me, Joel Carlson, the very astute Johannesburg lawyer who had made a specialty of representing Blacks accused of crimes against the state. The man was an expert on apartheid-type legislation. In no time, Mr Carlson had twisted my desire to defend my country into a defense of the apartheid system. It still makes me shudder to remember it. I behaved like the most crass debating society greenhorn and made the whole thing worse by losing my temper and attacking both Frost and Carlson in personal terms.

I'd forgotten that there is a difference between knowing of a conspiracy and proving it, especially to a live television audience which looked as if it had been handpicked to shout me down. Frost, quite rightly, stopped the show. It was only then when I realised what an easy mark I'd been. I went home to lick my wounded ego.

Bob Molloy continued:

In the end, the constant message of Barnard as playboy wore him down, and placed great strain on his marriage to Barbara [his second wife]. Despite his natural devil-may-care bent, he began to curb his public utterances and adopt a more conservative public image. But, as he discovered, he was damned if he did and damned if he didn't.

Chris Barnard has long since achieved his niche in medical history. Undeniably, he did it his way. But opinion in some media quarters is that he was their creation. As one reporter put it, 'He was nobody until we made him.' The media's love-hate treatment of the world's most famous surgeon has a more likely explanation. Having begun to believe their own hype, which reached absurd heights in the early days, they would have deified him if they could. Instead, finding themselves with too solid a mortal for divinity, they turned to rend him. A fanciful theory. It's a common theme in religious myths but what proof do I have in this case? None, except personal experience. I went to the Crucifixion.

Chris's former mentor, Walt Lillehei, however, did not think Chris had been treated too badly by the media. When I asked him whether he thought Chris had been treated fairly by the press, he replied:

I think so. Chris has had so much publicity. There have been thousands of articles—good ones and some bad ones. But I think the press, by and large, have reported his activities accurately. Of course, he was very disturbed by press coverage of some of his 'playboy' activities, particularly by the paparazzi—the photographers that were always around trying to catch him in an undignified pose. But that's part of the game if you're a celebrity. Yes, I think he was treated fairly.

Personally, I think the truth lies somewhere in the middle: between Mr Molloy's opinion that the media intentionally tried to 'pull Chris down a peg or two' and Dr Lillehei's assertion that Chris was treated fairly. There seems little doubt that the press built up Chris to an unbelievable level, creating a 'hero of our time', only to then highlight his frailties in order to 'cut him down to size.' Whether this was fair on him remains difficult to determine. His undoubted enjoyment in being the centre of attention certainly played into the media's hands but, without this desire on his part, he would not have been the Chris Barnard we came to know.

Chris later summed up his interactions with the media.

I suppose my problem is that, when I first came to world attention, I was simply a working surgeon. One day a name on the duty list at Groote Schuur Hospital, the next a celebrity, but without the build-up that prepares most people for the limelight. Nobody held my hand, combed my hair, checked my make-up, wrote my scripts, censored the film footage. I didn't have a manager to warn that words could be quoted out of context, that public occasions could be manipulated. Sure, I made a lot of mistakes along the way. But for a little Afrikaner boy from Beaufort West I don't think I did too badly.

# 27

# Putting Pen to Paper:
# A Secondary Career

Chris wrote three research dissertations and was author or coauthor of more than two hundred academic papers on his surgical work but, in addition, he wrote extensively for the layperson. For some time, he contributed a regular newspaper column, and his books included several advising the public on matters of health, but also four novels. It is these, and not his academic publications, that I would like to address here.

In my opinion, Chris's gifts as a writer have not been fully appreciated. His forte was to write on medical and health topics in a style that was understandable, interesting, and entertaining to the average man in the street. However, his interests extended well beyond the field of medicine, as illustrated by his books on euthanasia and the politics of South Africa.

I do not know many, if any, other leading surgeons or physicians (or indeed leaders in other professional fields) who have demonstrated the range of interests that Chris had, nor one who had the ability to capture the attention of the lay reader so successfully. Having written for the lay public as well as for my colleagues in the medical profession, I understand the challenge this can provide. To think that it is easy for an expert to make the topic of their expertise understandable to the uninformed reader is incorrect. Chris's ability in this respect has been under-appreciated. Just as he could pitch a lecture at just the right level for his audience, so he could do so with the written word.

However, he undoubtedly received help from professional writers and editors in preparing some of these books, and so it remains uncertain how much he contributed personally. In most cases, I suspect the ideas were his, but others did much of the 'legwork' in seeking out facts and in writing the first draft or improving his first draft.

As many of the passages in his articles or books that I quote below shed light on Chris as a person or on a recent episode in his life, I make no apology for including them.

## Chris as a Newspaper Columnist

Journalist Bob Molloy, who collaborated with Chris on his columns written for the *Cape Times*, which were syndicated throughout South Africa, collected a number of Chris's best articles together as *The Best Medicine*, published in 1979, and again in *The Best of Barnard,* published in 1984. Most of the articles in both collections make stimulating and interesting reading. As one might expect, many of them relate to matters of health, but others cover a wide range from lifestyle advice to comment on global problems as Chris saw them. Perhaps also not surprisingly, given his interest in the opposite sex, there was a sexual theme underlying several of them, which almost certainly appealed to many of his readers.

It is interesting that in an introduction to *The Best of Barnard*, Chris wrote not only that meeting a media deadline certainly concentrated his mind, but also that the articles were 'a product of a thought, an emotion or an experience which I felt compelled to put on paper.' True writers are often people who feel *compelled* to put pen to paper; the urge to do so is so strong they cannot resist. Chris wrote so extensively in his life— admittedly often with professional help— that I have come to believe that his urge to write was strong.

I have selected some abbreviated examples to provide a sense of his comments and style. Let us begin with some of his comments related to sex.

In 'The Benefits of Exercise', perhaps with tongue-in-cheek, he advocated sexual activity as a form of exercise.

> You expend about as much physical energy in an act of intercourse as in twenty press-ups, probably a good thing for many middle-aged couples who get no other form of exercise. Physicians nowadays recommend exercise for patients with cardiovascular disease. Sex would be a delightful way of achieving this ... An average act of intercourse consumes about two hundred calories.

'Aphrodisiacs' addresses another sex-related topic.

> In order of importance the best aphrodisiacs are youth (yours or hers), beauty (hers) and ... variety. After these come trappings of dress, posture, gesture, pleasant surroundings, good food, lighting, music, conversation and general lack of stress ... Any teenager knows that an expensive dinner is more erotic than a hamburger. As a peacock spreads his tail feathers to show the female what she's missing, so men flash their wealth. Take a look at the cars they drive, the clothes they wear,

the exclusive wristwatch and all the paraphernalia that says: 'Baby, I've got it.' Not surprisingly, they do get it, at least often enough to make the whole exercise worthwhile.

In a letter to the South African edition of *Time* magazine published one day after Chris's death in September 2001, he wrote:

> Laughter is very therapeutic. Anything that makes life less miserable, more happy, is good for you. That's why sex is good for the heart … Medicine today is injections, drugs, surgery and bills. How often do you go to a doctor these days and the doctor tells you, you must laugh more often, listen to some good music, sleep, relax, have sex, use Viagra if it helps?

His readers sometimes directed his attention to more mundane topics of health. One very irritated male reader asked him, 'You've written about women, sex, old age, death, superstition, capital punishment and even pollution—for heaven's sake, when do we get something on heart disease, or is that too boring for you?'

In an article entitled 'Heart Attacks', Chris responded by asking 'How could one avoid heart disease?'

> My thumbnail sketch of the person *least* likely to have a heart attack, or anything else, is briefly: an effeminate municipal worker, completely lacking in physical and mental alertness, without ambition, drive or competitive spirit and who has never tried to meet a deadline of any kind. A man with poor appetite, subsisting on fruits and vegetables laced with corn and whale oil, detesting tobacco, spurning ownership of radio, television or motor car, scrawny and unathletic in appearance, constantly straining his puny muscles by exercise, low in income, blood pressure, blood sugar, uric acid and cholesterol, taking drugs to regulate blood pressure, blood fat content and blood-clotting level ever since having his precautionary castration.

In 'Smoking and Drinking,' Chris appealed to the government to do more to prevent people developing bad habits that resulted in poor health, and pleaded particularly on behalf of children.

> How nonsensical … to shape an educational system aimed at producing children sound in mind and body while ignoring advertising campaigns which tell them how to find great adventure and become he-men and sophisticated women through smoking the right cigarette or drinking the right liquor.

'The Population Explosion', he claimed, was the single most important problem facing the world.

> Every other problem the human race has ever had fades into insignificance besides that of overpopulation. Most people would see this as a crisis. They are right, we are in the midst of the worst crisis mankind has ever experienced, yet nations the world over act as if they had more important things in mind. In South Africa, for example, we have a family-planning budget measured in thousands of rand while the defense budget soaks up cash to the tune of hundreds of millions of rand.
>
> What we can do immediately is to shake up our ideas on sex education, particularly for schools. At the same time contraceptive information and devices should be freely available to all, and I do mean all. Thereafter what is needed is a reversal of the tax burden from the childless single to the married or unmarried parent … Make no mistake, the breeders are killing us. Either we defuse the population bomb or we get wiped out in the population explosion.

He wrote about abortion in his book, *Good Life, Good Death*.

> For my part, a Calvinistic upbringing does not allow me to accept the idea of 'free' abortion, in which the fetus is aborted simply because it is not convenient for a woman to have a baby … On the other hand, it is clear to me that there are times when a doctor might conclude that a woman's life can be saved, or the quality of her life preserved, if she has an abortion. Or that by terminating a pregnancy … a child doomed to a life without quality would not, indeed, be born.

Chris was known for his love of youth—of children, of retaining one's youthful good looks, of fighting against the aging process. He would have supported George Bernard Shaw's statement that 'Youth is wasted on the young.' Yet, in an article he titled 'Gerontophobia', he defended the rights of the aging and aged.

> He questioned the 'unconscious assumptions that age is to be avoided and that the possession of youth is in itself a positive value. This is 'ageism'. Like sexism and racism, it is the setting apart of a selected group from the rest of the human race in order to discriminate against it in some way. Mandatory retirement, old age homes or 'age ghettos', inadequate health care, poor incomes and, not least of all, being the first choice for muggers, await those who cross the line between 'us' and 'them'.

Despite the continued existence of illness in the world, Chris reminded his readers of how well off they were in respect of the quality of life at the time. In 'We Never Had It So Good', he wrote:

> So next time somebody gives you the catastrophic line remind him that we may not be living in the best of all possible worlds but it is a long way off from the worst that has happened to us. If that doesn't impress him ask to see his mouth for dental caries or expose his pessimist's abdomen to show his appendectomy scar, then point out that at one stage in human history he would have lived in misery because of the one commonplace condition or died in agony from the other.

He expanded on this topic in a piece called 'Prescriptions'.

> Now, with the knowledge that complete cure of the nation's ills is not only unattainable but too costly, the bias is swinging towards prevention of ill-health—a concept already largely achieved by the work of the great nineteenth-century engineers. It seems strange to think that an engineer can have much control over your state of health, but it is a fact that the engineering and architectural departments of any university annually turn out more guarantors of the nation's health than any medical faculty. Modern sewerage, water supplies, housing, transport, agricultural advances and communications have done more to raise the health standards of mankind than Hippocrates and his entire pill-pushing crew.
>
> A single plumber probably achieves as much in the field of preventive medicine as most medics, while the ordinary health inspector, doing a boring routine check of take-away shops and corner cafés, saves more in terms of the nation's health budget than any topflight, nationally known specialist, myself not excluded.

In 'Looking at Leaders', Chris recommended assessing a political leader's ability to lead by not only assessing their physical health but also their mental health.

> Last month, a British doctor called for brain scans for politicians and national leaders as a check to ensure that they still have all their marbles. He pointed out that we often go along with the illogical behaviour of a national leader just because he or she is the boss, and when things go wrong we start looking for the problem among his opponents.
>
> I have always thought it an appalling oversight to choose a leader who has not been tested out as physically fit but I must admit that the idea of brain scanning for deterioration of mental function takes the idea a bit further.

Cases in point are John Stonehouse, a former British MP who faked his own death to avoid fraud charges and is now serving seven years as a guest of Her Majesty; President Nixon who made a mockery of the American presidency; and Idi Amin, the African buffoon whose rule made even the OAU [Organization of African Unity] wince.

While leaders concern themselves with their own selfish pleasures, they do little harm nationally. Louis XIV was a pampered fool who drained the nation's treasury but he did France a helluva lot less harm than the little Corsican whose dreams of empire wiped out a whole generation in the Napoleonic wars.

All this faded into insignificance with the power-mad old men who slaughtered hundreds of thousands healthy young soldiers daily as they played a four-year-long game called the Great War. It was only after this catastrophe that people began to suspect that perhaps the leaders were not always right.

Examples of his writing on topics outside of medicine, particularly in relation to the politics of South Africa, have been quoted elsewhere in this book, but I provide a couple of examples here. On the topic of 'Hardwork', he wrote:

Once you've identified the problem you can get on with the solution. It's no accident that the Japanese yen and the German mark are the hardest world currencies. Hard currency is produced by hard work from the top of our over-stuffed, expense account, executive sector down to Joe Blow. And the solution? To me it is so simple I wouldn't think of sending you an account; just extend your gluteal maxima, those large muscles in the buttocks. That should take your bum out of the butter long enough to get some work done.

For all the liberalisation that had taken place in the world, Chris was not convinced that the individual had any greater freedom than before. In an article, 'Freedom', he stated:

Today's urban youth are the victims of a carrot-rich upbringing. We wanted to give them freedom and we gave them license. In doing so we reduced the freedom of all. No one who lives in an urban environment, behind the locks, bars and burglar-proofing of modern housing, need doubt that he is less free than his grandfather. No businessman threading his way through the maze of bureaucracy could fail to be aware of the chains on private enterprise and no traveller remains untouched by the invasion of personal privacy enforced by security requirements.

The above passages are, I suggest, examples of a writer with the gift for making old topics of renewed interest, and of Chris's ability to capture the attention of his readers.


## Chris as a Writer of Books

Bearing in mind the examples I have quoted above, my first impression was that Chris was at his best when composing a short, pithy article— not exactly a 'sound bite', but the shorter the better—and did not have the patience or persistence to write longer pieces. However, he wrote or co-wrote (sometimes with significant help) a surprisingly large number of books, covering different topics.

There are three books—*The Body Machine*, *The Living Body,* and *Junior Body Machine*—in which Chris is listed as a 'consulting editor'. Each of them is a very well-produced, highly informative, and readable book on its topic. All three are profusely illustrated with many of the illustrations being in colour. I am sure all three books have been valuable to people who wanted to know more about the human body and matters of health. Chris wrote the introduction in each case, but how much else he contributed is uncertain, though I suspect not a great deal. His name on the cover raised the profile of the book in the public eye and I am sure engendered attention and publicity. *The Living Body* was primarily edited by Karl Sabbagh, who was at the time a leading medical journalist and television producer, and the book is based to a large extent on a television series of twenty-six programmes on which Chris collaborated.

There were, however, books in which he stepped outside medicine. I have addressed his discussion of the South African political situation, *South Africa: Sharp Dissection*, elsewhere in this volume (Chapter 28).

Although *Good Life, Good Death*, published in 1980, fell partly under the medical heading, it extended beyond it. In it, Chris discussed the topic of the book's subtitle: 'a doctor's case for euthanasia and suicide.' As this was a topic about which Chris clearly felt strongly, and not infrequently commented on, some mention of the opinions expressed in the book are warranted here.

He first commented on his own attitudes to death and religion.

According to the scientists, nature abhors a vacuum. The same is true for the theologians and the mythologists. Wherever the unknown yawns, man has theorised, mythologised, and storified to fill the gap ... That which is unknown has a greater component of horror than even the most threatening concrete event. Better by far to sketch its outline, give it a shape, and thereby evolve rules of coping. Man, as a sentient being in a nonsentient world, has great need to cope—to make order out of the chaos, to explain what looks like a cruel cosmic joke.

Although Chris had told me that he believed in some form of God and that he not infrequently prayed, the above comments suggest that his opinion was that much of religion was man-made mythology.

He defined dying as 'the irreversible deterioration of the quality of life that precedes the death of a particular individual.' His main message throughout the book was that when death cannot be prevented, the doctors' responsibility is to do their best to maintain the quality of life rather than attempt to prolong a life of miserable quality.

He pointed out that a survey indicated that in 1900, no fewer than two-thirds of Americans who died were under fifty years old, and most of them died at home, whereas at the time of writing this book, most Americans died when they were over sixty-five and usually in hospital or other institution. He emphasised that doctors, nurses and paramedics should attempt to 'cure sometime, to relieve often, to comfort always.' He quoted others to support his concept that 'in terminal illness, the primary aim is no longer to preserve life, but to make the life that remains as comfortable and as meaningful as possible. Thus, what may be appropriate treatment in an acutely ill patient may be inappropriate in the dying patient.'

Although he recognised that the concept of medical euthanasia (the termination of a life as an extension of the medical treatment of a dying patient) had never had much public support, he put forward his reasons for believing that there is a place for it in medical practice. He differentiated active euthanasia, 'in which life is ended by direct intervention, such as giving a patient a lethal dose of a drug', from passive euthanasia, in which death results 'from withdrawal of life-support systems or life-sustaining medications.' He suggested that there was little 'morally indistinguishable' between a deliberate act of omission, when death is the goal or purpose, and a deliberate act of commission.

One example close to his own experience was when, at the conclusion of an open heart operation when the heart fails to recover, the surgeon decides to turn off the heart-lung machine that is sustaining life. Although it could be claimed that the surgeon had killed the patient, it could equally be claimed that the surgeon had given 'the patient, who could no longer have a good life, a good death.' He added, 'Few people realise the total loneliness of the surgeon when a patient, as the expression goes, "dies on the table." There is a feeling of complete inadequacy as the doctor pulls off his gloves and mask and walks out to the waiting room to explain to the relatives what happened.'

Chris made no excuses and asked no forgiveness for admitting that he had practiced passive euthanasia for many years.

> In fact, I gave instructions to the doctor attending my own mother in her last illness that she should receive no antibiotics nor be tube fed. At that stage, she was in her ninety-eighth year, suffering from her third stroke and unconscious with pneumonia. I am convinced that is what she wanted. During the eleven years after her first stroke, as she lay bedridden with repeated bladder and lung infections, she told me on occasion, 'I wish God would come and take me away.'

He also recounted an incident when he and his brother had attended the dying moments of a patient whose death was miserable.

> When Marius and I walked away from his bed, shaken by our inability to comfort our patient, we turned to each other and vowed that each of us would help the other if we found ourselves in similar circumstances. We agreed that this could be done either with the administration of a fatal overdose (if the sufferer was incapable of helping himself) or by leaving within reach enough tablets so that the sufferer could take his own life.
>
> I cannot speak for anyone else, but in my case it is not pain I fear. As a chronic arthritic, one learns to live with pain. What I fear most is becoming depersonalised—the ending of life that may come before death, the phase in which I would no longer be in control of my environment.

Fortunately, Chris was not faced with this in the event of his own death, which was unexpected and mercifully sudden and rapid.

Although Chris never practiced active euthanasia (though as a young doctor, he had clearly considered it [Chapter 3]), he had 'often stood at the bedside of a dying patient and realised the need for this service.' His opinion was that anyone who claims that 'one can always alleviate the suffering of the dying has either not had enough exposure to the problem or is lacking in a simple quality—compassion.'

He compared the attitude of the human race to war, often enthusiastic, with that of providing assistance to a person to end unbearable suffering.

> Consider that, for as long as man has inhabited the earth, he has accepted with few reservations the right to kill and be killed on the battlefield, even when this leads to not only his own but multiple deaths. The decision to enter into such mass killing is usually taken by a country's rulers. The individual, as such, has little say in the matter, and not infrequently

the reasons given for killing total strangers are seldom clear to those compelled to kill. Illogicality is compounded by the fact that it is not the aged, the crippled, and the socially defective who are selected to kill and be killed, but the very flower of the country's youth—the young and the healthy. Refusal to accept battle training can result in a jail sentence. Refusal to kill on the battlefield can earn a court-martial and, in some cases, a death sentence. The whole process of mass killing between opposing groups is carried out with great patriotic fervor, the trained killer being sent off to the sound of martial music and waving flags. And with great pride, the death toll of the opposing group is headlined in the daily newspapers. The trained killer who kills more than others is often decorated for his courage and skill in achieving what is seen as something meritorious, and a hero's welcome awaits him when he returns.

He compared this attitude with the 'outcry of horror [that] is heard when a doctor asks for the right to actively end the suffering of a terminally ill patient.'

He also highlighted the public's attitude (at least in some countries) to capital punishment.

In my own country, and in many other civilised countries, we accept the right of a judge to condemn another human being to death for a capital offense and to request the government to carry out the sentence. Great care is taken that such a death is quick and clean. Yet what a furor when someone suggests giving the dying patient a similar right to a quick, clean death.

Another example he put forward was the community's acceptance of abortion.

In the past ten years the demand for more liberal abortion laws has resulted in a human wave of aborted fetuses. Thousands of lives are almost literally washed down the drain. But consider what happens when there is a request for the right to terminate a life that has lost all quality.

Finally, he commented on the great difference in society's attitudes to humans and animals.

I have always wondered at the kind of person who would mercifully end the life of a suffering animal yet would hesitate to extend the same privilege to a fellow being.

In his book *Heart Attack* (see below), he again expressed that life should not merely be measured by quantity, but also by quality. Chris suggested that society should expect doctors to be 'humanitarians and not merely scientists, that life-support mechanisms ... not be used where there is no hope; and that when the patient is suffering from severe pain it be relieved by medicines even if this means shortening the life of the patient.' He repeated a favourite phrase of his. 'Death is not the enemy. Inhumanity is.'

He went on to state that 'where there is no more joy in living, no further hope of joy, and no wish to continue, then there can be little problem in arriving at a decision [to help the patient end his or her life].'

One may not agree with all of his arguments, but one has to admit that he put his case clearly and logically. I certainly found the logic of his opinions to be influencing me. It is of interest that the subject of euthanasia forms a basis for his second novel, *In the Night Season* [see below].

*Heart Attack: You Don't Have To Die,* published in 1971, appears to have been written solely by Chris, although he does acknowledge very considerable help from Dr Eugene Dowdle, then the professor of clinical science at the University of Cape Town, and credits several other sources of information. However, it is quite reasonable to believe it was written by Chris because it relates to the heart, which was, of course, a special interest of his. It is a relatively short book of about 170 pages, written for the public to inform them of the reasons why one develops a heart attack (or, in medical terms, myocardial infarction) and what one can do to prevent it or to live after it.

In writing for the layperson, the writer has to find the correct level of information to direct to the reader (not too much detail) and has to make that information readable and, if possible, entertaining. In my opinion, this book fulfilled its aim extremely successfully. The information that Chris gave the reader was, as far as I could discern, entirely accurate; also, the book is highly readable and, in places, quite entertaining. I believe it would have been a valuable source of information and opinion to anyone suffering from heart disease, or wishing to prevent it. Chris emphasised that medicine had much to offer for patients with heart disease.

First, there are important differences between the doctor's responsibility to scientific inquiry and his responsibilities to his patients ... Second, I do not subscribe to the view that the aim of every doctor should be to conquer death ... In my opinion, the principal aim of the doctor should be to help the patient to achieve a physical and mental state of health that will enable him to indulge his own private concept of being alive. My third point expresses what I believe to be a very important principle. It is quite simply that patients must be kept informed.

Chris took pains to emphasise the medical profession's limited knowledge on many aspects of heart disease. For example, when discussing the thickening of the arteries, known as atheroma, that occurs in many patients—particularly of the coronary system—he wrote (with humility):

> But, tell me, doctor, why does the atheromatous plaque form in the first place? Answer just that one little question. If I were a really clever man instead of just a surgeon, I would write many thousands of wise words in answer to that question. I would present the theories and weigh the evidence for all of them. I would quote this experiment that proved one thing and that experiment that proved another, and I would probably stare into the distance and say something very profound, something that would make you feel that I know the answer, but that you are not quite smart enough to understand it Unfortunately, I am not that clever, and all I can do is admit that I don't know ... It is far better to admit our ignorance than to pretend with arrogance that we know more than we do.

Chris expressed a disdain for physicians and scientists who do not keep an open mind, but who 'do research to sustain their theories rather than to examine them. They react to criticism with snarls and anger because their theories contain such a strong element of their emotional selves that they interpret any attack on their theories as an attack on their persons. These are the con men of science and medicine, and, generally speaking, they are a pain in the neck.'

He also warned against treating diseases, rather than patients. He felt strongly about this. 'For as doctors, we treat patients. We don't treat coronary arteries. It is the patient who is sacrosanct—not his heart.'

In this book, as in several of his others, Chris maintained the reader's attention by leavening the text with occasional anecdotes and humour.

> I once sat next to an elderly gentleman in an airplane and, as we were about to land at London's airport, we were given the usual immigration forms to complete. In the space next to the word 'Name' he dutifully printed his name. On the next line, in the space marked 'Sex', he wrote wistfully 'occasionally'.

On the topic of coronary artery disease, Chris pointed out what he mischievously saw as an inconsistency in doctors' advice regarding a patient's life-style. 'Stress, which increases the heart rate and elevates the blood pressure, is considered bad, whereas exercise, which also increases the heart rate and elevates the blood pressure, is considered good.'

He sometimes played down the complexity of medical practice. Most of medicine, he wrote, 'is basically very easy to understand. So easy, in fact, that we often use long words to make everything appear more difficult— for it would never do to have the public realise that we deal with matters that lie within the easy comprehension of even the slowest.' Although these words perhaps illustrate Chris's humility, I do not believe they are true; medicine is often a complex subject.

On occasions, he also took pains to recount the mistakes he had made, whereas I know many eminent surgeons who would not wish to damage their aura of infallibility in this way.

Many years ago, before we had pacemakers, there was no really effective treatment for heart block, and patients often suffered periodic short-lived attacks of ventricular standstill during which the blood supply to the brain was temporarily cut off, resulting in sudden loss of consciousness— the patient appearing, to all intents and purposes, dead. I blush to recall an episode from my younger days when a woman experienced an attack of this nature while I was examining her. Convinced that she had died, I left her bedside to inform her relatives of her death. I didn't appear very clever when the grieving relatives went to pay their last respects and found her 'resurrected' and very much alive.

Overall, Chris's book was well-balanced and surely helpful.

Chris's last book was *50 Ways to a Healthy Heart*, published in the year of his death, 2001, by which time it had already been translated into twenty-four languages. It is full of good advice, simply stated. His advice includes the usual messages about good nutrition (and dieting, if necessary), reducing stress, taking exercise, avoiding smoking, and thinking positively.

For example, after pointing out that he had been privileged to have never been overweight, and thus never needed to go on a diet - the most he ever weighed was 85 kg (10 kg more than his weight in 2001) and, therefore, at a height of six feet, he should be considered 'thin' - he proceeded to impart some home truths. 'My mother gave me the best dieting idea in the world: "Stop eating when you're still hungry".'

He prophesied that obesity would become 'the greatest health problem of the twenty-first century', and to date he has been proven right. He suggested people should: 1. be wary of dieting ('most get-thin-quick diet programmes only reduce the size of your wallet'); 2. use their common sense ('losing weight takes time [and] attaining a bikini figure in two weeks only works in magazines'); and 3. train themselves ('a healthy diet is like jogging; practice a few times and it will come naturally'). He recommended drinking red wine ('alcohol plays the role of Dr Jekyll and Mr Hyde; it is a killer, but it can also promote our health') and eating plenty of fruit and vegetables (as he said he had done as a child).

He advised that 'a sensible diet has to ensure that the body fat amount is reduced while simultaneously building muscle. This is the reason why a diet without exercise is something for the dustbin. Exercises or sport help to stimulate the metabolism; weight-loss diets do the opposite. When you become active your body suddenly stops storing fat and begins to burn it—you begin to lose weight.' He continued that 'virtually no one manages to lose weight and keep it off.'

Chris also discussed the role that stress might play in relation to heart health. He admitted to personally being under stress only three times in his life. 'All three times had to do with people who were very close to me.' The first was when his father died unexpectedly. 'It caused me a great deal of grief. He was a very charismatic man and we were very close.' The second was when André, as a boy of ten, could suddenly not breathe because of an obstruction of his windpipe; fortunately, he quickly recovered. The third was when his second wife, Barbara, divorced him: 'it was a new and painful experience: separation from a person can sometimes cause more stress than their death.' It is perhaps surprising that he did not include the occasion of André's untimely death.

However, elsewhere in the book, in discussing grief, he lists three periods when he experienced profound sorrow in his life. These again included the death of his father, but also the deaths of André and Barbara.

Chris recommended to his readers that they should avoid what he called 'techno-stress', for example, not being a slave to a cell phones, computers, or emails. Indeed, he worried that in medicine, 'the use of technology is greatly exaggerated. In many hospitals doctors and nurses no longer watch over patients but rather leave that to high-tech devices. Machines, however, cannot give love.'

He admitted, however, that he did not believe he would have become a good doctor without a certain amount of stress.

> I always wanted to be there 100 per cent for my patients. If someone was ill in my clinic, I could think of nothing else all day. The pressure I was under allowed me to care even more intensively for my patients. I wanted to know everything about their illness. Therefore, stress was, in my job, a kind of engine that drove me to do better and more. [I believe many conscientious surgeons and physicians feel the same—I know I did.]
>
> ... [There was] no patent remedy for the right recreation after work. Everyone has to find out for him- or her-self what the right method of relieving stress is for them. Some people enjoy sport, others like to

meet up with friends or just relax with the family. I always enjoyed gardening. The times I felt under pressure I found it soothing to see how my tomatoes were doing or what fruit tree was blooming. If I were more talented I would paint; fortunately, I also had the ability to write. But as it is, gardening fulfills all my requirements for relaxation.

One interesting aspect of the book is his comments on the role sex might play in life.

Sex is and always was a very important part of life for me. Sex always meant many things to me: love of my partner, pleasure, relaxation and activity—much better than all that mindless jogging … Sex is not some new type of competitive sport. It is the most beautiful experience in the world.

He recommended that one should always have sex when there is 'a natural need for it', but never if it 'feels like a chore.' Furthermore, one should never have sex outside the bedroom, never have sex in strange beds, and never pay for sex.

I am more of a romantic lover. Perhaps many will laugh at this description, but I believe it and refer exclusively to personal experience: I never just 'needed' sex enough to pay for it. I can even recall a very unpleasant experience concerning this subject back in 1963. I had just arrived in the city of light, Paris, from a very depressing Moscow during Cold War times. As I was walking along the Champs-Elysées I encountered an attractive woman who gave me a friendly smile. We got conversing and suddenly, out of the blue, she asked me to come to a hotel with her. I agreed and we went to a small, clean and discreet hotel. It was so discreet that I almost didn't notice the 'spy' who was observing us in the foyer through a keyhole in a wooden door.

Upon entering the room, the attractive young woman immediately began undressing. I said: 'No, no, that's not the way I want to do it. I would like to talk with you some more first.' She replied: 'Talk? Well, OK, but that will cost you more.' I quickly left the room. Even the 'spy' was surprised. He opened his door and yelled after me: 'That was the quickest session we ever had in this house!'

This story, recounted to illustrate that Chris was not prepared to pay for sex, is very revealing. At the time, he was married, and yet willingly went with the young woman to a hotel (I suppose he must have imagined she was a visitor to Paris, like himself) and appeared very willing to have sex with her, but not the way she wanted to do it. It is not a story that most of us would be willing to recount about ourselves, even many years later.

He admitted that he had had 'a lot of sex' in his life:

> The older I got the more important it became for me. However, I believe that sex should always be in the context of a love affair—however short-lived or minor. This may sound a bit strange coming from a man who has always been described by the media as a kind of 'womaniser'. But I ask you to believe me when I say that a married man should try to be faithful. That is my firm conviction. I realise today that my marriages never ended because of unfaithfulness but only because I neglected my partner at the time.

I am not at all sure that this 'spin' Chris puts on the factors contributing to his divorces is in any way true. He continued his advice on sex:

> It's important for couples to keep sexuality 'alive', never stop being creative and never stop making sex interesting. Many couples no longer enjoy sex because they have stopped making it interesting or trying to think of something new to stimulate themselves.

Yet he had just advised his readers to 'never have sex outside the bedroom' or 'in a strange bed'—surely not a very innovative way of keeping a couple's sexuality alive. Furthermore, in the story he recounted above, he seemed perfectly willing to have sex in 'a strange bed.'

Despite some of these contradictions, like his earlier book on heart disease, the excellent advice he gave in this, his last book, must have been valuable to many of its readers. Although most of the advice he gave was already well-known at the time, coming as 'the definitive guide from the world's most respected doctor' (as the cover stated), his straightforward and entertaining writing frequently put the advice across in a novel and meaningful way.

Some years previously, Chris had published a similar book, *Christiaan Barnard's Program for Living with Arthritis*, for patients with any form of arthritis, but particularly with the form from which he suffered: rheumatoid arthritis. This book, published in 1984, was written with Peter Evans. I am not sure whether Peter Evans was a medical journalist or had expertise in the field of arthritis, and so he may have contributed as much or more than Chris to the preparation of the book. However, Chris's opinions clearly run through the book, and I suspect that the general outline of the book was conceived by him, but with research being carried out by Peter Evans to fill all of the gaps. The research effort put into writing the book must have been considerable.

This again is a book for the public on a topic of which Chris was not a trained expert, but of course with which he had considerable personal experience through his prolonged affliction with rheumatoid arthritis, with which he lived for more than forty years.

On the cover page, the following words precede the title: 'The preeminent physician of our time relates his personal experience with arthritis and offers compassion and hope for sufferers who can learn to live with arthritis.'

It is again a book that is well-written, informative, and readable. Chris explained the various forms of arthritis, the various types of treatment that were available then, including drug therapy and surgical procedures, and went on to discuss the problem of living with pain. Suggestions were made as to how life could be made easier when one is a rheumatoid arthritis patient. Although I am not by any means an expert on arthritis, I once again believe that the information given to the reader was accurate, and the suggestions on how to live with arthritis were reasonable, balanced, and helpful.

Chris again called on his personal medical experiences in providing anecdotes to illustrate the points he wanted to make.

All surgery is physically as well as mentally demanding, imposing enormous strains on the surgeon as he stands for long periods carrying out delicate manipulations. With heart transplants there are added complications ... You really have two 'patients': the person whom you are fighting to save, and the precious heart, which must remain viable. In this complex medical setting, populated by large teams of surgeons, physicians, anaesthetists, nurses, and auxiliaries, one needs to perform with maximum efficiency—which is not so simple when pain is crippling one's feet and legs, and one's hands are swollen and sore in practically every joint.

He explained how he suffered from the mental pain of rheumatoid arthritis as well as the physical pain.

The worst diseases, I feel, are those where people around you see you have got it. If you have a hole in the heart, nobody is aware of it. So it's not as bad as having a faceful of acne that other people can see. These are diseases that greatly reduce the quality of life. That is why I see nothing wrong with having face lifts and bags under the eyes removed surgically and things like that. I would have had myself done if I felt my quality of life would be improved by it. At my stage now, it is difficult to cover up the fact that I am crippled, and it hurts my pride. I cannot generalise. I must speak only for myself. Some people don't mind it very much, but I do mind it very much. I also mind when my children see that I am struggling. There is something in the way they look at me which I cannot bear. So as far as diseases are concerned, the worst ones for me to have are those where you are not only suffering from it physically but you have the emotional trauma that other people see you have the disease.

He emphasised how rheumatoid arthritis had limited his interaction with his children, robbing him of the chance to play with them as often as he would have liked. However, he took pains to advise such patients not to feel too sorry for themselves—not to dwell on what they could not do, but to appreciate what they could do in life—to concentrate on what one had left. He believed that a patient's mental attitude towards his or her disease was important, and a 'real willingness to get better plays a definite role in recovery, and that is true whether the treatments being given are orthodox or unconventional.'

His final conclusion on his personal battle with rheumatoid arthritis can perhaps be summarised by the following passage.

You will have realised by now that temperamentally I have never felt 'suited' to being the victim of arthritis. It is too much like being taken over by decrepitude and immobility at a time in one's life when one wants and needs to be active. At the same time, and in complete opposition to this, I have done my best work, toiled for long hours, and had an immensely rewarding life, despite being a sufferer. So who am I to lapse into self-pity at having a disease which is not, after all, life-threatening, merely exceptionally inconvenient?'

## Chris as a Novelist

On the second occasion that I visited Cape Town (in 1973, when I was a cardiac surgical resident in Cambridge in the UK), I again spent some time with Chris at GSH. Now, six years after the first heart transplant, he was at the peak of his career, and so I was surprised when he told me that he was carrying out fewer operations because he was spending some of his time writing a novel. This must have been *The Unwanted*, published in 1975.

My understanding from those close to Chris is that he was first stimulated to consider writing a novel through his experience in putting together his autobiography, *One Life*, with professional writer Curtis Bill Pepper. He would ask Dene Friedmann to type out the pages and would be forever pestering her to see whether she had completed them or not. He would also ask her what her opinion was of the chapter. If she said it was not very good, he was very depressed and upset.

Between 1975 and 1996, Chris wrote four novels, three in collaboration with Siegfried Stander, already a relatively successful published novelist in South Africa. Evidently, Chris, who knew it was his name on the cover that would sell the book, was a hard businessman when it came to making deals with Mr Stander, who did most of the work. With each novel, Stander had to argue his case to obtain an increased percentage of the profits. Although their first book was a publishing success worldwide, the subsequent novels did relatively poorly. Mr Stander died of a heart attack (following several previous ones) in 1988. His widow claimed that he realised that he had made a professional mistake in collaborating with Chris, and made very little money out of their work together.

To provide an indication of what Chris thought would capture a reader's attention, and how imaginative he was in writing fiction, I provide a brief critique of each novel.

## The Unwanted

This was Chris's first novel (the title of which I understand was suggested by his wife, Barbara) and, like many first novels, is very autobiographical. The story is based on a man, Deon van der Riet, whose boyhood was spent on a sheep farm owned by his father near Beaufort West. Although Chris was not brought up on a farm, he must have had friends in Beaufort West who were. One of the workers on the farm was a coloured man whose son, Philip, was very friendly as a child with the hero of the book, Deon. Despite their different ethnic and social backgrounds, the two boys spent a great deal of time together. For example, they embarked on a jaguar hunt in the desolate hills around the town, killing the jaguar with their bows and arrows. Chris never mentioned such a hunt in his autobiography nor to my knowledge to any of his colleagues or friends, but it is quite likely he heard the story from adventurous school friends in Beaufort West. Philip's father dies, and so Philip and his mother move to Cape Town where she becomes a domestic servant. Moreover, Philip is academically gifted and does very well at school.

Deon enters medical school in Cape Town, and finds that Philip has also won a place there as one of the very few non-white students attending the university. His fees are secretly being paid by Deon's father, and it eventually becomes clear that Philip and Deon are actually half-brothers, as Deon's father illegitimately fathered Philip.

During medical school, Deon gets a university student pregnant and there is a realistic description of her undergoing an illegal abortion. Whether this is based on a true experience of Chris Barnard—he never mentioned such an experience to me—or possibly on the experience of a fellow student, is unknown. The two young men, Deon and Philip, graduate together and both are appointed to house jobs (internships) at the hospital before they finally part company. Philip emigrates to Canada where he becomes a world-famous geneticist, even being nominated for a Nobel Prize, although his nomination is unsuccessful. He later returns to Cape Town when his mother is dying.

Deon becomes a cardiac surgeon, and there are several very accurate descriptions of him carrying out heart operations (where Chris is obviously drawing on his immense personal experience). In the laboratory, he carries out a head transplant in a dog (just as Chris had carried one out in real life).

Several other characters may be based on Chris's colleagues at Groote Schuur Hospital. For example, the chairman of the department of surgery may well be based on Professor Jannie Louw, though his character has been modified. They have something of a love-hate relationship (and so the real-life comments of Chris's brother, Marius, in this respect may have been correct). Deon has a close colleague with whom he eventually falls out, and I suspect that this character may have been based loosely on Marius. Deon finally falls out with his boss, and his junior colleague (the Marius figure) is appointed head of surgical research. Deon feels his long-standing colleague has worked against him and has not been loyal to him.

Although descriptions of surgical operations obviously have an appeal to some, I would have thought there are too many details to be of interest to many lay readers. However, the descriptions of the operations are good, including the thoughts of the surgeon as he overcomes barriers or is faced with defeat and failure.

Chris clearly called on his medical experience throughout the book. There are vivid descriptions of a casualty department with dozens of dehydrated babies receiving treatment, and of a child of eighteen months who had been raped. Chris also repeats several other episodes that he writes about in his autobiographies. One is that Deon is doing research on cooling the inside of the stomach to treat gastric ulcers, which was a project Chris explored in Minneapolis. The second is that he repeats the story of the two little boys, racing around the wards on a trolley (which has been described in Chapter 16).

Deon breaks up with the girlfriend who had undergone the abortion, and hits it off with a blonde girl from a very wealthy family whom he meets at a party. As the book was published in 1975, while Chris was married to Barbara, although she was a brunette, the wealthy young girl may to some extent have been based on her. He eventually marries her and they have two children: an older daughter and a younger son (just as Chris had with his first wife).

The teenage daughter is taking drugs and her life is in a mess (which, although perhaps reminiscent of Chris's own first son, André, may not have been based on André's experience as in 1975, he was aged only twenty-four and may not have developed his drug habit at that time). Clearly based on Chris's own mother, Deon's mother is in an old people's home as she has had a severe stroke. Deon does not visit her very often (just as Chris did not visit his own mother very frequently).

We eventually learn that Deon's wife had previously had a very brief affair with Philip before the marriage. Although there is a hint she might leave Deon and get together with Philip again, I see no real reason why this liaison should have been written into the story although it does demonstrate how the apartheid policy affected the everyday lives of people in South Africa. It contributes to the picture of Philip being the 'unwanted' in his country.

Several years later, the first girlfriend shows up again with a son, who has Down's syndrome, and it is hinted that this was caused by the previous abortion (although I do not think there is much evidence that this would have occurred). She brings her son to Deon because he has a rare birth defect of the heart, tricuspid atresia, that had never been corrected surgically before. Deon works in the animal laboratory to design a novel surgical technique to correct this cardiac defect. Before he carries out the operation, however, he hears that French surgeons have designed the same operation. This is clearly a Fontan procedure, named after the French surgeon who developed it in 1971, and may have been in Chris's mind at the time. Whether Chris actually developed the operative technique in the laboratory before Professor Fontan is not known, but I think unlikely. However, the French have not yet carried out the corrective operation in a patient. Deon does so, and saves the boy's life.

While Philip is in Cape Town temporarily, he sets up a laboratory to carry out some research on *in vitro* fertilization. He has a problem with a staff technician, who reports him to the newspapers because he is fertilising women's ova (eggs) that Deon has obtained for him from a gynaecologist using his own spermatozoa. Fertilization of a white woman's egg with a coloured man's sperm was against the apartheid laws in South Africa at that time, where mixed marriages were prohibited. This causes a scandal, and Philip begins to think that he will give up his career in genetics research and move back to Beaufort West where he would plan to become a general practitioner for the coloured community. To me, this career move seemed unlikely because he would be much more likely to return to Canada where he is an established and internationally recognised professor of genetics.

The story is well-written and many times reminded me vividly of living in Cape Town and of working as a cardiac surgeon at Groote Schuur Hospital. The book is very readable and it kept me interested until the last page or two when I was disappointed that there was no definitive outcome for any of the main characters. The ending of the book was, to me, unsatisfactory as we do not learn what Philip finally decides. Deon is considering divorcing his wife and marrying the girlfriend on whose son he has operated. A weakness of the story is that we do not get a sense of a burning desire in him to spend the rest of his life with this woman. It would appear that she does not wish to marry him and he also becomes ambivalent, but we are left in slight doubt. Deon's troubles with his boss in the hospital also remain unresolved.

Due to his ethnicity, it is presumably Philip who is the 'unwanted' of the title but, as he is treated so amicably by many of the hospital staff, including Deon, this point is not hammered home. However, his biological father did not really want to own him, although he secretly supported him financially, and Philip clearly represents many of the educated coloured and black population in South Africa at that time, who were not given full opportunities in their own country.

Like most popular modern literature, however, the story leaves little lasting impact in one's mind, and the plot and characters are readily forgotten. So, it is an okay novel with an intriguing storyline, but certainly not a great one. There are so many autobiographical aspects to the story that I strongly suspect the story line was Chris's, with Mr Stander putting it on paper.

## In the Night Season

This novel—Chris's second—was again written with Siegfried Stander; published in 1978, it also has a medical basis. The main character is a fifty-year-old country doctor, Charles de la Porte, who has also trained in surgery and so carries out some surgical procedures in a town a couple of hours drive from Cape Town (possibly based on Chris's time as a general practitioner in Ceres). Like Chris, Charles de la Porte had trained in medicine and surgery at the University of Cape Town. One of his patients is another doctor, a woman whom he finds has cancer of the breast that has already spread to the bones of her back. He therefore deems she is incurable and that no operation will be of benefit to her. Rather than give her the bad news, he believes it will be in her best interests to tell her that the biopsy of the breast he has taken is negative, and that she has nothing to worry about. Telling her the true situation would lead her to worry about her health during the few remaining months she has to live.

Some weeks later, she finds out the truth, and she and her husband decide to sue de la Porte in the courts for malpractice. She consults another local surgeon who believes she should be treated aggressively with all of the surgical procedures and other therapies available to him that might slow the progress of the disease and prolong her life, even though the side effects of these procedures may make the quality of her remaining weeks very poor.

The story is complicated by the fact that de la Porte had had an affair with the patient many years previously when he was a surgical trainee and she was a medical student. He was married to his first wife at the time, but the girl was unmarried. She was a headstrong young woman who, although white, was involved with an underground anti-apartheid group of coloured and black people, working towards undermining the South African government by terrorist activities. Our hero becomes peripherally drawn into this intrigue and is forced to protect her, and subsequently one of her activist colleagues, from the police.

The plot is further complicated by the fact that de la Porte's first wife, with whom he has a small daughter, became suspicious (if not confirmed in the fact) that he was having an affair. When driving the child over a mountain pass, the wife drives the car off the side of a road and the occupants plunge to their deaths several hundred feet below. Charles de la Porte is uncertain whether this is an accident or whether she purposely committed suicide because she was distraught about his affair.

Before the malpractice case comes to court, however, the patient's health has deteriorated to such an extent that her husband comes to de la Porte and begs him to persuade the other surgeon to discontinue all treatment and let her die a humane death with some dignity. The two surgeons discuss the pros and cons of how the patient should be managed. This part of the book is rather artificial in that it becomes an argument between two men on the responsibilities of doctors and whether passive euthanasia should be carried out or whether every effort should be made to prolong life even if it results in a deterioration in the patient's quality of life.

While the book is generally well-written, like *The Unwanted*, the ending was, to me, unsatisfactory. Some of the loose ends relating to the complicated plot are not tied up.

A major weakness of the story is that one would have imagined that de la Porte would have at least told the patient's husband that the outlook was poor. Furthermore, he surely would have felt obligated to give the patient some indication of the seriousness of her condition while, importantly, leaving her with some hope, as Chris himself had experienced when being given the diagnosis of rheumatoid arthritis

The story is well-told and there are several throwbacks to Chris's own life. First, he was a general practitioner in a town about equidistant from Cape Town as the town in the novel. Second, some of the research he is described as doing as a surgical trainee is actually the same research that he was doing at the University of Minnesota when a young man. Showing a distinct lack of imagination, this research is the same as discussed in *The Unwanted*, namely on the topic of healing gastric ulcers by cooling the inside of the stomach. Third, although this is purely conjecture, perhaps de la Porte's situation in having an affair with a younger woman while married is based on Chris's personal experience during his first marriage. Whether any other aspects of the story are related to his own personal experiences, such as being involved in underground terrorist activity (even peripherally) seems unlikely.

The story generally maintains the reader's interest and, although it is not a book that you are reluctant to put down, it is every bit as good as many novels that have been on the bookstands in the last forty years. Again, I suspect that the story was primarily Chris's, but that much of the writing was by Mr Stander. However, like *The Unwanted* and all but the most outstanding novels, I found the story was easily forgotten.

## The Faith

This was Chris's third novel, again written in collaboration with Siegfried Stander, and first published in 1984.

Again, it is a good stab at writing a novel, although in my opinion, it has several weaknesses. The story is perhaps more complicated than either of his previous two novels, and revolves around a surgeon, Dr Brand, at a hospital in one of the South African homeland states. The homeland is supposedly situated north of South Africa (probably based geographically on Botswana). The story revolves around a hospital ship called *The Faith*, which has been developed from the wreck of an old paddle steamer that had been used for entertainment purposes in the past. The surgeon is faced with an outbreak of a lethal haemorrhagic fever (similar to the Ebola outbreak that occurred in recent years in West Africa) that has affected some patients and some of his staff.

As a medical detective story, this alone would have sufficed as the basis for an intriguing novel, but the authors were much more ambitious. They bring in a love element in the form of one of the surgeon's junior colleagues, a young doctor of Cape Malay origin who had worked in both London and the Far East. The story also involves South African military activity that was going on at the time in the states north of South Africa, such as Namibia, where insurgents (terrorists or freedom fighters, depending on your political persuasion) are trying to take over the country. Even this is not sufficiently complex for the authors, as they also link the secretive activities of an international charitable foundation (that funds the hospital) with East German criminals.

The story becomes increasingly unlikely in that, towards the end, the female love interest is raped by the terrorists, and then, to save her life, has to undergo an emergency operation performed by the surgeon on the boat under extremely difficult conditions. To my mind, the proceedings become too farfetched.

The story is far too detailed to summarise easily, but the description of the areas in which the events take place (the wetlands of southern Africa) are convincing in most respects. However, some of the characters are not as fleshed out as one would like, and one does not get the sense of commitment to them that a reader should have. Despite their adventures, I found myself not caring greatly whether they lived or died.

As with his previous two novels, I found the ending less than satisfactory as there were so many loose ends that remained, and I was left with a sense of desertion by the authors. For example, the relevance of the East German criminals is not made clear, at least to me. The story has the makings of an adventure movie, but for someone with his feet on the ground, it would seem all a little over the top, and I do not believe the ending would be satisfying to the majority of film-goers.

There are occasional hints as to Chris's own opinions. His relative disdain for medical administrators and 'pen-pushers' raises its head: 'At what stage, Brand wondered, did a doctor become a bureaucrat? Was it when papers became more important than people?'

The writing is generally good, but towards the end, there are short passages that seem to me to be very amateurish, which surprised me in view of Siegfried Stander's reputation as a published novelist. An example of a passage that is unusually and surprisingly poor is when Dr Brand has just operated on, and saved the life of, his female love interest:

Is there any mark on me, he thought, to show the abundance I found within myself as my hands laboured within the body of the woman I love?

Say it, he thought. Let them hear it and scream their condemnation if they wish. She is of another race and colour and God knows there are overwhelming obstacles between us. But she is the woman I love.

'I think she's going to be all right,' Da Costa said.

'Of course she's going to be all right,' Brand said.
'You're a hell of a surgeon, doc,' William said.

I am surely not alone in finding this passage quite dreadful.

## The Donor

This final novel was written entirely by Chris Barnard, apparently without professional help, although he does thank Bob Molloy for encouragement and assistance. He also expresses his gratitude to certain professional colleagues, presumably for advice on some of the medical aspects of the novel, and it is clear that Chris did much research before putting pen to paper. The novel was first published in 1996, well after his retirement from UCT, which was in 1983.

In an author's note, Chris writes:

The search for knowledge and truth should never be curtailed but the ways in which the findings are used certainly call for control. Like the veneer of civilization which overlies human savagery, the ethical barriers between the pure scientist and misapplied research findings remain thin. This story is one of good intentions gone wrong, and some of the myriad ways in which we can mislead ourselves.

Chris demonstrates a good novelist's skill by immediately capturing the reader's attention with his opening two sentences. 'Rodney Barnes had never seen a real hangman's rope before, much less fixed around a human neck. The body hung, suspended below the open trap door of the prison gallows, turning slightly.'

Like his previous novels, it is a complicated story, again being based to a large extent on his personal experience, but with considerable embellishments. The lead character, Rodney Barnes, is a thirty-eight-year-old heart transplant surgeon in Cape Town whose 'name is known far beyond the world of medicine', who lives in a luxury apartment in Table View, which looks back at Table Mountain from the other side of Table Bay. For a period of his life when separated from Barbara, Chris had the same view from his home in Blouberg.

Rodney Barnes (clearly based on Chris himself) is an unmarried, internationally renowned surgeon but who, unlike Chris, apparently does not lose his temper with his colleagues in the operating room or in the wards. He has a senior research colleague named Kapinsky, who I am sure was based to some extent on my former GSH colleague,

Dimitri Novitzky, in that he hails from Eastern Europe (as did Dimitri's parents) and has similar research interests. Indeed, at one point when the police are searching for Dr Kapinsky, they mistakenly identify him as a 'Dr Novitsky'. Although based loosely on Dimitri, the comparison goes no further because (of course, unknown to Rodney Barnes) Kapinsky is a former Nazi who was involved in some of the Second World War concentration camp work.

Barnes and Kapinsky are trying to overcome the shortage of donor hearts for transplantation, and are approaching this problem in several different ways. First, Barnes arranges with the authorities in Pretoria that hearts can be removed from prisoners undergoing capital punishment (hence the hangings) and then flown to Cape Town. Second, Kapinsky is genetically engineering baboons so that their organs will not be rejected by humans. Third, he is storing human hearts by transplanting them into baboons until they are required for a patient. Fourth and finally, Kapinsky and Barnes determine that the heart of a brain-dead human donor ceases to function within a few days because of the loss of control of the brain.

This latter work is clearly an extension of the work that Dimitri Novitzky carried out on using thyroid hormone to stabilise brain-dead donors before the heart is excised (outlined in Chapter 21). In the novel, they take this a step further and believe there are other products from the brain that circulate in the donor that can maintain long-term stability of the donor's circulatory system. They connect the head of a baboon to a brain-dead donor so that the products of the baboon's brain maintain circulatory stability of the human donor. They set up an intensive care unit in the hospital for the long-term management of these brain-dead donors (with their attached baboon heads).

Although there is some factual basis for all of their approaches, the author takes them well into the realms of science fiction. The plot is further complicated as, unknown to Barnes, Kapinsky funds his research by producing illegal drugs in the laboratory, which he sells to underworld dealers in Cape Town. He is also in a relationship with one of his laboratory technicians, who is a dominatrix to whom he submits himself at relatively regular intervals.

Kapinsky has used his own spermatozoa to impregnate a female baboon, and she delivers a son, who is part human and part baboon. Kapinsky is excited to have a son of his own, and eventually purchases a large, secluded mansion with extensive grounds so that the son may live there out of the public eye. Furthermore, one of the baboons that has been given the heart of a human murderer behaves in an aggressive and 'criminal-like' manner.

Rodney Barnes has a love affair with a young woman who is a transplant nurse-coordinator at the hospital. Unfortunately, when out riding with him, she is thrown by her horse, and loses their unborn child. She suffers severe brain damage, and is finally placed in the intensive care ward attached to the head of a baboon, officially as a potential organ donor. However, his hope is that she will eventually recover her own brain function (although this seems exceedingly unlikely). As he wants her to bear them a son, when he is alone in the unit with her, he personally impregnates her (which I found rather distasteful). However, this possibility is also complicated because Kapinsky secretly also impregnates her with baboon spermatozoa with the aim that she will deliver a human-baboon child.

The plot, therefore, is exceedingly complicated, and I have only touched on parts of it in this brief summary. The story ends with Kapinsky and his dominatrix dying suddenly as a complication of their sexual activities. The child that the brain-dead lover is carrying is about to be born by Caesarian section. We are interested in the outcome, but we are left at the end (as with the previous novels) frustrated as some of our questions are left unanswered.

Although passages are well written, for me, the story was far too fantastic and far too complex. I must admit that I am not somebody who enjoys fantasy in any form, and to my mind, the science fiction in this book was beyond the realms of possibility. I, therefore, found the latter part of the book, where the story became increasingly preposterous, to be disappointing. However, for those readers who enjoy science fiction, possibly as put forward in the work of doctors Robin Cook or Michael Crichton, the book may be more appealing.

Nevertheless, the story does entail numerous aspects of research work in transplantation that have been explored previously or may even be on the horizon in clinical practice. For example, the idea of storing human hearts in non-human primates has been around for many years, but never eventualised. The use of prisoners as (living) kidney donors was carried out some decades ago, in particular by Tom Starzl, and you will remember that Denton Cooley suggested the use of hearts from executed prisoners when he attended the Cape Town conference in 1968. In recent years, executed prisoners provided large numbers of donor organs in China, a practice that was heavily criticised on ethical grounds by many in the West. The approach of making humans immunologically tolerant to tissues from animals, such as baboons or pigs, has been discussed and researched for many years. The potential of the brain supplying substances that maintain cardiovascular stability was certainly indicated by the research of Dimitri Novitzky, and there may be more secrets still to be discovered in this respect. Indeed, it clearly must have been Dimitri's work that suggested this topic as a subject for Chris's novel. Furthermore, in the book, in an effort to save a patient's life, Barnes carries out a heterotopic (piggyback) heart transplant using a heart from a baboon, which is something that Chris Barnard did himself (as we noted in Chapter 19).

One of the laboratory assistants in the story is a black man whose story is clearly based on that of Hamilton Naki (Chapter 11). He comes from one of the homelands, obtains work at UCT as a gardener, is promoted to be a janitor in the laboratory, and eventually is taught how to do numerous operations and becomes a key member of the laboratory research team. This character is given the nickname of 'Boots', which was the nickname of one of the real-life coloured research technicians, Frederick Snyders (but not that of Hamilton Naki).

There are, therefore, many overlaps between Chris Barnard's real life and the various intermingled stories in the novel. I suggest, however, that the various storylines are too complex and that not all of them contribute to the story in a meaningful way. If the story had been simplified (instead of being so complex), I believe it would have made more impact on the reader and would have lost nothing.

Although I have been perhaps unduly critical of all four novels, I admire Chris's literary ambition and his determination to bring them to fruition. The ideas behind all of them were imaginative and exciting, and not without considerable merit. With some restriction and focusing of the story (as is necessary when a novel is made into a movie), each of them would be as successful as most of the Hollywood and television films of the period.

Chris's relatively prolonged effort to write novels, extending over more than twenty years, was perhaps primarily driven by a desire to augment his income; in this respect, he was only modestly successful. However, my friend, the surgeon and medical historian David Hamilton, has suggested that Chris may also have been stimulated by a desire to entertain people, and possibly by an underlying need to embellish his own life (eventful and exciting, as it was) by blurring fact and fiction, and thus living his own life even more vividly in his novels.

# 28

# Was Everything Black or White?
# Chris's Opinions on Apartheid

Chris's personal attitude to race and colour, inherited from his father, was passed on to his children. Deirdre recollects:

[As a child, I] grew up in a house where the door was always open to anyone who chose to walk through it. It didn't matter what colour they happened to be. There was always enough in the pot to offer a plate of food. That was how our family lived then. It's how we live now. Perhaps it's only a very small thing but it's the only way we know. We have accepted comfort and support when we've needed it and offered it, in our turn, when we've been able to do so. I know this doesn't make us in any way exceptional. I say it only because it is, always has been and always will be our way.

Certainly, in his personal life, I do not believe Chris discriminated against anybody on the basis of race or colour. Deirdre's comment that their house was open to everybody supports this conclusion.

In my own experience during the several years I worked with him in Cape Town (and Oklahoma City), I never witnessed any discrimination on his part in the care of the patients (or staff) in our department at Groote Schuur and Red Cross War Memorial Children's Hospitals. Patients were treated on the basis of need alone.

Dene Friedmann, who worked with Chris for far longer than I did (approximately twenty years) recollected:

Chris insisted that all his patients, no matter what ethnic group or gender, would be nursed in the one ICU where he had the most experienced staff, and all should receive the very best treatment. He went against the hospital authorities and the government, but got his way to do this,

saying if anyone [i.e. any patient] didn't like it they could go elsewhere
for their heart operation.

Similar changes did not take place at most other comparable hospitals in
South Africa in those days. My close colleague and good friend, Dimitri
Novitzky, had joined Chris's department after a year working in the
equivalent hospitals in Bloemfontein in the Orange Free State, another
of the four provinces (states) in the country. In Bloemfontein, there were
separate hospitals for black and white patients. On one occasion, the
operating rooms in the 'black' hospital required closure for renovation.
During these few days, a patient presented who required urgent open
heart surgery. Dimitri requested that, as an exception to the rule, the
operation should be carried out in the 'white' hospital. His request was
initially turned down but, after some argument and negotiation, the
authorities agreed the emergency operation could be performed in the
'white' hospital.

The patient was transferred by ambulance, and the operation was
carried out successfully. Dimitri then asked for the patient to be moved
to the ICU for immediate post-operative nursing and recovery, but was
told that this had not been part of the agreement, and that the patient had
to be transported back to the 'black' hospital. No amount of argument
could change this decision, and so the patient, still anaesthetised, with
drainage tubes coming out of his chest, monitoring equipment attached,
was taken from the operating room to an ambulance and, in this critical
state, driven back to the 'black' hospital. Fortunately, he survived the
hazardous journey.

This was obviously quite a different situation from that at GSH and the
Red Cross Children's Hospital, and Chris must take credit for changing
the system in Cape Town many years previously. Chris would never have
agreed to work under the conditions that Dimitri faced in Bloemfontein.

Lest this story appears to be too critical of South Africa, it is worth
remembering that open heart surgery in any hospital—black or white—
would not have been available to a patient in any other sub-Saharan
African country. In this respect, the patient was very fortunate to live in
South Africa.

From my personal experience of working as a surgeon in Cape Town,
where the majority of my patients were coloured or black, I felt I was
contributing significantly to the well-being of ethnically and economically
disadvantaged groups.

Perhaps to give some perspective to the situation in South Africa,
Eugene Dong, a highly productive Chinese-American medical researcher
who joined Shumway's team at Stanford in 1960, found it difficult to

rent an apartment because of discrimination against people of his race. As is well-known, Muhammad Ali (then Cassius Clay), an Olympic gold medalist in 1960, was barred from eating in many restaurants in his home town of Louisville, Kentucky, because of his ethnicity. Furthermore, at that time, Australia still followed a 'whites-only' immigration policy, and there was significant discrimination against the Aborigine population.

There are two aspects of apartheid that we shall consider. The first is how heart transplantation and apartheid were viewed in 1967, and the second is Chris's personal attitude to apartheid.

## Heart Transplantation in the Land of Apartheid

A discussion on race, colour, and politics can hardly be avoided when commenting on any event that took place in South Africa in the 1960s or even in subsequent years until apartheid was abolished with the installation of Nelson Mandela's government in 1994.

Following the first and second heart transplants in Cape Town, there was much discussion on the medical, moral, ethical, philosophical, religious, and political aspects of transplantation, both in the South African and foreign media. These discussions ranged from the those of the 'man in the street' who might state that the churches should condemn interference in God's will—if someone is destined to die, humans have no right to prolong life—to the opinions of 'experts' in every field.

There were numerous comments in the South African newspapers, many written by religious leaders. Almost without exception they agreed that, in principle, transplantation was a good thing. The rabbinical authorities stated that the transplant of the heart from an Anglican Christian girl into a Jewish man did not transgress the laws of the Jewish religion.

Several authors discussed the ethical questions raised by the transplant, questions that had been discussed years earlier when both dialysis and kidney transplantation began to become available to patients with kidney failure. For example, given the limited supply of donor hearts, who should receive one? Should it be prohibited to a child or young person? Should a leading member of society, such as a political leader, a scientist, an eminent businessman who provided work for thousands, take precedence over someone who is perhaps contributing less to the community? Should the organ be given to the man with many children to support?

The topic of apartheid was, of course, of particular interest—at least to the media—when an organ was transferred from the body of a person of one race to that of a person of a different race. In South Africa, where the official government policy was separation of the races, would some white people object to receiving an organ, particularly a heart, from a non-white person? It is perhaps surprising that there were no official criticisms of Chris and his colleagues when they later carried out heart transplants across the racial divide, or when they had performed the transplantation of a black kidney into Mrs Black or of Denise Darvall's white kidney into a coloured boy. A similar sort of medico-racial dilemma could potentially arise in other parts of the world, where discrimination ran deep, or possibly in India. Would an Indian of high-caste accept an organ from an 'untouchable'? Would a high-caste Indian donate an organ to an 'untouchable'?

Chris and Val Schrire had discussed the possible reaction of the Nationalist government if a transplant was to be carried out between a 'black' donor and a 'white' recipient. They had come to the conclusion that, although some of the politicians 'might be horrified by the idea, they wouldn't utter a murmur in public as the heart transplant programme was the only positive news coming out of South Africa at that time.' They were proved correct as there were very few criticisms from the politicians. An American newspaper article claimed that the South African government was planning to introduce legislation prohibiting organ transplantation between the different ethnic groups, but this claim was unfounded.

Various foreign newspapers, such as the liberal (or left-wing) *The Guardian* in the UK, questioned whether the laws in South Africa allowed a white man to live with a coloured man's heart within him, as Dr Blaiberg did. Could he sit on a park bench restricted to 'whites only'? There was some basis for such comments as the early heart transplants made nonsense of the petty apartheid laws. South Africa House in London was inundated with questions as to how heart transplants impacted apartheid.

It is of interest to note that the outside world's obsession between heart transplantation and apartheid continued well into the 1980s. For example, in 1984, I attended a congress of The (international) Transplantation Society in the UK to present a scientific paper. Although the number of heart transplants carried out in Cape Town remained relatively small, we had statistically analyzed which factors were associated with a good outcome and which with a poor outcome. These might include the age or gender of the patient and donor, the underlying cause of the heart disease, and many other potential factors. One point we had observed was that the very few white patients who had received a heart from a 'black' donor (as opposed to a 'coloured' or 'white' donor) survived statistically longer than those who received hearts from white donors. Although we had no evidence at the time, this was probably related to tissue typing; perhaps the black donor lacked certain tissue (white blood cell) antigens that might stimulate rejection in a white patient. It was an interesting observation among many other more important observations we had made.

Unknown to me, the organisers of the congress had allowed members of the press to attend the scientific sessions, which in my experience is very unusual at medical congresses. After my presentation, I was immediately approached by a journalist from a British newspaper whose only question related to this point and not to the many other points I had discussed. On the following day, the headline in his newspaper announced 'Black Hearts Are Best, Say South Africans.'

When asked this question, I had admitted that we did not know why, but I had also mentioned to the journalist that I hoped this would not be the only point from my presentation that he would report, as several other observations were far more important from a medical perspective. In his article, he stated that I had tried to persuade him not to publish the fact that 'black hearts were best', which was certainly not the case. This was a small personal example to me of how the press can twist one's words. Interestingly, when I returned to Cape Town, although the news item had filtered through, I found that nobody seemed to have taken any interest in what the journalist had written.

The absence of strong feelings about race in relation to heart transplantation in South Africa at the time was exemplified by many of those personally involved in the donation of organs or as recipients of those organs. Chris and Marius were encouraged by the fact that not only was Denise Darvall's father readily willing to donate her kidney to a coloured patient, but that Clive Haupt's family was equally willing to donate his heart to a white man.

The publicly and vehemently anti-apartheid Marius Barnard said:

> For me, particularly, as a South African, this operation [the first heart transplant] has a lot of significance. Here we have a case where the heart of an Anglican Christian girl [Denise Darvall] was placed in the body of a Jewish gentleman [Louis Washkansky] and her kidney in the body of a coloured child. This is a significant thing for all the world, being in the state it is in today. It makes me feel that there is some hidden force behind all this.

Dorothy Haupt, who had lost her husband after only three months of marriage, expressed the opinion that race and colour were unimportant in matters of life and death. 'I am glad that my husband's coloured heart could save the life of a white man,' she is reported to have said. 'I am also glad because it has changed the whole idea of apartheid. Now everyone can see that all of us—White, Black or Brown—have the same heart.'

Ms. Haupt's views reflected those of Chris himself. He often said that, when he looked beneath the skin of a patient, 'no matter what colour the skin, everything looked the same.'

Chris's views on apartheid were summed up when he wrote that Clive Haupt's family 'agreed without hesitation, without anger and hatred for the whites who had humiliated and degraded and deprived him for so long.'

South African journalist and author of *Heart Transplant*, Marais Malan, reported that the mother of Jonathan van Wyk, the ten-year-old coloured boy who had received a kidney from Denise Darvall, felt strongly on this topic. 'It is wrong of the people to drag apartheid into Professor Barnard's great achievement,' she said. 'Just like all the coloureds who have come here to encourage us we have never thought about it that my son now has a 'White' kidney. We don't even discuss it. Apartheid has nothing to do with us as human beings. We are all human beings, and I think most of the Whites feel the same way.'

Mrs Black, Chris's first and only kidney transplant patient who had received a kidney from a black donor, felt similarly. According to Mr Malan, she only found out months after the operation that she had received the kidney of a Bantu.

Blood transfusion is similar in many respects to organ transplantation, and so the views of the South African population on this topic are of relevance. Tissue typing expert, M. C. Botha, who ran the blood transfusion service at GSH, pointed out that, of about 25,000 blood transfusions given each year at the hospital, only about one patient would take any interest in determining from whom the blood had been donated. Furthermore, in his experience, though rare, it was as common for a non-white person to express a concern about a transfusion from a white donor as it was for a white to express reservations about blood from a non-white. He also pointed out that, in South Africa, more blood donated by whites was transfused into non-white patients than blood donated by the non-white population. 'This is because the Bantu are still not used to the idea of donating blood freely while a certain amount of superstition has made the task of the blood transfusion service difficult.'

## Chris's Personal Attitude to Apartheid

It is important that we try to differentiate between Chris's patriotism (for South Africa) and his attitude to apartheid. Throughout his later life, and particularly during the twenty years after the first heart transplant, he remained an unofficial spokesman and ambassador for South Africa, attempting to present a balanced view of his troubled homeland. From my personal observations and from statements Chris made throughout life, it is clear that he opposed the policy of apartheid. However, he would defend other, sometimes controversial, actions of the South African government if he believed they were right for his country.

In one of his newspaper articles, Chris addressed the topic of patriotism.

I've had my patriotic instincts equated with racism by television interviewers who seemed to think that I was some sort of a monster for trying to defend my country, another twist to confuse any uncommitted youngster who wants only the best for his homeland ... Patriotism for me, for this country at this time, isn't narrow sectarianism, it isn't some kind of totem pole to which I bow before I start thinking. And it certainly isn't a set of rigid tribal rules.

I am an Afrikaner. My forefathers have been in this land for more than three centuries. My blood, like the rest of my tribe, is a mixture of Dutch, German, French, British and a medically proven percentage of Black, Coloured and Malay race groups, according to research by an Afrikaner who also happens to be one of South Africa's leading haematologists.

In his book, *South Africa: Sharp Dissection*, Chris wrote:

I want to stress that I am just as much an African as Hamilton Naki, the Black African with whom I have worked for many years in the laboratory at Groote Schuur. I am as much an African as Dorothy Fisher, the Coloured African who was perhaps my most successful heart transplant patient (to that time). The colour of my skin may be white, but my roots are as deep in this great continent of Africa as those of the Black and Coloured youngsters with whom I grew up in dusty Beaufort West.

It is said that blood dictates patriotism. If that is so then it dictates my wish to preserve a country we have fertilised with our dead, made wealthy by our living and, if called on, will maintain by our dying. It also dictates that I try to make that country livable for my children and that means ultimately for the children of all who live here.

It is no secret that after my first heart transplant—on Louis Washkansky on 2 December 1967—I was inundated with offers of positions at overseas hospitals and clinics, including six from American medical institutions, within a month of the first transplant. These, as well as similar offers I had received as a cardiac surgeon before the news media made a sensation of the heart transplants at Groote Schuur, would have been more lucrative than the professional position I enjoy in Cape Town. Yet, despite the temptation, there is something that anchors me to the country of my birth where my family and friends are. There is a magnet that draws me back to South Africa, no matter where my travels take me.

Those in the South African government and diplomatic service quickly and fully realised what a positive impact Chris could make on South Africa's image abroad. Walt Lillehei recounted an occasion when he was accompanying Chris when they met the South African consul in New York City. The consul, Pik Botha (later to become foreign minister in South Africa), had not previously met Chris.

> He said to Chris: 'Dr Barnard, you have done a great thing for South Africa. Most of the people in this country and around the world think South Africans are living in mud huts and wearing grass skirts—a very primitive society. I encourage you … talk to many people, meet as many people and spread the message not only of the heart transplant but of the cosmopolitan society in our country.' Chris was listening, of course, nodding his head, and I must say in later years he took that very literally … He did a lot of good work, I think, for South Africa by trying to neutralise, at least in part, the very bad image that South Africa had at that time.

Without wishing in any way to defend the iniquitous concept of apartheid, there is no doubt in my own mind that when I was in Cape Town in the 1980s, at a time when international sanctions against South Africa were beginning to have a detrimental effect on the economy, South Africa sometimes received an undeservedly bad press. Let me give you two small examples of the media bias against South Africa in the 1980s.

When I worked there, the GSH cardiologists would regularly travel to the Eastern Cape, several hundred miles from Cape Town, where they would examine any patient referred by the local physicians. Many of the patients, if not the vast majority, were black. If one of them had heart disease requiring sophisticated investigation or an operation, the patient would be transported (often by air) to Cape Town, admitted to GSH, and fully investigated by the best cardiologists in the country (and, indeed, in my opinion equal to any in the world). If an operation were indicated, the patient would be seen by Chris or one of his colleagues, operated on, and given the best post-operative care that could be provided in South Africa at that time. When recovered, the patient would be transported back to his (or her) home in the Eastern Cape, where he would be followed up by his local physician and by the GSH cardiologists during their visits.

For most of these patients, who came from poor backgrounds, the costs of all their attention would be covered by the provincial government, and the excellent treatment they received would therefore cost them nothing. I do not believe there was anywhere else in Africa (certainly sub-Saharan Africa) where a man or woman could obtain this sort of superb medical care. From this perspective, I would far rather have been a black or coloured South African—at least in the Cape Province—than an African from any other country on the continent at that time.

Chris was clearly proud of the health care the Cape Provincial government provided for all its population. Without intending his comments to be associated with race, he asked, 'Are there any comparable achievements to be found in Black Africa?' Where else in Africa could a poor patient receive healthcare of the quality at such low (or no) cost, he asked?

I am not sure whether a poor African in any of the other provinces in South Africa (Transvaal, Natal, or the Orange Free State) would receive such excellent attention (without discrimination). I think possibly not in every province, but certainly in the Cape Province it was available, and I believe to a large extent in Natal and Transvaal. Such access to medical care was not available at that time to millions of people who could not afford healthcare insurance in the USA. Even today, some may be excluded. This type of information was not generally known outside the country's borders. I would go so far as to state that many of South Africa's political critics did not want to know this information.

Very few black Africans underwent heart transplantation, but this was not because of any discrimination on the part of Chris and his colleagues. It was, unfortunately, a consequence of the fact that so many of them lived in poor conditions that would have doomed the transplant to failure: remote geographic locations (making it difficult to obtain continuing advanced medical care), inadequate support by those (such as family and friends) who could understand the relative complexities of immunosuppressive therapy, inadequate sanitation, and so on. Yet this was not the fault of Chris Barnard, who was always committed to giving patients—any patient—the best treatment that could possibly be given if it had a realistic chance of success. One of Chris's famous quotes was, 'A life is important, and you can never buy that life. Therefore, there is no limit to the amount of money that can be spent to save a life.' This surely must have put fear into the hearts of the politicians and administrators who had to find the money to pay for the health services.

The second small example of media bias confirms my opinion stated above that many members of the media did not wish to hear anything good said about South Africa. It relates to the wife of a colleague of mine who had recently arrived from Europe to work in Cape Town. She was a journalist, and made enquiries of various newspapers and magazines in her home country as to whether an article on her first impressions of South Africa might be of interest. At least one editor wrote back inquiring what she would say. When she submitted a balanced view of her impressions of the country, both the good and the bad, the editor lost interest; the article would not be sufficiently critical of South Africa to fit with his political views.

## Chris's Relationship with the South African Government

For someone who did not support their apartheid policy, Chris had an ambivalent relationship with the South African government. This is perhaps surprising in that he had been brought up in a house in which his father was vehemently opposed to the Nationalist party. Relatively late in life, for a short period of time, he actively campaigned for a new opposition party, the Democratic party. However, he opposed economic sanctions when South Africa was subjected to them by much of the outside world. So depressed was he as to the future of his country during this period (the late 1980s and early 1990s) that he met personally to express his views with the then president, F. W. de Klerk—a small illustration of the influence he still had in South Africa.

I never spoke to Chris in detail about his political views. Although relatively rarely outspoken in public, Chris was at times openly critical of the apartheid policy, even when addressing diehard supporters of the policy. On the first occasion, he threw caution to the wind when addressing the Cape Town Afrikaans Chamber of Commerce, to whom he had been introduced as one of the 'greatest Afrikaners'; he directed some very pointed questions at his audience. Deirdre recollected this speech in her memoirs.

> Did it not occur to them, he asked, how strange it was that [white] children who were lovingly raised by black women, and other women of colour, could not be cared for by them if they happened to find themselves in hospital? My father went on to say that whenever he went abroad there were a great many questions fired at him and he was now wondering whether these great movers and shakers in his own country, at present seated before him, had any answers for him. He asked if they had ever asked themselves why white children played with black and coloured friends in their little towns, yet when they grew up were not allowed to compete with each other on the sportsfield.

To say the least, his comments were not well-received. One member of the audience provided an answer of sorts. 'If that's the kind of question you get asked when you're out of the country, then you can tell them we do these things because it's our business, not theirs. If you think it's so wrong, you can go and join them if you like.'

For the first time in his life, Chris was hissed and booed, though Deirdre reported that this did not 'worry him at all'. His comments directly contributed towards the withdrawal of the VIP privileges he had hitherto enjoyed at South African airports. Several of his former friends felt they could no longer be seen to associate with him.

In the early period after the first few transplants, however, Chris had taken advantage of the opportunities his new-found fame and popularity provided him. He became quite close to some of the country's leading politicians.

Marius addressed this subject in his memoirs.

By the late 1960s, not only was Chris one of the best-known figures internationally, but he was an excellent speaker, a good debater and had a 'miracle-man' image all over the world. If the government could recruit him to their cause, they could use him in many guises for their own sinister purposes. They could not fail: Chris's personality made him a pushover for such a ploy.

One of Chris's most charming features was his willingness to please everyone. It was also his biggest weakness and resulted in numerous disastrous adventures. When one was in his company or when he was addressing an audience, Chris had an uncanny ability to sense what people wanted to hear or what they would approve of. He could, for example, be a liberal or a conservative at the appropriate time, when it suited him.

In public, Chris was a hesitant liberal, pointing out the evils of apartheid and creating and nursing this image of himself. In private, he certainly did not display the same sentiments and had many fierce arguments with me. He disliked the Progs (the liberal Progressive Party, which opposed the Nationalist Party [Nats] government) with a passion. I never knew whether this was due to our policies or because they had asked me, and not him, to become one of their MPs.

My first realization of Chris's increasing political involvement was when he called me to his office and showed me a large pile of documents. He had been invited to a debate with one of the Nationalist government's most hated men abroad, Peter Hain, on a televised BBC broadcast. Hain was a former South African who had become a political refugee in the United Kingdom. A so-called radical, he had fled South Africa to become a very vocal and successful anti-apartheid campaigner—and a thorn in the side of the Nats.

The documents that Chris showed me were lengthy, pages and pages on Hain, this 'enemy of South Africa', compiled by none other than the government's infamous and sinister Bureau of State Security. Chris had been given the file so that he could prepare himself adequately for the debate with Hain. I was shocked and refused to look at the documents. I left perplexed, but with a broader understanding of what was going on. I could not believe that Chris was allowing himself to be used by the Nats as a form of secret agent.

According to Marius, several of Chris's overseas trips were 'well-disguised attempts to break the sanctions imposed on South Africa at the time.'

Soon new and ominous faces started to appear in the passages of Groote Schuur Hospital. Dr Eschel Rhoodie, his brother and others of the now-infamous Department of Information [soon to be embroiled in a major political scandal that led to their downfall] became regular visitors to Chris's office, which was close to mine. Although Chris was certainly under no obligation to report his activities to me, I felt compelled to warn him of the dangers of consorting with these men ... Poor Chris. I think few people were as used and abused as he was. [It appears that Chris had received travel expenses from government sources, and the implication was that he would do what he could when he was abroad to defend government policies.] After this, his enthusiasm to act as an envoy to polish the tarnished image of the government waned.

I have no knowledge of what happened later, as I resigned from Groote Schuur Hospital soon afterwards, in 1980, but Chris told me over the phone in 1986 that he had been offered a post of ambassador and that his suggested preferences were London or Washington, D.C. He was very excited about this prospect; I am sure he saw himself as 'Mr Ambassador'. In fact, I believe that Chris, with his boyish charm and excellent public-speaking ability, would have made an excellent foreign representative. But the bubble soon burst. Chris's dreams were dashed when the best the government could offer him was Rome or Athens. He felt that those appointments were beneath his dignity, and he declined them.

Given how much Chris enjoyed his visits to Italy and Greece, where he was always very popular, I am surprised to learn that he turned down this opportunity. The ecstatic welcome he usually received at Rome airport illustrates his popularity in Italy. Many years earlier, Chris told me that he always enjoyed visiting Greece, and indeed he had been made an honorary citizen of that country. He greatly valued the honour the Greeks had bestowed on him and, because of the limitations of a South African passport at that time, he always travelled internationally on his Greek passport. One small reason why he enjoyed arriving in Athens was that one of his former surgical trainees in Cape Town, Mike Bonoris, always met him at the airport (a small example of the love and loyalty of some of his trainees), which Chris appreciated very much.

## Chris's Personal Views on the South African Government's Policies

It was not always easy to be sure what Chris's real views on the policies and politics in South Africa in the later part of the twentieth century were because he relatively rarely made his views fully known even to colleagues and friends who were fairly close to him. Rodney Hewitson, who had worked with Chris for many years, could not really tell me what Chris's politics were, but it seemed that both he and Father Tom Nicholson (in many respects Chris's father confessor) thought that they were fairly neutral—neither very positive nor negative with regard to apartheid.

However, Chris took the trouble to write a book on this topic, *South Africa: Sharp Dissection*, published in 1977, which at least demonstrates his very considerable interest in the topic. Although relatively brief, it is well-written, very readable, and explains his arguments clearly. It makes interesting reading, and I suspect reflects the views of many white South Africans at that time—perhaps the silent majority. There is some evidence that members of the South African government offered to help Chris write such a book, but I am convinced that the book he published expressed his own personal opinions.

To some extent he was stimulated to write the book from a feeling of guilt. In his memoirs, *The Second Life,* he commented that, at one stage of his life, he felt he 'should play a much bigger part to overthrow this wicked regime—and be unafraid of the consequences.' But, he lamented, he 'sat on the fence … Like Gary Player [the well-known golfer] … the Oppenheimers [the wealthy mining magnates], and many other Afrikaners like myself, I only did enough to assuage my conscience but not enough to rock the boat. Very few of us were prepared to stand up and be counted. We were all cowards, taking care of our own safety and comfort before anything or anyone else.'

Therefore, those who perceived him as being (in practice) politically neutral were probably correct.

In *South Africa: Sharp Dissection*, Chris lucidly put forward the good and the bad about his country, the mistakes that the government had made, and his tentative solutions to the problems South Africa faced. He wrote:

> In retrospect, the Nationalist Government made three mistakes, and today we have to look at the situation recognising and realising that these mistakes were made. The first mistake they made was actually as a result of their honesty. They told the whole world that South Africa was practicing discrimination on the basis of colour of skin.
>
> The second mistake they made was as a result of our isolation, and therefore, was a result of ignorance. We are really a western civilization removed seven to nine thousand miles from the next western civilization, and as a result of this I think they misjudged the trend of the world in that after the Second World War racism was no longer tolerated and the world tried to move away from racial discrimination. Therefore, we went in the worst direction and that is that we increased racism in this country.
>
> The third mistake that they made was that the whole system was not practical; it could never work in this country. And therefore, unfortunately, although they honestly believed that they would have separate but equal facilities for the other groups, it was never like that. The facilities were separate but never equal. In most cases they were inferior. But I must point out, and I think this is very important, that because the government really intended for the facilities to be equal, they have done a tremendous amount in the form of education, in the form of medical treatment, in the form of housing for the coloured and the black man and their achievement in South Africa is in many ways better than in any other country in Africa.
>
> Now I think today all South Africans realise that we've made these mistakes and that this has had a tremendous consequence which is that the western world brought all its mass media and propaganda media against South Africa.

## Crossroads

Chris's criticisms of the South African government were not confined to their policy of apartheid, though this troubled him most. In a newspaper column entitled 'Orwell's *1984*', he tackled the government's efforts to censor what the public read or heard (which was still very much in place when I lived in Cape Town in the 1980s).

I looked up the censorship figures and found that in one year we had managed to place more than a thousand [book] titles out of reach of curious South Africans. I didn't bother to check plays and films, took it for granted that our morals were well protected on telly by the blue pencil, and ignored the gibes from various quarters that we rewrite the history books. And the conclusion was still painfully obvious that we are building a generation with a cockeyed view of the world and a contradictory value system.

SATV [the South African television network] has learned the lesson well and our news broadcasts have become a parade of Cabinet ministers telling us what our opinions should be while well-chosen news clips keep crime, grime and gore out of our living rooms … Do you really believe that we can ignore more than a thousand titles a year in contemporary literature without it having some effect on us? Is it possible that 'offending words' in the soundtrack of a film can be bleeped out or some dubious piece of behaviour excised without giving a somewhat unbalanced view of where the rest of the world is heading?

I object to censorship in the service of a political ideology but hold no brief for unlimited license. Somewhere there must be a middle ground between the needs of the State and the creative urges of the artist or writer, a space between the upper and nether millstones.

In another article, 'Porn', he had more to say on the true meaning (to him) of the word 'pornography'.

Look around you. While the hypocrites mouth clichés about protecting your loved ones from pornographic filth you are surrounded by obscenity. We wallow in it. It is a fact of life. And I'm not talking of South Africa. I speak of every country. Where there is a starving child, a lonely old person, a brutal oppressor, unmerited violence or anyone living or dying in pain or fear, you have true obscenity. Sex cannot sicken me, make it as lurid as you will. Suffering and violence do.

In what can only be described as a diatribe against capital punishment, which was still carried out in South Africa until the apartheid policy was abolished, Chris pointed out that 'In the past ten years we have sent over seven hundred souls to meet their Maker at the end of a rope. In one month there were one-hundred-twenty wretches waiting in Death Row. Perhaps that is our problem, a purely economic one. It is cheaper to hang and flog than to educate, employ and house.'

# Freedom and Tolerance: the Politics of Hypocrisy

Chris addressed the criticisms of South Africa by the outside world and the pressure being put on his country to change its political system. He was particularly critical of bodies such as the United Nations (UN) and the Organization of African Unity (OAU).

> The United Nations has abused consistently and with growing abandon its position of trust by adopting double standards in international affairs ... The founders of this organization wrote into the constitution a firm resolve to eradicate racialism around the world. But they promptly went ahead and singled out for condemnation South Africa, later Rhodesia and for a while, Portugal ... but a blind eye was turned to violations of human dignity and gross instances of racialism elsewhere in the world.

There is considerable truth in this. A colleague with whom I trained in the UK, who later worked in Malawi (where he originally intended to spend his career), told me that there were two major tribal groups in that country. One ruled and discriminated against the other group. The discrimination, he claimed, was every bit as bad as in South Africa. Yet one never read about this 'apartheid' in the Western press.

Chris complained that one never heard of some other countries being condemned at the Organization of African Unity or in the United Nations General Assembly for being racist or a minority, let alone for the racial atrocities committed during recurring episodes of genocide.

He drew attention to those who demonstrated in places such as 'Trafalgar Square, protesting the people killed in rioting in South Africa', but who turned a 'blind eye to the death of half a million Cambodians in a single year under Communist repression.' Chris continued: 'I am the last person to deny the existence of racialism and political intolerance in my country. I have often taken a stand for racial justice and tolerance in South Africa.' However, he pointed out:

> Since World War Two there have been two major racial incidents in South Africa: in 1961 when sixty-seven people were killed at Sharpeville, and in 1976 when an estimated 300 lives were lost in township unrest. Yet, in the same period, more than ten million people have been killed around the world as a result of racial, ethnic and cultural violence and intolerance. In a single country, the Sudan, half a million people have died because of a deliberate policy of genocide.
>
> The irony of it all is that there is more racial discrimination, more denial of basic human rights and more dictatorship in Black Africa than

there has ever been in South Africa or in Rhodesia. The experts will confirm that only six of the forty-eight Black and Arab African states are democracies; but even there 'democracy' has taken on a meaning far removed from the original. For the rest, there is military and civilian dictatorship, often tyrannical and always totalitarian and intolerant.

Several Western countries came in for particular criticisms.

Americans, of course, are prone to preach to South Africa by virtue of the fact that Americans have removed racial discrimination from their law books; that the treatment has been ineffective and the disease left undiagnosed does not deter them. Racialism does not need to be institutionalised in order to create explosive situations.

As an aside, it is of interest to note Marius's experience when living in the US in the mid-1960s. When Marius was training in Houston in Texas, he experienced prejudice there, just as in South Africa. He recollected this experience in his memoirs.

During the Labor Day weekend of September 1966, I hitched a lift to Richmond, Virginia, where Chris was working … Near New Orleans, we were stopped by the police for speeding, and my traveling companion was arrested. Being from New York and a Yankee at that, was perhaps a greater offence than the speeding. We were taken to the local prison, where he was placed in jail. But, being in the Deep South, when they discovered I was from South Africa I was treated like royalty and given food and Coca-Cola. Racial bigotry was still very much alive in the southern parts of the USA—clearly the Civil War had not been forgotten.

Chris also drew attention to laws in Australia that discriminated against the Aborigines. He concluded that they made apartheid 'look positively benign by comparison.' Australia had a 'whites only' immigration policy that was not finally repealed in totality until 1973, but that country received little criticism from the outside world.

## The Assault on Freedom

One politician to come in for particular criticism by Chris was Dr Henry Kissinger, then the American Secretary of State, who he described as one of those 'who is guilty of this application of double standards through blind commitment to "majority rule".' In April 1976, after Kissinger visited

Africa and 'propagated the "majority rule" view,' Chris felt it necessary to write to him.

'What puzzles me,' he wrote, 'is why you do not insist on the same criteria for a selection of governments in other African countries?' He referred to Angola and to Mozambique, where minority groups [sometimes with backing from foreign powers] had assumed power without elections. 'As was to be expected, I did not get a direct reply from Dr Kissinger.' The best that the Acting Assistant Secretary of State for African Affairs could manage in his reply, on behalf of Dr Kissinger, was an admission that the 'opposing side' in Angola represented the majority of the (Angolan) population, but that the United States Government had been unable to give active support to this majority 'due to the unwillingness of the U.S. Congress to provide the necessary additional funds.'

Chris's interpretation of this response was that 'the United States demands so-called "majority rule" in a country such as Rhodesia, but is not prepared to insist on majority rule in that country's immediate neighbour, namely Angola ... It appears that discrimination, in the eyes of the democratic powers of the West, works only one way; if it is practised by a dictator with a black skin it is perfectly justifiable, but if the perpetrator has a white skin then it is an intolerable infringement of basic human rights.' Chris considered this double standard to be 'racialism in reverse'.

What he found distressing was the refusal of intelligent men and women in civilised communities to consider the South African situation in an objective way.

> It appears that in Africa a Black man's suffering is only recognised by the Press and government if he suffers at the hands of a White man... Disease and hunger to the point of starvation is ignored when it occurs under Black rule, but how much praise is given to White rulers who prevent such misery?

## The Competitive Spirit

Chris also addressed what he considered the failings of another international organization, the International Olympic Committee (IOC), which he believed was also guilty of adopting double standards. At the time, the IOC and some other world sporting organizations did not recognise world records achieved by South African athletes. Furthermore, the IOC did not allow South African athletes to participate in the Olympic Games. He commented:

The IOC does not, as it purports to do, arrange world games to find world winners. It kowtows to political pressure certainly ... It awards the winners gold medals. But when the flags are lowered and the crowds go home, those medal-holders are not the kings of the castle. We have our own kings of the castle. And until we can all play in the same castle nobody can claim the international crown.

## Prisons of the Mind

It was not only the UN, the OAU, and IOC that came in for Chris's criticism. Amnesty International, an international body concerned with the rights of political prisoners, asked Chris to look into the conditions of political prisoners in South Africa. He readily agreed and, perhaps surprisingly, the South African authorities gave him permission not only to visit political prisoners (provided the prisoners gave their permission), but also to take a television crew of his choice with him.

'Why not expand the whole thing?' Chris thought. 'Every country had political prisoners; we could do an in-depth survey of the problem as a whole. In a mood of high enthusiasm, I wrote to Amnesty by registered mail, outlined my revised plans and asked their help in also gaining access to political prisoners in other countries.'

My understanding is that Chris never received a reply.

## Interactions with Political Leaders

Due to his high profile and frequent travels, Chris had several opportunities to meet influential leaders worldwide, and he used these occasions to discuss their countries' attitudes to South Africa. He provided two examples.

When he met with Mrs Indira Gandhi, the prime minister of India, he challenged her to visit South Africa to examine the conditions there herself. She felt she could not accept the invitation. Chris responded saying:

You see, Mrs Gandhi, it's impossible for you to accept my challenge because if you were to send a delegation to South Africa on a fact-finding mission you would be terribly unpopular and, secondly, if this delegation should leave South Africa and say anything good about it, then you would really be in trouble, because you know as well as I do that you choose your friends not because you believe in their systems, or their outlooks, but because it suits your international political image.

Chris received the highest civil decoration that can be awarded in the Philippines, the Golden Heart Award, and by Presidential decree he was made an honorary citizen of the Philippines. He and Barbara were invited to accompany the Filipino delegation, led by Mrs Marcos [the President's wife], to the crowning of the King of Nepal in Katmandu. On the basis of these gestures of goodwill, and after discussion with the South African prime minister, Chris extended an invitation to President Marcos to visit South Africa, all expenses paid. 'It was immediately clear to me from the President's reaction that he did not share my enthusiasm.'

Chris concluded that 'The politics of hypocrisy has become so pervasive in the conduct of international relationships that the freedom to express a view contrary to that dictated by the articulate advocates of these politics, is all but suppressed.'

## South Africa: Chris's Views on the Road Ahead

Chris went on to give his own views on how he would try to resolve South Africa's racial problems.

> The political solution in this country must fulfill three criteria. First it must be a just solution. That is, it must be morally acceptable. Secondly, it must not endanger the survival and future of minority groups in this country [the whites, coloured, and the Indians—i.e. those whose families originated in the Indian subcontinent, for example].

Furthermore, he pointed out that in South Africa, there were people from no fewer than nine different black nations, 'and the one is completely different from the other, and doesn't tolerate the other. They are often greater enemies than with the white man!'

Lastly, he emphasised that any political solution 'must make certain that the country [and the running of this country] remains in the hands of capable people.'

He suggested that 'very little will happen to South Africa if we abolish discrimination overnight. And I've actually told the Prime Minister that this is what he must do ... First, we must abolish social apartheid (by which he meant all of the myriad of laws that regulated where people of different ethnic groups could live, where they could eat, who they could marry and have sexual relations with, and so on).' In Chris's opinion:

> Change must be dynamic, but evolutionary and not revolutionary ... Against this background, the immediate and urgent priority for

South Africa is the abolition of what has become known as 'petty apartheid', those pin-pricks which daily dehumanise the life of so many people in this otherwise wonderful country and which generate so much unhappiness, bitterness and hatred. Petty apartheid takes many forms: separate entrances at public post offices and other government buildings, signposts which indicate separate bathing areas for different races, notices on buildings which allocate separate entrances or lifts for 'goods and non-Europeans', the taxis and buses labeled 'second-class' when they are reserved for Blacks. These and numerous other instances of petty apartheid must be done away with immediately.

Too much of the discrimination based on race in South Africa is utterly indefensible from a Christian point of view, let alone from the point of view of a profession or trade. In my own field, I have often expressed disgust at the discrepancy in salaries paid to White doctors and nurses, and those paid to non-Whites. The argument is that Black people need less money to live on. This is no argument at all. It makes matters even worse, for it shows up the inferior living conditions Blacks are forced to put up with. I have always maintained that it is ridiculous to pay medical staff who have the same training, and do the same job, different salaries because of the colour of their skin.

Billions of rands must have been spent on erecting the trappings of petty apartheid, billions that could have been used more profitably to provide educational facilities, health services and better jobs for the developing peoples of this country.

Chris quoted a top South African financier who believed that South Africa's gross national product would be about fifty per cent higher without the costs associated with apartheid. In a newspaper column, he wrote, 'Statistics published recently gave the projected annual per capita personal income for whites as R2,716; Asians R752; coloureds R633; and blacks R307. There is no need to labor the point that groups who earn such disparate incomes must have equally disparate lifestyles.'

The researchers who published those figures also listed the hardships attendant on living at the bottom of the heap; poor nutrition, inadequate housing, lack of clothing, heating, training, transport, recreational opportunities and amenities, as well as insufficient access to health services and facilities ... Load luxury goods if need be. Bury booze beneath a surcharge. Tax tobacco back into the ground. Raise groans ... but, for pity's sake, leave the poor alone.

## 'There's the Rub', as Hamlet Would Say

So far, his criticisms and solutions would be acceptable to most liberals in the Western world as well as by many black Africans. However, his further solutions differed greatly from those who demanded majority rule. 'Secondly, we must properly consolidate the black homelands and try to give them a solid government as we've done in Transkei [the first homeland].'

The problem with this was that the homelands, although usually areas of land that were the traditional homes of the various black tribal groups, were largely situated in regions of the country where there were few natural resources or infrastructure developments. As a consequence, there were few decent jobs for the inhabitants. Most black South Africans had to migrate to the cities or mining regions to find work, usually necessitating leaving their wives and families behind. The family would only be together for perhaps one month each year. Consolidating the homelands was an absolute non-starter with black Africans and white liberals the world over.

He pointed out that in South Africa:

We have a situation where an illiterate man can be given a vote to elect the Government of the country, but a professor with a string of degrees behind his name is denied that vote, simply because the former has a white skin and the latter a black or brown skin. This, to my mind, is the height of absurdity.

Chris claimed that he had 'nothing against black majority rule as long as that black majority is capable of ruling this country and that's where the problem lies.' He clearly did not think there were enough well-educated and experienced people within the black community to trust to run the country. While members of the black majority were achieving the level of education and skills he felt necessary, he recommended—temporarily—a 'one-party' state. The government would consist of people from all racial groups who all had the education and expertise to help run the country—a meritocracy. The problem at that time was that the majority of young black people did not have an equal opportunity of attaining the necessary education as those of other ethnic groups, particularly the whites. However, Chris had thought of this.

White South Africa does not want to give up the dynamic society it has built up. There are White South Africans who think that they can keep it all for themselves for ever; this is foolish. The Whites have to be prepared to draw others into their society, but then there must be some kind of selective process that will ensure that those who are drawn in will be able to help sustain that society, not destroy it ... This one-party state must be run in such a way that it gives everybody, irrespective of colour of skin, the right to obtain all the facilities to reach the top, in any profession. But in the meantime, while they are being educated, the country must remain in the hands of capable people and therefore the selection of government must be made on merit only, not on colour of skin, religion or any other aspect.

However, Chris's knowledge of the way many African countries had—sometimes quietly, without much criticism from Western leaders—lapsed into dictatorships influenced his thinking.

Is South Africa really expected to exchange its admittedly imperfect society for the horrors of a one man, one vote situation which will inevitably turn into a one man, one vote only once situation? It is the ordinary Black man, woman and child who would suffer most; a small clique of rulers imposes tyrannical dictatorship.

He asked a rhetorical question.

Would White Americans have applied their advice to South Africa to themselves if they had a four to one majority of American Indians in their midst instead of a minority negro group? Would they then still have insisted on 'majority rule' in the USA?

The same question can readily be posed in respect of Australia: would their labor leaders apply such advice to themselves if the Aborigines outnumbered the White Australians four to one? Would White Americans and White Australians not look for built-in protection against the majority before handing over power?

And let it be noted that in the great democracy of the United States, special laws protect minority groups like the Negroes, for instance. If laws are needed to protect a minority group in America, why not in South Africa?

Chris's solution to his country's problems would certainly not have been acceptable to the ethnic black South African or to the international community. He wrote:

The reality of ethnic separation cannot be ignored and we must make provision for the distinctive national groups within our population to decide whether they will form sovereign states [with individuals having the choice of deciding on their own citizenship], or remain within the present White-dominated South African political framework, or become separate and autonomous states with an umbrella link with the larger South African grouping.

An individual from one of these independent homelands who has resided in South Africa for less than five years, would still be a citizen of his homeland. When he has been living legally in South Africa proper for more than five years, he should have the choice to either become a homeland citizen or a citizen of South Africa, depending on a citizenship qualification examination. If the standards demanded in such an examination are sufficiently high, we will have an orderly transition to a society in which merit, not colour, is the criterion. Under such a system of gradual and evolutionary advancement to a multi-racial society, and eventually a majority government, no White person need have any fears about his or her future.

Basing his suggestions for the future on the black homelands (reviled by most critics of South Africa) as Chris did, was certainly naïve, and immediately rendered his proposals unacceptable.

Chris's book, *South Africa: Sharp Dissection*, was written in 1977. Subsequently, I believe Chris's views became modified, maybe from necessity, when he saw the 'writing on the wall' for South Africa in the late 1980s and 1990s. He certainly seemed to admire the qualities Nelson Mandela showed as the country's first black president. However, I suspect he had an underlying fear of deterioration in the management of the economy as has sadly occurred in several other sub-Saharan countries. Only time will tell whether South Africa degenerates into a dictatorship or not.

I conclude this chapter with some paragraphs that I suggest, despite his flawed solutions, sum up Chris's opposition to apartheid—indeed, his passionate opposition. In one of his newspaper articles, he wrote:

South Africa, in fact, hasn't got any Black problems. We have a major White problem, and one of its most peculiar aspects is that we don't simply want bread and butter like any other nation. We want cake too, with jam on it, and we want to eat it.

We want cheap Black labor in White areas ... But we don't want the natural side effects of wives and children. So we invent the pass system. In this way the family stays at home and the husband migrates to where we want his labor. Every year or so he migrates home again.

Who do we think we are fooling with our glib talk of stemming the flood of Blacks into White cities? What we have done is to create an iniquitous, self-serving system for a self-serving people who still have the gall to sit in church on a Sunday and mouth pious words. [Yet his solution, based on the 'homelands', would almost certainly have resulted in this 'iniquitous' system being continued, at least for several years.]

You can page through your law books for ever. You can prove that our actions were legally clean. You can even show that—in terms of the screen of legislation that we have built around us to block out reality—it was a legal necessity to ensure that the law was obeyed. You can do what the hell you like! But no amount of legal posturing will wipe out the fact that we have created an immoral system and whatever we do to enforce it is but an extension of that immorality.

# 29

# The Nobel Prize:
# Should Chris Have Received It?

One question frequently raised in the months and early years after the first heart transplant—at least by the public, if not so often by those in the medical profession—was whether Chris Barnard should have been awarded a Nobel Prize for his breakthrough in surgery. Marius Barnard certainly believed his brother should have received this recognition. After all, heart surgery, particularly open heart surgery, was one of the great medical advances of the middle and later part of the twentieth century, as was organ transplantation. Transplanting a human heart combined both of these great advances in a very dramatic manner. Let us examine whether Chris had a realistic claim to such a prestigious award.

The Nobel Prize for Medicine or Physiology is awarded each year by the Nobel Foundation, the recipients being selected by the faculty of the Karolinska Institute in Stockholm, the premier medical centre in Sweden. Having received numerous nominations from institutions and individuals from around the world, the professors at the Karolinska make the recommendation each year. Up to three people can share the prize, but it is never awarded posthumously. Of course, there are innovations in many different fields of medicine that claim the Nobel committee's attention, and the members of this committee therefore have to make difficult decisions selecting from several disparate fields.

The terms of Alfred Nobel's bequest stated that the prize should be awarded for a 'discovery' during the previous twelve months. As it is difficult to assess the true importance of any discovery so quickly, the Nobel committee often waits several years before awarding the prize in order to be sure the innovation has been proven to be of lasting benefit. Even so, they sometimes make the wrong choice, which, if they had waited longer, they would have realised. So, they have come to be cautious.

The perennial problem with the Prize has been the interpretation of the word 'discovery'. What is a discovery in medicine that could justify the award? Some advances are obvious. For example, when Sir Alexander Fleming observed the ability of penicillin to kill certain bacteria, that observation was considered as a 'discovery'. However, when he was awarded the Prize, he shared it with two other scientists. One, Howard Florey (later Lord Florey), had developed a method of producing penicillin in large amounts, making it available to very many patients (without which it would have been of only limited value in medicine). The other, Ernst Chain, had clarified the chemical structure of penicillin, allowing it to be produced much more readily. Were Florey and Chain's contributions really discoveries? One might claim they were—the discovery of methods to produce penicillin in large amounts—but many would see these as 'developments' rather than true discoveries.

This point has been of relevance to the assessment of advances in both heart surgery and organ transplantation in relation to the Nobel Prize. Some have asked, 'What was the "discovery"?' Was Gibbon's development of the heart-lung machine a discovery? Did the work of Lillehei and his colleagues in developing, first, cross-circulation and, second, a much simpler heart-lung machine constitute a discovery? Some would say 'yes' and others 'no', but surely the essential point is that each of these advances proved to be of immense importance in advancing medicine and in improving the health of the world's population; surely, this should be the purpose of the Prize.

I would suggest it should be awarded to recognise a major fundamental breakthrough or 'truth', which may have taken time to achieve, and may not necessarily be by a single discovery, but will have a major impact either directly or indirectly on the health of the population.

The other problem with the Prize is that the members of the Swedish Foundation have relatively rarely awarded it, in the words of the late Stockholm heart surgeon Clarence Crafoord, 'in recognition for work performed in the fields of clinical medicine or surgery.' The selection committee seems to be over-endowed with basic scientists who place too much weight on basic scientific advances that may, or may not, be ultimately translated into the realm of clinical medicine, and too little weight on advances that clearly improve the health of millions of patients.

US kidney transplant surgeon, Arnold Diethelm, told me that the opinion of the late Carl-Gustav Groth (a Karolinska Institute transplant surgeon who once acted as chairman of the selection committee) was that the Prize was awarded for 'new ideas, but not for the refinement of old ideas'. Diethelm agreed with this view, but felt that the introduction, for example, of liver transplantation or of a drug that prevented rejection, were examples of new ideas and thus deserved recognition. Surely, the successful introduction of a heart-lung machine was also a new idea that deserved recognition.

The Prize has been awarded for several discoveries in basic science or clinical medicine that unfortunately to date have made little or no impact either directly or indirectly on the health of the population. In contrast, open heart surgery has literally saved millions of patients' lives worldwide since it was introduced in the 1950s, and that would include the thousands who have benefited from heart transplantation. It could be argued that it has had far more relevance to the average citizen's everyday life than has the landing of men on the moon.

## The Nobel Prize and Heart Surgery

It has always amazed and disappointed me that none of the heart surgeons who are mentioned in this book won a Nobel Prize for their contributions to medicine. I particularly have in mind recognition for the development of open heart surgery, which really was a quantum leap in surgical technique since it involved not just a large number of new operations, but a dramatic new concept—the development of a machine that would support life while the heart was stopped. What can be more innovative than that?

I discussed the Prize in relation to heart surgery in my earlier book, *Open Heart*, and so will only provide a brief comment here.

Perhaps a majority of those with whom I discussed this topic believed that the Prize should have been shared between John Gibbon, Jr., for his early and prolonged studies demonstrating that a heart-lung machine was feasible, and Walt Lillehei, who, with his several colleagues, established that open heart surgery could be performed using the cross-circulation technique, and subsequently greatly simplified the heart-lung machine so that it was available to surgeons worldwide (Chapter 4). There would seem little controversy if these two had shared the prize. However, the Swedish group, particularly Clarence Crafoord and Ake Senning, who soon followed Gibbon's lead and equally soon surpassed him, could certainly claim to be included for consideration.

Thus, I would suggest we can reasonably conclude that the Nobel Committee failed miserably in its responsibilities in this respect.

## The Nobel Prize and Organ Transplantation

What about the field of organ transplantation, rather than open heart surgery? Has it fared any better in the eyes of the Nobel Committee? It has, but only just, and with some controversy. In 1990, the Nobel Prize was shared between Joseph Murray, whose contributions were summarised in Chapter 8, and Donnell Thomas, who was one of the pioneers of bone marrow transplantation, which is carried out in patients with malignant conditions of the cells in the blood, usually white blood cells, such as leukaemia.

At the time of this award, Swedish organ transplant surgeon Carl-Gustav Groth was chairman of the Nobel Committee determining who should be awarded the Prize in Medicine. Carl, who was later to become a good friend of mine because of our shared interest in cross-species organ transplantation (Appendix I), had trained under Tom Starzl in Denver in the very early days of liver transplantation. Thus, Carl was in an ideal position to assess the relative contributions of the several surgeons and physicians who could realistically expect to be considered for the award. Presumably, he had around him several colleagues on the committee who also had insight into this field of medicine.

Therefore, why did they select Joe Murray and not others who were clearly in the running? My understanding from Tom Starzl is that, at first, three names were being put forward: Murray, Calne, and Starzl. Many would have supported the selection of this group. David Hume, also a strong contender, had already died, and so could not be considered. The French innovators of Küss and Hamburger were other potential candidates.

Murray had carried out the first successful transplant between identical twins, though he had used the surgical technique largely introduced by René Küss (Chapter 8). In general, however, the problem of kidney transplantation was not the surgical operation. It was rejection that was the overwhelming barrier to successfully developing organ transplantation in the clinic. This, of course, was not a barrier when the recipient and donor were identical twins, and so this transplant did not address the real problem that had to be overcome. Indeed, several years earlier, Küss had suggested this would be the case. Nevertheless, this transplant did much to stimulate the field of kidney transplantation at a time when little progress was being made.

Murray then went on to carry out the first successful transplant between fraternal (non-identical) twins. Although the rejection response between non-identical twins would not be anticipated to be as strong as between completely unrelated donor and recipient, this was the first step in overcoming the immune barrier, which was fundamental to the success of organ transplantation if it were to be performed on large numbers of patients.

Murray's group was quickly followed by Hamburger's group, who actually published the results of their transplant before Murray.

Furthermore, the recipient in both cases was treated with irradiation therapy (in an effort to reduce the rejection response), with which both Hamburger and Küss had experimented previously. Third, and perhaps most important, Murray had carried out a successful kidney transplant between two unrelated people, again using irradiation therapy, and again quickly followed by similar operations by Hamburger and Küss.

It should also be remembered that Hamburger and Küss had begun their kidney transplant programs as early as 1951, and Hume had performed a series of nine transplants between 1951 and 1953. Murray had not become involved in the kidney transplant studies until Hume's departure to fulfill his US military commitments in 1953. It could therefore reasonably be anticipated that, if the Nobel Committee were searching for the true (surviving) pioneers in the field in 1990, they might have shared the Prize between Murray, Küss, and Hamburger. Henri Kreis, a physician who worked with Hamburger for twenty years, told me that the French medical profession was certainly disappointed when neither the French surgeon nor physician shared the Prize with Murray.

Sir Roy Calne commented to me:

> The Nobel Prize is such an extraordinary prize, it has become very unsatisfactory because advances in life sciences are now nearly always from a multitude of people working maybe in more than one department, more than one company even [and we could add more than one medical centre]. Perhaps the Prize should be shared for the discovery, rather than pinned on a person's shoulders.

Yet the story of organ transplantation does not end with Murray, Küss, Hamburger, or even Hume. The problem of rejection had certainly not been resolved. Even though irradiation enabled a handful of patients to survive long-term, it was less than satisfactory as a means of preventing or treating rejection. It was not until immunosuppressive drugs were introduced that kidney transplantation became more than an occasional success. Those involved in the development of immunosuppressive drugs have contributed to saving hundreds of thousands of lives through organ transplantation during the past fifty or more years.

Surely it is for contributions in this field that the Prize should have been awarded. If so, who were the leaders in this respect?

It was Roy Calne who, following up on an observation by others that 6-mercaptopurine (6-MP) might suppress the immune system, demonstrated its beneficial effect in prolonging kidney graft survival in dogs (Chapter 8). It was also Calne who requested other similar drugs from George Hitchings and Gertrude Elion, and tested the drug that became known as azathioprine, which became a standard immunosuppressive agent in patients for almost twenty years. Chris Barnard's first heart transplant would not have been possible without azathioprine.

It was also Calne (and his colleague David White) who picked up on the potential of cyclosporine, which proved much more potent than azathioprine, and replaced it in the 1980s, bringing about a sea-change in the results of organ transplantation. Calne also introduced rapamycin, which, if not as important as cyclosporine or tacrolimus in the development of organ transplantation, is another drug used commonly today. If those contributions are not sufficient, he also played a major role in introducing yet another biological immunosuppressive agent, alemtuzumab, known as 'Campath' (developed by his colleagues in the department of pathology at Cambridge University) into clinical practice.

Even with azathioprine, the results of kidney transplantation remained relatively poor and depressing until Tom Starzl combined its use with high-dose steroid therapy in the early 1960s. It was also Starzl who, by combining steroids with cyclosporine, enhanced cyclosporine's important role in transplantation. Finally, Starzl persevered with an even more potent drug, tacrolimus (originally known as FK506), until it largely replaced cyclosporine in the 1990s.

Neither Calne nor Starzl produced any of these drugs. Americans Hitchings and Elion synthesised 6-MP and azathioprine (while searching for drugs that might be beneficial in the treatment of malignancies, and for which they were awarded a Nobel Prize in 1988). It was Jean Borel of the Swiss pharmaceutical firm, Sandoz (now absorbed into Novartis), who discovered the immunosuppressive properties of cyclosporine. It was scientists at the Japanese pharmaceutical firm Fujisawa (now Astellas) who discovered tacrolimus. However, it was the combined efforts of Calne and Starzl that tested several potential drugs and demonstrated their effects, first in experimental animals and subsequently in patients. Cyclosporine and, even more, tacrolimus allowed the transplantation of organs that had hitherto been found very difficult or even impossible to transplant because of their susceptibility to rejection—organs such as the liver, lung, pancreas, and intestine.

Even heart transplantation was associated with only an approximate 40–50 per cent one-year patient survival until cyclosporine was introduced. Rejection became much less of an ogre, its incidence and severity being greatly reduced, and patients could leave hospital after their transplants much more quickly. Whereas Dr Blaiberg remained in hospital for seventy-four days, which was not uncommon in the 1970s and early 1980s, by the 1990s, I cared for some patients in Oklahoma City who were discharged home on the fifth or, in one case, even the fourth post-transplant day.

In addition to their immense contributions to immunosuppressive therapy, Starzl (in the USA) and Calne (in Europe) were the first to establish liver transplant programmes, a much more complex surgical procedure than kidney transplantation. Surely, these contributions are more than sufficient to warrant a Nobel Prize.

It could, of course, be argued that all of the drugs utilised by Calne and Starzl, including corticosteroids, had been discovered by others before them, and therefore they discovered little. Yet applying these agents to overcome the specific problems of organ transplantation was very important; this was their great contribution.

So why was the original proposal to share the Prize between Murray, Calne, and Starzl shelved? According to Tom Starzl, his understanding was that those in the field of bone marrow transplantation felt that one of the pioneers in this field should be included, and they had put forward the name of Donnell Thomas. That meant that there would now be four potential awardees: Murray, Calne, Starzl, and Thomas—one more than allowed by the regulations governing the Prize. Yet others felt that Norman Shumway should be included, making five. However, Shumway's claim was less strong than either Calne or Starzl since (like Barnard), although he had played a major role in establishing heart transplantation, he had not contributed to the development of immunosuppressive therapy, but had simply used the drugs made available by the research of others. It is noticeable that Barnard's name does not appear to have been considered at this time.

It was inconceivable to all concerned that it would be fair to award the prize to Starzl but not Calne, or *vice versa*, and so what to do? In their wisdom, the committee decided to make Murray and Thomas the laureates, thus, in my opinion, excluding the two surgeons who most clearly should have been honoured. The answer would have been to award a separate prize (perhaps the following year) for bone marrow transplantation, which presents significantly different problems from organ transplantation.

According to several of those I consulted on this topic, if Hume had been alive, the award should possibly have been shared between Hume, Calne, and Starzl. Hume's work at the Brigham had preceded that of Murray, and so he is considered by many to be an earlier pioneer in the field than any of the others, with the exception of the French.

## Chris and the Nobel Prize

Chris received many academic and public honours, most of which are listed elsewhere in this book (Appendix II), but it must be noted that few of the world's most prestigious universities or medical schools acknowledged his contributions to surgery. Was this because they did not believe his work was significant, or was their response influenced by his public image and flamboyant lifestyle? The answer is probably that his activities and status as a celebrity (even a playboy) diminished his achievements in the eyes of many of his peers. This is possibly a reason why the Royal College of Surgeons of England bestowed an Honorary Fellowship on Norman Shumway, but did not honour Chris similarly.

Nevertheless, in the late 1960s, some of the public expected that Chris might be awarded the Nobel Prize. Although his work in initiating heart transplantation was an important development in both heart surgery and organ transplantation, it was largely based on the work of others before him. As such, in my opinion, it was not original or fundamental enough to warrant the award of the most prestigious prize in medicine. An award of the Prize to Chris in the euphoric months after the first heart transplant when public opinion lauded him for the step he had taken, particularly when Dr Blaiberg was making such good progress, would have perhaps been understandable, but might well have been a mistake.

I can perhaps compare it to the award of the Nobel Peace Prize to Barack Obama within a year of his inauguration as President of the USA when, at that time, he had really done nothing to deserve it. Whatever his intentions—good as they undoubtedly were—and no matter how poorly the previous president was viewed at the time (rendering Obama 'a breath of fresh air' to American and European liberals), the award to Obama was precipitate and unjustified. An award to Barnard in 1968 would have been equally precipitate and certainly unjustified.

It would seem that Chris would agree with me. In his book *Christiaan Barnard's Program for Living with Arthritis*, he addressed the question of whether he should have been awarded the Prize. In a section on the benefits of taking corticosteroid drugs, such as prednisone, to suppress the features of rheumatoid arthritis, he wrote of the discovery of these drugs that have such immense anti-inflammatory capacity.

These compounds were introduced with considerable fanfare ... [and] widely hailed as 'miracle medicines' and 'wonder drugs' by enthusiastic doctors and their patients. They had been developed by three researchers—Edward C. Kendall, Tadeus Reichstein, and Philip S. Hench—who in 1950 shared a Nobel Prize for showing that these hormones would suppress symptoms of inflammation and allergy. Now, more than once it has been suggested to me that I have earned a Nobel Prize for being the world's first heart transplant surgeon. But I have always found that idea ridiculous. Mine was undeniably an achievement.

It needed certain skills and techniques. I had to enthuse, inspire even, and lead a large team of people, each with a specialised role to play. I had to do the actual surgery. But when I think of the intellectual and imaginative power of people like Kendall, Reichstein, and Hench, I see my own work in perspective. I appreciate that if there are to be such institutions as medical prizes, then the highest honours should go to people who advance mankind solely by the power of thought.

Therefore, it appears that even Chris did not believe his contribution to medicine, as important as it was, deserved recognition by the award of the Nobel Prize, unless his written comments did not truly reflect his private thoughts. Some have claimed that he privately complained that he had been overlooked and, furthermore, that he believed he would have received the Prize if he had been a black South African, rather than white. Due to the influence of politics in the world, even the world of medical prizes, this is a possibility. However, over many years, I never heard him make any statement to this effect or any comment that contrasts with his written opinion.

On a much lighter note, Chris tells the story that a journalist once advised him that his flamboyant lifestyle, in particular his being seen with a stream of beautiful young women, had alienated the Nobel committee. If it had not been for this flaw, the journalist said, he might have been awarded the Nobel Prize for carrying out the first heart transplant. If he had his life again, the journalist asked, would he make changes to his lifestyle? Chris thought carefully for a few moments. If the journalist were correct, he replied, and if it truly came down to a choice between the Nobel Prize and the company of beautiful young women, then he had to admit that, if he had his life to live again, he would still choose the beautiful women.

# 30

# Old Age and Death

*Growing old is humanity's greatest tragedy.*

Chris Barnard

Chris Barnard died suddenly during what was reported to be an asthma attack (although there remains some doubt about this) on 2 September 2001, at the age of seventy-eight. Reports vary on when he suffered his first asthma attack, with one report stating that this was as early as 1976, but it does not appear to have been a major health problem to him until quite late in life. Dr Johan Brink, head of the clinical cardiac surgery service at GSH who advised Chris on health matters on occasions during his later life, does not remember asthma being a problem during the 1990s, fewer than five years before Chris died. Even late in life, with proper medication, the attacks relatively rarely curtailed his lifestyle, though he would on occasions suffer a severe attack, particularly when he was 'uncontrollably' laughing, which was frightening to him. These attacks became rather more problematic in his last few years.

During and after the break-up of his marriage to Karin, Chris went through what must have been the worst period of his life. He wrote, 'As I write this book [*50 Ways to a Healthy Heart*], the divorce from my third wife is affecting me particularly deeply, and I have had great difficulty falling asleep over the past few months. Most of the time it has been impossible for me to get to sleep without taking a sleeping pill.'

Not only was he separated to a large extent from his two young children, Armin and Lara, but his health was steadily deteriorating, as it does in many of us as old age approaches. In Chris's case, this was associated with a loss of his good looks, which must have been a huge blow to him. He had always valued youthful good looks and, indeed, this is what had led him to undergo at least two facelifts as he aged, and to tint his graying hair. To make it worse, as a result of surgery for skin cancer, the facial changes that became obvious to all who saw him were insensitively reported in the press.

During this period, he spent a considerable amount of time in Europe, particularly in Austria, working with a publisher who planned a book on health written (at least largely) by Chris. In 2000, he undertook a hectic tour of radio and television stations in Europe, promoting the book. Chris remained well-known in Europe, but in the preceding decade, he had steadily fallen out of the limelight elsewhere, except in South Africa where he and his family had something of the Kennedy aura about them. Almost everything that happened to Chris or his extended family was newsworthy in his homeland.

In Austria, where, by the way, he was awarded citizenship, he lived in a hotel, which he found lonely and impersonal. Even the companionship of a blonde female medical student, almost fifty years his junior, was insufficient to fill the void opened by the absence of his family and close friends. Every few months, he would phone me in the USA, which was a great pleasure for me, but I did not fully realise at the time that his calls were an indication of how lonely he felt. He had always been so sociable and outgoing that I found it difficult to believe he was actually really lonely. In retrospect, his phone calls were a sign of this loneliness.

He did not call me very often, but the calls were very different from those a few years earlier, when he had still been positive in his outlook on life. For example, he had real happiness in his voice when we spoke soon after South Africa had famously won the Rugby World Cup in 1995, the event portrayed in the movie, *Invictus*. Chris was obviously very pleased that the South African team—the underdogs in the final to the powerful All Blacks from New Zealand—had emerged as champions, but what particularly thrilled him was to see Nelson Mandela (Figure 30.i), the president of the country, appear wearing a Number 6 shirt, the shirt of the captain of the (predominantly white) South African team, Francois Pienaar. Chris clearly had immense respect for President Mandela, and I believe he saw this event as providing hope of a great future for his beloved country. This was in marked contrast to his attitude to Mandela many years earlier when, like most Afrikaners, he had considered Mandela to be a 'communist'.

This happy event faded into a sea of depression and despair that surrounded him most of the time in his last couple of years. He related his problems to me: the break-up of his marriage to Karin, how he missed seeing his two young children, and Karin's efforts—despite the fact that she had signed a prenuptial agreement—to take him to court for alimony (which Chris blamed on the influence of others on her). There was considerable acrimony and unpleasantness associated with this, his last divorce. I know he found the experience stressful; perhaps he was less able to cope with the stress it imposed on him than when younger.

Perhaps his major problems were physical. His rheumatoid arthritis continued to trouble him—and pain can be immensely stressful—and he had developed a skin cancer on his face, encroaching on to his nose.

I wrote to him at intervals between the telephone calls, hoping my letters would perhaps help distract him from his many problems. It was during this period of time that I asked him to write some words in my copy of his second memoirs, *The Second Life*, which had been published in 1993. I mailed him the copy, and on 24 August 2000, a little more than a year before his death, he wrote:

> To David Cooper,
>     My colleague and friend with happy memories for the times we had together. It is sad that this is something of the past. With lots of love to you and your wife,
>     Chris Barnard.

On re-reading his words, his relative unhappiness comes through. The message is that he is faced with the prospect—nay, the reality—that the many good times of life were over.

Away from his family and friends, Chris was clearly suffering from a profound loneliness. In a newspaper article, 'Starlight and Poppies', he had written of the loneliness that can affect people of any age, but particularly the elderly.

> Loneliness and the despair of age are two faces of the same coin— spiritual death. It is an instinctive reaction to flee from death, to be where the noise and the people are. From that arises the unspoken belief that if there are enough people to reassure one of existence one can stave off loneliness. If one can surround oneself with youth, one can stave off death. If the lonely are desperate enough, and if they have the means, they will try to buy what they cannot have. Hence the gigolos and gigolettes, the face-lifts, the booze, and drugs and the parties. People respond negatively to loneliness. They avoid it, making the lonely [even] more lonely. Yet they criticise the lonely for trying to get closer to the fire, for behaviour which is simply substitution for what is lost.

In another article, he commented, 'Big populations have led to more loneliness, not less. Too many people mean too many faces. In the end all become faceless.'

Chris also reached out to his estranged brother, Marius, during this period of loneliness. Marius addresses this in his memoirs.

My brother then became very lonely and felt rejected. He was of the opinion that his great contribution to medicine was no longer appreciated. I believe that at that moment, after years of estrangement, he made a sincere attempt to repair our poor relationship. He started to phone me regularly to complain bitterly about his personal problems and the way the media and others were treating him. He started to open his heart to me and I listened but gave nothing in return. My attitude was dismissive. 'When you were in the limelight, you turned your back on me,' I thought. 'I have now had my own life without you for twenty years and I am content.'

Today, one of my greatest regrets is that I did not respond to his endeavour to restore our relationship. I kept him at a distance. Since the heart transplants, he had disappointed me so often that I could not forgive him. But I am now convinced that he was crying out for help, and I failed him.

Chris had discovered that rejecting his roots and relishing in fame could not preserve his good looks—his handsome, boyish features, which he tried so hard to maintain, became disfigured from cancer and surgery—nor provide him with the affection and compassion of a loving family. The people he considered loyal turned on him, but he found love and care with Louwtjie [to whom he had become partially reconciled] and Deirdre. The wheel had come full circle.

Unfortunately, it seems Chris delayed treatment of the skin cancer for too long, despite Deirdre urging him to get it dealt with. The cancer was a basal cell carcinoma, which, unlike most other cancers, is rarely serious in respect to spreading to distant sites in the body, but which can spread locally. Exasperated by his procrastination, and before she could 'bite off my tongue and stop the words jumping out,' Deirdre told him he looked like the 'Elephant Man' [the greatly deformed man described by the London surgeon, Sir Frederick Treves, in his 1923 book, and portrayed in the 1980 film by actor John Hurt]. Chris evidently accepted this remark with good grace, and it prompted him to consult a surgical colleague.

Sadly, by the time he decided to undergo treatment, his surgeons found it more difficult to remove the cancer completely than they would have done at an earlier stage. To ensure it did not recur, they had to excise it widely, which necessitated covering the site with a skin flap taken from elsewhere on the face, mainly from the forehead. This resulted in a less-than-perfect cosmetic result. It was followed by irradiation therapy to ensure killing any remaining cancerous cells, which also took its toll on the surrounding tissues. The surgery impaired his previous fine features (Figure 30.ii).

Subsequently, in Austria, he fell and broke his hip bone and required an emergency operation. This was not totally successful and so he returned to Cape Town to undergo a second surgical procedure. These physical stresses, when added to the many emotional stresses he suffered at this time, undermined his usual positive and optimistic approach to life. What may have compounded his sense of depression was the fact that some journalists appeared to take pleasure in drawing his physical decline to the public's attention.

As an example, in her memoirs Deirdre points out how William Sanderson-Meyer, the writer of a column called 'Jaundiced Eye', in South Africa's *Saturday Argus* newspaper, wrote about 'Passing Your Sell-by Date':

> Last week I saw pictures in the newspaper of a seedy looking fellow with a few thin strands of lank hair plastered in neat agricultural rows across his balding head. His lumpy, large nose looked as if a dyslexic kindergarten pupil had put it together out of play dough. He had mottled skin and haunted eyes. It was only when I read the caption that I found out that it was the world-famous heart surgeon and one-time playmate of the Hollywood stars, Dr Christiaan Barnard, who was commenting on some new research in combating heart disease. It was horrific.

Whomever the subject, such gratuitously cruel comments as these are unforgiveable, and authors of such words should be deeply ashamed. They are beneath contempt. Mercifully, it is unlikely that Chris ever read this particular article as he was abroad at the time and it was published less than a week before he died.

Deirdre points out that some members of the public take a perverse interest in someone once beautiful who loses those looks, and the media seem to love it. They publish the worst photographs they can find. Her father was now vulnerable and exposed, and she felt protective towards him. When one considers that, at the peak of his career, some magazine editors had considered him to be one of the 'world's greatest lovers', it must have been an immense blow to him when he lost his good looks. According to author Donald McRae, Norman Shumway met Chris at a medical congress in Paris in 2000 (approximately a year before Chris died), and felt only compassion for him, knowing how much his appearance meant to him.

Perhaps the only way for beautiful people to avoid this fate is to die young. We remember the delectable Marilyn Monroe, the handsome and charismatic John F. Kennedy, and the elegant Princess Diana as they were at their peak. We cannot imagine them as elderly, failing people, and so their youthful, glamorous images will remain with us forever. As an aside, Chris had met Diana on several occasions and they had enjoyed each other's company (Figure 30.iii).

While in Austria, Chris was invited to present an award at a major function. This was the award of sports personality of the century to Muhammad Ali, the great American boxer. Like Chris, Ali was another icon of the twentieth century now well past his prime, debilitated by a Parkinson-like neurological disease from injury to his brain. The photograph of the two of them together on that occasion is in many ways one of the saddest I have ever seen (Figure 30.iv). With their glory days well behind them, only further deterioration and death awaited them. However, unlike most of us, they at least had experienced many glory days during their lifetimes, and in varying ways had contributed massively to the enjoyment or well-being of the lives of others. Chris told me that, when presenting the glass trophy to Muhammad Ali, because of Ali's tremor, he was very worried that Ali would drop the trophy. Fortunately, he did not.

Nevertheless, Chris's personality could still distract from his physical imperfections. Deirdre reported:

> People would stop him on the street to talk to him—they always did that—and even when he looked his worst he was always willing to stop and chat, and he wasn't a fool. He could see that people took notice of what he looked like and were probably thinking: 'Haai, shame, and he was such a nice looking man in his day.' He talked his way through it. If you were with him you could actually see him doing it and he was able to do that, just as he always had been, because no matter how he looked, he was still himself. Only the outside had changed and it was the inside people responded to. I suppose in a way some of them might have missed that old glamorous package, but no one ever went away after speaking to him feeling unsatisfied or let down.

When Chris's marriage to Karin was ending, despite the efforts of Father Tom Nicholson as a counsellor to both parties, Chris set up home on his own. The ever-loyal Deirdre—she who, when informed of her parents pending divorce, had immediately asked her mother 'who would care for [her] father?'—became his main carer for the rest of his life. She realised she could not fill the void that had opened in his life and that she worried and fussed too much over him, but she happily made every effort to open up new avenues to him, many of which he never wanted to follow.

She telephoned friends who were still important to him, urging them to visit him and cheer him up, and presented him with brochures for cruises, none of which he chose to take. She even suggested an old friend he might consider making 'wife number four', but, much as he liked the friend to whom he had been close for many years, he was in no mood for another wife. Deirdre, who even thought he would benefit from some psychological counseling, plied him with self-help books, but he was uninterested. He told her he knew what she was up to and, if she did not mind, he would prefer it if she skipped 'all that psychological stuff'. He would claim that he was capable of looking after himself, and the last thing he needed was 'an anxious daughter forever on the doorstep, checking that the house was in order, whether the cupboards were full, wanting to make tea or see that he was eating properly.' Considering how impatient and temperamental he could be, Deirdre was surprised how patient he was with her efforts to stimulate him out of his depression.

As with many people in their declining years, caring for him even in seemingly little ways could at times be a major undertaking. Deirdre recollected some of their rituals together.

> I'd go with him when he went swimming in the pool in the townhouse complex where he lived. It was quite a caravan. There was my father in his bath-robe and me behind, talking, carrying the towel and a book and looking for the keys so we wouldn't get locked out, while he worked through the checklist. Did I have the towel? Did I remember to bring the keys, and what about the asthma pump? I would have to show him I had it just so that he could be sure. Through the garden we would go, past the gardeners, with me talking and doing the 'hullo, hullo' thing to anyone who happened to be there, and looking for a nice spot where my father could spread his things out and I could set out a 'chaise' so that he could be comfortable, while the blue pool blinked in the sun and the Kreepy-Krauly sucked its way around. After his swim it would be the same thing all over again. My father would go into the sauna, I'd go into the sauna with him and I'd read to him.

One of the books Deirdre read to him was *Angela's Ashes* by Frank McCourt. One statement from the book that remained in her mind was 'Children love their parents unconditionally.' She thought, 'Yes … That's how it's been for me and that's how it should be.'

Deirdre, who was closest to him in those last months, believed that, although he put on a good outward show, inside he was worn out.

> He was unused to being alone: he liked people around him and he loved home life. He was used to a house where there were children: he missed Armin and Lara. This was the third family he'd lost. There

are some who might say that in a sense my father managed to self-sabotage, to destroy all those things that were precious to him, and perhaps there's an element of truth in this. The fact is that the moment when it happens, whatever the causes may have been, the pain is real enough.

It hurt her to see his underlying sadness, as well as his physical problems: his disfiguring cancer and the relentless pain of arthritis, which, like his asthma, was always with him. She 'could not bear to see him so alone and in such distress.' Even though he put on a brave face for most of the time, Deirdre could sense that he was a broken man. She wondered 'if, after all, this is what all the glitter and stardust amounted to in the end.'

At times, Chris was reduced to sitting quietly in his new townhouse listening to music, often with Deirdre as his companion. Kris Kristoffersen's 'Lover Come Back' was a favourite. Sometimes, he was moved to tears, such as by the traditional Afrikaans song, 'Skipskop'. It is a song about the forced removal of a fishing village, the disintegration of a community, and the irretrievable loss inherent in that. It seemed to Deirdre that he wept not only for the sadness of all that had happened in South Africa, which he loved dearly, but also for some of the sadness in his own life: 'A piece here, a piece there, the pieces of my life lie everywhere.' According to Deirdre, he cried every time he heard it. There is pathos in this picture of him in his last days.

Probably through Deirdre's machinations, Louwtjie, his first wife, was enrolled to help, and it is greatly to her credit that she was able to some extent to put the painful events and bitterness of the past to one side and help support Chris in his last years. Deirdre wrote:

> Towards the end, they began to spend time together. The old sparks of attraction between them were still there and in their old age they formed an uneasy, potentially volcanic alliance ... I can't imagine my mother not having been there. In his last interview with Time magazine, my father said of my mother, 'All the credit must go to Louwtjie, my first wife, who took the strain and stood by me when we were young. She married me because she loved me.'

Louwtjie even shortened the trousers of a new dinner suit he wore at the last function he attended in South Africa, a fundraising dinner for the Organ Donor Foundation of Southern Africa. It was the day before he left for Israel on his last fateful journey abroad. He evidently seemed to enjoy telling people of the help Louwtjie had given him. Deirdre commented:

[It] was like coming full circle, all the way from those long-ago days when she [Louwtjie] had fine-stitched those heart valves for him in that time of their young married life. It was during the time when André and I were small and she used to make our clothes. We were a long way from the high life in those days and she also sewed to earn extra money. The truth is that the journey of my mother, Aletta Louw, who married her freshly qualified country doctor in 1948, didn't end in a shower of fire. It ended on a small domestic note, something which, I am sure, neither of them could ever have imagined all that long time ago when they first met.

As the oldest of Chris's children, Deirdre also took it upon herself to take the lead in organising family events, although my understanding is that her half-brother, Frederick, has also done much to keep the various members of the family together. Her half-siblings and their children sometimes called Deirdre the 'BBC'—the 'Barnard Broadcasting Corporation'. With so many wives, children, and grandchildren around him, she sometimes likened her father to the king in *The King and I* with all of his family. The family was of the opinion that they did not have a family tree but instead a 'creeping vine'. At family gatherings, for example, at his last birthday party held at the Castle in Cape Town, where all the members of the family sat at one long table, Chris sometimes referred to them as the 'Full Catastrophe', probably taken from the story of *Zorba the Greek,* who referred to his own large family in this way.

## Christiaan Barnard Foundation

Nevertheless, Chris still took pleasure from some of his activities. After the first heart transplant, children from all races came from all over the world seeking treatment at Groote Schuur or the Red Cross War Memorial Children's Hospital. The Cape Provincial Administration and the South African government deserve credit for providing medical and surgical care free to many of these young patients. As far as I am aware, Chris never charged a personal fee for his services, no matter what demands were made on him.

It is perhaps not surprising that, with his great empathy and love for children, Chris should consider that one of his greatest achievements was to master the surgical techniques necessary to correct life-threatening defects of the heart in young children. He found it difficult to understand how God could allow a child to be born with such a serious abnormality that threatened to curtail their life at such an early age.

In later life, therefore, he set up a foundation to provide funds to facilitate children coming to Cape Town for operations to correct their heart defects. It is said that he was influenced to take this step by Princess Diana, who encouraged him to do so. Chris no longer carried out the operations himself. These were done by younger surgeons, such as Dr Susan Vosloo, who had trained at GSH and the Red Cross Children's Hospital. The operations were carried out at a private hospital in Cape Town originally named City Hospital and recently renamed the Christiaan Barnard Memorial Hospital (Figure 30.v).

With his Christiaan Barnard Foundation, he wanted to make a contribution towards a more humane twenty-first century. The Foundation aimed to help improve the living conditions of children and mothers, particularly in poorer countries. It aimed to do this by addressing the population explosion, particularly in Africa, by disseminating the message of birth control; improving preventative health care by creating primary health-care facilities, including mother-child care centres; and helping children in need, particularly those with heart disease and those exposed to psychological trauma, such as through war. The Foundation could clearly not achieve all of these laudable aims itself, and so it planned to collaborate with several internationally renowned organizations, local organizations, and committed private individuals.

The last child during Chris's life who came to South Africa as a beneficiary of funding from the Christiaan Barnard Foundation was a little boy from Russia. One of the last great joys of his life was meeting the mother and child. The operation was successful, which was immensely satisfying to Chris as the boy could now return home with no disability to prevent him from leading a full and happy life.

Deirdre recorded that Chris received a fax from Mikhail Gorbachev, the former president of of the USSR, extending his warmest wishes and thanking the Christiaan Barnard Foundation for choosing a Russian boy for this life-changing operation.

Dear friend!

I am happy to know about this successful surgery and recovery of the little Russian boy. This saved life and returned happiness to the family are possible only because of your generosity and nobility, the high professionalism of the doctors of your clinic and the effectiveness of your assistants from your Foundation. We are sincerely grateful to you and proud of you. Hope to continue our co-operation and to see you soon.

Gratefully, Mikhail Gorbachev.

Chris also continued to provide help and advice to any friend (or friend-of-a-friend) in need, doing his best to advise even on medical conditions outside his area of expertise. Deirdre wrote:

> My father was always very good about things like this. He always kept up to date on what was happening in all facets of his profession. He was also very willing to put things into layperson's terms where he could and to help people. He knew very well that these informal questions were put to him not in the expectation of a formal diagnosis but simply by people seeking some kind of reassurance.

As Chris grew older, of course, the media were prone to ask him to look back over his life and assess its undoubted ups and downs. In the last television interview he gave in South Africa before his death, he was asked what he considered the greatest sadness of his life. Of the many sad, even tragic, episodes in his life he could have selected, he chose the fact that his father had died a month before he performed the first open heart surgical procedure at Groote Schuur Hospital after his return from Minneapolis, thus initiating the first truly successful heart surgery programme in Africa. Chris knew how proud his father was of the achievements of his sons, and how much he would have enjoyed hearing of this major step forward. Chris always became emotional when he spoke of his father, whom he admired for his Christian simplicity and goodness, and whom he continued to feel he had failed by not seeing him frequently enough in his later years.

## The Last Goodbye

The last time Deirdre saw her father was when she drove him to Cape Town airport. He was going on a visit to Israel and then for a short holiday in Paphos in Cyprus. Israel was to be a working visit to learn details of some new medical research, about which Chris was excited. He was then to spend a few days relaxing in Paphos. He had visited Cyprus previously and had enjoyed it. Deirdre hoped he would be happy there again, and that the holiday would re-energise him. Her description in her memoirs of his departure from Cape Town airport is poignant and moving. With her permission, I record it here in her own words.

> I had a sense of something out of place. I'd done the airport drop-off so many times in these last months of his life. My friends used to joke with me about it and ask why he couldn't take the shuttle like everyone else did. It would have been much easier. Certainly, when it's a crack of dawn

flight, as his last flight out of South Africa was, it would have made far more sense. The truth is that I liked taking him to the airport. I liked the drive out and the two of us alone in the car. I'm tempted to say it was like old times, and it was in a way, and then again it wasn't.

We had our way of doing things. I'd draw up in the five-minute drop zone, he'd get a trolley and then we'd say our goodbyes and I'd go back to town. [But on this occasion] I got out of the car and left it just where it stood and went back, dashed back if you must know, looking for my father. I just had to see him. It was as simple as that.

He was walking slowly, pushing his trolley as if it held all the burdens of the world in it, and he didn't see me and I stopped right where I was and just looked at him. An old man hunched over his trolley walking very slowly as if every step hurt. I just couldn't bear it. I knew how much his arthritis hurt. When he was on 'public display' he made every effort to hide the pain, but the truth is that he was in pain almost all the time and on that morning there was no attempt to hide it at all. I felt so sorry for him. I felt my heart shrink and slide up into my throat. I felt the way you feel when something terribly sad happens.

People moved between us and he still didn't see me. I watched him move painfully into his place in the queue and then I forced myself to be myself and just rush up to him. It wasn't the way we usually were, but if he thought it was odd, he didn't comment on it. 'It's nothing,' I said. 'I've just come to say goodbye to you. That's all.'

What he did was something he rarely did. He turned to me and put his arms around me and they were the strong, safe arms of my childhood. I could see his hands, his famous hands gnarled now by arthritis. I could smell him and feel the rough texture of his jacket under my cheek and I could close my eyes for just a moment and feel complete. 'Thank you, Didi,' he said. 'Thank you for everything. I love you.'

It was the last thing he said to me.

Deirdre never saw her father alive again.

# Death

Chris Barnard died in Paphos, Cyprus, on Sunday, 2 September 2001. Deirdre heard the news as she and her husband, Kobus, were driving towards Saldanha Bay on the west coast of South Africa to attend the funeral of a close family friend. Her mobile phone rang and a voice said, 'Deirdre, I am sorry, but I have very bad news for you ...' Kobus pulled the car to the side of the road and Deirdre cried like she had never cried before. 'I didn't know I could cry like that,' she later wrote. 'I didn't know I had so many tears in me.'

After the death of his son, André, Chris had said that 'grief is pain beyond description'. It was a pain so unbearable that a new special word was needed to describe it because 'pain' by itself was insufficient. Deirdre, for whom her father had in many ways been the light of her life, experienced that special pain.

In Paphos, Chris had been staying at a hotel for a few days' rest. He went to sit by the swimming pool and, by all reports, suddenly died. The circumstances suggested a heart attack, or possibly a pulmonary embolus (a blood clot that blocked the major artery to the lungs), but a *post-mortem* examination in Cyprus found that his heart was not diseased and there was no evidence of a pulmonary embolus. It was concluded that he had died from a sudden asthma attack; reports vary as to whether he had forgotten to take his asthma pump with him to the pool (which Deirdre had always ensured he had with him at home) or whether he could not employ it quickly enough. The consensus is that his asthma pump was close by. If he had it with him, it would have been an unusually rapid asthma attack that would have killed him so quickly. A pulmonary embolus seems more likely. His body was flown back to Cape Town, where a second autopsy confirmed the findings of the first. Evidently, his heart was in reasonably good shape, and so that was not the cause of his death.

I must say my suspicions were that he had suffered a heart attack, but that this fact may have been covered up by the publishers of his new book, *50 Ways to a Healthy Heart*, as his death from a heart condition might clearly have impacted sales. It seems my suspicions were unfounded.

However, a pulmonary embolus remains a distinct possibility. Chris had undergone two operations for his fractured hip earlier that year, and surgical procedures and immobility predispose to the development of a deep vein thrombosis in the legs or lower abdomen. A clot can break off and travel in the blood stream to the lungs (as a pulmonary embolus). A large embolus can be instantly fatal. If the embolus had been missed (or dislodged) in Cyprus, it may well not have been picked up when the organs were returned to Cape Town for the second *post-mortem*.

If, however, he had died from an acute severe asthma attack, then questions were raised as to whether he had purposely not carried his inhaler with him (or had purposely not employed it urgently) as perhaps he had a suicide wish. Chris's father confessor, Father Tom, confirmed to me that Chris had been very depressed by his many problems that year, and they had sometimes discussed the subject of euthanasia—what was passive euthanasia and what was active euthanasia. On the evening before

Chris left on his final journey, he had spoken at a fundraiser for the Organ Donation Foundation in Cape Town. The evening proved stressful for him because Karin and her boyfriend were in the audience, yet he overcame some initial nervousness and received a standing ovation. Later that evening, Tom telephoned him to wish him well on his travels, and was worried by the fact that Chris mentioned that he was 'going away for a very long time.' These words led Tom to become suspicious that perhaps Chris had wanted to die.

Personally, I think it is unlikely that Chris would have taken this step. Even if a massive pulmonary embolus had not killed him almost instantly (in which event an asthma pump would have proved useless), it seems more likely that, on vacation by himself, in a depressed state of mind, and without the loving attention of Deirdre, he had either forgotten to take the inhaler with him or, in a panic, became too confused to find it quickly enough. A severe asthma attack can be so frightening to the patient that I think it is very unlikely Chris would have purposely not reached out immediately for the inhaler.

## 'Lara's Theme'

Soon after Chris died, a letter addressed to 'Dr Barnard's Daughter' was handed to Deirdre, who soon realised that it was actually intended for her little half-sister, Lara (Chris's youngest offspring who, at that time, would have been four years old). The letter was from the pianist at the hotel where Chris had spent the last night before he died. The pianist wrote that Chris had asked her more than once to play 'Lara's Theme' from the film score of *Dr Zhivago*, and that she had been happy to do so. As the real-life Lara was still too young to have spent much time with her father, the letter will always remind her that Chris had her very much in his thoughts the evening before he died.

In the US, the public interest in Chris's death was only modest, but it was noted much more in Europe and several other parts of the world (Figure 31.iii). Some years previously, I had been invited by the British newspaper, *The Guardian,* to write Chris's obituary—evidently, these newspapers plan ahead—and this was published with those in many other newspapers around the world. Denton Cooley invited me to collaborate with him in writing an obituary on Chris for the leading medical journal, *Circulation.*

Both Nelson Mandela and Thabo Mbeki, his successor as president of South Africa, praised Chris's contributions to the country, with Mandela commending Chris for speaking out on apartheid.

# Coming Home

Chris's family and two very close family friends were at Cape Town airport to receive him home.

Chris had often told me that he was never as happy as when he returned home to South Africa after his trips abroad. He once described it as 'a joyous experience, an inner glow, a feeling of elation that lasts for days.'

I can well believe that. During the seven years I lived and worked in Cape Town, I was always filled with joy when I returned from overseas. There is something about Cape Town that is so inspiring and uplifting— the combination of fine weather and beautiful scenery is captivating, simply wonderful. Even though I was born and brought up in London and have lived in the US now for thirty years, I have never felt quite the same when returning to these homes. I am sure Chris, to whom Cape Town was very much more home than it ever was to me, would have been pleased to be 'coming home', even under these tragic circumstances.

Deirdre also emphasised Chris's love of his homeland. 'My father always liked coming home. No matter where he'd been in the world or how exciting his adventures, coming home was the best part of all. He'd said so. I would have liked him to see it, to see for himself this last homecoming.'

At the airport to greet his simple wooden coffin were Deirdre and her husband, Kobus; Chris's two sons from his marriage to Barbara, Frederick and Christiaan, Jnr; and his third wife, Karin, and their young son, Armin—almost the 'Full Catastrophe', as Chris would have called them. Supporting them were two very close family friends.

One was Dene Friedmann, whose father had been a good friend of Chris for many years—perhaps his best friend. Dene had water skied with Deirdre all those many years before, and subsequently worked for Chris as one of his heart-lung pump technicians for almost twenty years, and indeed had been a member of the team for the first heart transplant operation. The other was Father Tom Nicholson, who had supported Chris and his family through all of the upheavals of their lives. He had counseled Barbara when she was contemplating divorce and while she was dying. He had been a confidante of André. He had counseled Chris after the break-up of his marriage to Barbara and after the death of André. He had officiated at Chris's wedding to Karin and at the funerals of both André and Barbara. He had been there for every crisis in the Barnard family. Deirdre acknowledged Father Tom's constant support to all of the family. 'The Barnards are not the greatest communicators in the world, but we could always talk to Father Tom and when we did, he always listened.'

Two indications of the regard in which Chris was still held in South Africa were the fact that his family and friends waiting to welcome him home were invited to use the VIP lounge at the airport, and that a local funeral parlor requested what they considered the privilege of organising all arrangements relating to Chris's cremation and memorial services without charge to the Barnard estate. They wanted to make this gift to Professor Barnard, and the family greatly appreciated this kind and generous gesture.

In her memoirs, Deirdre wrote that she did not want Chris's coffin to be carried in a black car; to her, this would not have been in keeping with his love of 'laughter and energy and light', but she did not feel she could mention this to the undertakers who were so kindly making all of the arrangements. To her joy, they sent a white car. She was also pleased that the Greeks in Cyprus had sent him home in a plain wooden coffin because, despite his fame and even notoriety, she was sure that her father still saw himself 'as a plain man, and a simple wooden coffin would have suited him just fine.'

## Laying Chris to Rest

The family was overwhelmed with telephone calls and condolence letters that arrived from all over the world, full of kindness, sympathy, and even love. In Deirdre's opinion, South Africans 'wanted to show that at the end of it all, my father, with all his powers and with all his frailties, had been a major public figure in this country. I think people wanted us to know they acknowledged this and respected him for it.' Letters arrived from heads of state, ambassadors, famous people, former patients, and many from those who had never even met Chris.

Chris had been clear that he wished to be cremated and his ashes returned to the place where he had been brought up: Beaufort West, in the Great Karoo. He had stated publicly that 'I would like a Karoo stone brought in from the veldt where I walked as a boy. I want it placed in the garden of the house in Beaufort West where I grew up. On it I would like a plaque saying, "I've come home again".' He was clearly a romantic at heart, with a sense of nostalgia.

Deirdre looked on this as his wish to 'complete the circle of his life and lie at the end in the place where his life began.' Chris and his sons, as well as his grandson, Adam (André's son), had on occasions enjoyed hunting expeditions in the wilderness outside Beaufort West. 'In the Great Karoo the sky is immense,' wrote Deirdre. 'The air is thin and clear and people come and go from the landscape and live on in the stories that those who come after tell about them, or in the few words engraved on the headstones in the little churchyards outside towns. That's how their passing is noted, while the land just goes on. It's right that my father should have returned.'

Chris's body was cremated, and there were memorial services at GSH and in Cape Town's historic and beautiful City Hall, the building from which Nelson Mandela had addressed the world after his release from prison in 1990. The well-known South African singer, Anneli Cilliers, sang 'Skipskop', the sad song of which Chris was so fond.

The celebration of his life then moved to Beaufort West, where Chris's ashes had been taken in a coffin, and where a second memorial service was held in the Old Dutch Reformed Mission Church where Chris's father had ministered to his flock of coloured folk and Chris had pumped the bellows for the organ which his mother played.

This church building had seen many changes since Chris was a boy. The coloured congregation had been displaced to a building on the outskirts of the town and the church converted into a sports hall. Chris had been outraged that the white population of the official Dutch Reformed Church had allowed this to happen and said he would have nothing to do with 'men of God' who turned a blind eye when the Nationalist government disobeyed the second most important of the Ten Commandments, which was to 'Love thy neighbour as thyself.'

'It offended everything in him,' wrote Deirdre, 'that men who wore the cloth as his own father once had did nothing to stop apartheid, but instead kept their heads averted while they combed the Bible to find suitable passages to make a dreadful wrong look like God's will.'

Times had changed in Beaufort West for the better. The church had been returned to its former simplicity (rather than glory), making Beaufort West acceptable to Chris again. A local guesthouse offered the mourners accommodation. The evening before the service, a party was held under the stars in the cold night air of the Karoo. Deirdre noted that her 'father would have loved it. I just wish he could have seen it.'

The following morning, 14 September 2001, the little church, filled with flowers from the surrounding veldt (selected by Karin), was packed and there was an overflow of congregants outside. A rose had been named after Chris and, at his son Christiaan's suggestion, a big bowl of these was displayed at the entrance of the church so that each churchgoer could take one and put it in a vase in front of the pulpit. The memorial service proved a joyous occasion. Chris's ashes were handed to Deirdre in two small caskets on which were engraved plates. Armin, Chris's youngest son, carried one of the boxes and Barbara's son, Christiaan (named for his father) carried the other.

The funeral service was led by the loyal Father Tom Nicholson, who had officiated on so many Barnard family occasions. That a Roman Catholic priest should lead the service in Adam Barnard's former church would surely have shocked and greatly displeased Chris's father, who hated what he termed the '*Roomse Gevaar*' (Roman Danger). However, Chris had often said that, if his father had ever met Father Tom, he would have held a different opinion of the Catholic church.

Chris's death drew Marius out of his relative seclusion to commemorate Chris's life. At the time of the Cape Town memorial service, however, he was ill, but he and his wife, Inez, attended the funeral in Beaufort West, which took place in his father's former church. 'It was strange to be back,' Marius recorded. 'I knew this church intimately from my childhood and associated it with my father in the pulpit and my mother at the organ. It had now been converted into a museum.' At Chris's private funeral in Beaufort West, Marius felt he was among strangers.

> Most of Chris's family, with whom I had nothing to do either professionally or socially, seemed like strangers to me. With the exception of Louwtjie and her family, Chris's relatives weren't part of the original Barnard family that to me were associated with that little Dutch Reformed missionary church from years ago.

Although Marius participated in the activities, there clearly remained some resentment in his heart to all but Chris's original family with Louwtjie.

'Chris's more recent family,' he wrote, 'had made no contribution to the historic transplant nor the fame and fortune that went with it. But here they were in the front seats, while poor Louwtjie and her family were essentially ignored. Louwtjie, who had made so many sacrifices to support Chris—particularly during the hard times—looked understandably out of place in their midst.' These comments are divisive, in contrast to those of the all-encompassing Deirdre.

Marius's last thoughts about Chris's funeral were that 'the man who at one time didn't want to set foot in Beaufort West again ended up leaving his ashes, interred in a cask, in the town. They are buried in the garden of the old parsonage in Beaufort West next to a little monument, on which is inscribed: "I came back home".'

Later, Marius admitted that, 'these days, I think of Chris often—mostly about what could have been. I wish that I could relive the last few years of his life. I would certainly welcome him back into the real Barnard family with open arms. But it is too late now. Chris was my brother, but we were always strangers to each other. He was a great doctor and a brilliant scientist, but he had feet of clay. Fortunately, I am now at peace with him and have forgotten the bad times. Today I only remember, with love, being his young *boytjie*. Sorry, Chris.' By using the Afrikaans slang term, *boytjie*, in this context, Marius probably meant 'little brother'.

Before his death, Chris had realised that, 'I have no regrets. At almost seventy-nine, people ask me: where do you go from here? I say to them I'm on the waiting list. I don't know exactly where I am on that list or where I'm going, but I'm on it.'

Chris had occasionally written about death in his *Cape Times* columns. One death that affected him emotionally was that of Princess Diana, whom he had met on more than one occasion and had corresponded with over a period of time. 'One tragic death that really shocked me was Princess Diana's,' he wrote.

> I had been an ardent admirer of hers. It still gives me great pleasure today to know that I was reasonably well acquainted with her. Just two months before her death she had invited me to a private dinner at Kensington Palace. I still honour the present she gave me on that occasion, and I wear it only on special occasions—a dark blue silk tie with an African pattern.

On another occasion, he wrote of a meeting with an elderly Bushman from the Kalahari Desert whose simple philosophy of life impressed Chris very much. 'Was he afraid of death?' Chris asked the old man. 'Men die, animals die, plants die,' the Bushman replied through the interpreter. 'But always there are the children, the new ones.' He held his fingertips a fraction apart. 'Death is a little thing,' he said. Chris believed that he had 'never seen such dignity in a man.'

If Chris had had any warning that his life was near its end, how would he have faced his impending death? Would he have welcomed it (as he would have welcomed euthanasia) as the quality of his life had deteriorated so much, or would he—as a man who had always lived his life to the full— have fought against it as long as possible, hoping for happier times ahead? Although his last years were by no means his happiest, I believe he would have gritted his teeth and fought on, just as he gritted his teeth when setting out those buoys on Zeekoevlei those many years before.

In one of his newspaper columns, he had expressed his attitude to death by quoting passages from Dylan Thomas's famous poem, 'Do not go gentle into that good night'. Chris had written the following:

> 'Do not go gentle into that good night', a famous Welsh poet told his dying father in a poem which is now almost a classic affirmation of life in the face of death. The poet was Dylan Thomas whose own flame of life was such that he burnt himself out in his early thirties, but not before he had left behind a wealth of poetry and prose that praised the life force in all its forms.
>
> The real enemy, according to Thomas, was not death. It was all those creeping, petty betrayals of good, well-rounded living: the greedy lives

of middle-class respectability, the neatly ordered mind of the bureaucrat, the drunken and disorderly mess of existence lived by the truly poor, and, in fact, anything that inhibited a gut reaction to life and love.

I never met Mr Thomas who died some time during the fifties but I know I would have liked a man whose advice to the terminally ill was to 'rage against the dying of the light', meaning not a niggling, complaining whine against illness but total defiance of all death can do until the last defeat pulls you down.

I suggest this was Chris's own attitude to death, and that he would have raged 'against the dying of the light.'

I give the last words in this chapter to Deirdre, the daughter who was so important to Chris throughout his life and to whom, in turn, he was equally important—from their water skiing days to the care she gave him in his final months—and from whose memoirs I have freely drawn.

There's something infinitely sad about this. When my father died that essence that made him the man he was died too. There are no letters, diaries or stories recounted that can even begin to capture the tiniest part of all those energies that surge together and make a human being quite unique and different from their fellows. That is what the sadness of death is really all about. That unique spark is gone and the fragile essence that makes up the person can never be recounted or recaptured no matter how hard we try. That is the pity of it.

What can I say about him that hasn't already been said? Except that, in my opinion, it isn't the beginning or end of his life that's important. What's impressive is its scope. He had a huge life and it went far beyond superficial glamour. He's gone now, but while he was here he made magic. Even looking back, I can see him. It was as I remembered it. There was something really special about him. At least there was for me. While he was here he shone ... he shone with a light so radiant it could make you feel sad.

These words perfectly sum up the Chris Barnard I knew. For all his failings, he had a 'huge life' that was 'impressive' in its scope, and there certainly was 'something really special about him' that enabled him to shine with a 'radiant' light.

# 31

# Looking Back

*It is not enough to die; one has to be forgotten as well.*

Samuel Beckett

Chris Barnard was one of those controversial characters who were either loved or derided—perhaps seriously disliked by some—who balanced on the fence between being an international (and my personal) hero and a fallen idol. If he had not been such a controversial personality, books such as this one would make much duller reading or would not be written at all. It was the contrasts of his character and behaviour that made him of special interest to us and that intrigued us.

Personally, I look on him as I look on Walt Lillehei: as a hero in a Greek tragedy who, to some extent, was responsible for his own downfall. He was the archetypal hero who was placed on a pinnacle by his peers and the public at large, lauded and praised, adulated and honoured, and then, because he did not always behave in the way expected of the standard professional man or scientist, those who had placed him there stepped back and watched, awaiting his fall. Some expected, and even hoped for, a catastrophic fall; others prayed that he would not let them down but would cling to the pinnacle for all he was worth, even if at times he balanced there somewhat precariously.

It may be that Chris was placed on the pinnacle rather hastily and that, in relation to his achievements, the pinnacle was rather too high. After all, what did he do to warrant the public recognition he received? He took out a diseased heart from one human being and replaced it with a healthy heart from another—a remarkable, even miraculous, achievement, one might say, particularly in 1967 (Figure 31.i). Yet the surgical technique had been worked out previously in experimental animals by other surgeons, and had clearly been shown to result in good cardiac function. Methods of attempting to prevent the acute rejection that would almost inevitably occur had been in use in patients with kidney transplants for several years before the first heart transplant was performed. In many ways, it could be argued that Chris's historical operation added little to what was already known.

Chris was, of course, aware of the experimental work that had taken place, and had practiced the relatively simple surgical technique in the laboratory until he had mastered it. He had also prepared himself with regard to management of the immunosuppressive drugs used in transplant patients by spending time with David Hume and Tom Starzl, and by performing one kidney transplant on his return to Cape Town.

## Courage and Conviction

So what did Chris contribute? He contributed courage and conviction: courage to take that first bold step, and conviction in believing in what he was doing. In a relatively rare compliment to his brother, Marius said he 'could never understand why the first human heart transplants were performed in South Africa. In Europe and the United States, cardiac surgeons had far better equipment than we had and their surgical ability was certainly not inferior to ours. Looking back now, I am certain that the major reason for our performing the first ever human heart transplant was Chris Barnard.'

Furthermore, Chris deserves credit for continuing to believe in heart transplantation when complications arose, at a time when most surgeons at other major heart surgery centres were throwing up their hands in dismay and giving up the fight. For example, as we have seen, the board of governors of the Massachusetts General Hospital in Boston, the major hospital of Harvard Medical School and a hospital with a stellar research history that included the epoch-making introduction of anaesthesia for surgical operations in 1846, did not allow the initiation of a heart transplant programme until 1985, almost twenty years after Chris's pioneering first effort.

Chris himself rather downplayed his surgical achievement. 'The heart transplant wasn't such a big thing surgically. The technique was a basic one. The point is that I was prepared to take the risk. My philosophy is that the biggest risk in life is not to take a risk.'

There were, of course, others with the same combination of careful planning and courage, but very few. The Stanford group of surgeons in California, led by Shumway, was undoubtedly ready and extremely well prepared, as were two or three others. Soon after Chris's first transplant, however, there proved to be many other surgeons with courage, but, without the essential planning and preparation, such courage might uncharitably be interpreted as foolhardy and rash.

There were similarly very few indeed—apart from Chris—who had the conviction to continue a transplant programme after initial failures; Christian Cabrol and his colleagues in Paris can have their names honorably added to those of Shumway of Stanford and Lower of Virginia and their respective associates.

Undoubtedly, Chris had a clear vision of the future. He foresaw the ultimate success of heart transplantation, the great need for such a procedure to try to save those patients whose hearts were irreparably damaged and unsuited to any other form of surgical intervention. Indisputably, Chris was successful in what he undertook.

Although his first patient, Louis Washkansky, died within three weeks of the transplant procedure, the operation was technically successful and convinced many doubters that it could be done; a suitable donor heart could be obtained and maintained in a viable state while being transplanted, and a very sick patient could be brought successfully through those first difficult post-operative days. Furthermore, Mr Washkansky was in severe heart failure at the time of his operation, and the transplant proved conclusively that the new heart would rapidly reverse this condition.

Chris's friend in Minneapolis, John Perry, wrote:

> Christiaan Barnard has had his critics in scientific and lay circles. He did not develop the heart-lung machine. He did not develop the technology to transplant the human heart. He never claimed to have done either, nor has he ever claimed to be more than a hard-working human who enjoyed some of the good and desirable things in life. He was, however, a visionary who was able to put it all together and bring about the first successful transplantation of the human heart.

Denton Cooley stated that 'to describe the event requires the use of adjectives such as stupendous, startling, and electrifying, none of which could be considered excessive.'

Chris's second attempt was a spectacular success, the patient, Philip Blaiberg, becoming the first heart recipient to be discharged from hospital, and the first to lead a substantially normal life after such a procedure, which he continued to do for more than eighteen months. The great potential of heart transplantation had been demonstrated.

As we have seen, four of Chris's first ten patients lived for more than a year, and two lived for more than twelve years, one of whom remained alive for more than twenty-three years—an absolutely remarkable achievement for such a pioneering effort. Almost all other surgical groups abandoned their transplant programs in the face of disastrous experiences. He then went on to introduce heterotopic piggy-back heart transplantation, an innovation with some advantages in that early era. Again, his initial results were remarkable with two of the first five patients living for more than ten years.

Is this achievement, this contribution to medicine, sufficient alone to warrant the acclaim Chris was given, the honours he was awarded, the popularity he achieved, and the acknowledgement he received?

The answer must surely be 'no'. Although his achievement, particularly his courage and vision, must never be underestimated, the first heart transplant was, as Chris readily admitted, just one more step forward in the progress of surgery. It was certainly no greater step forward than the first open heart operation—arguably a much more significant 'giant leap for mankind'—or the first successful kidney transplant, the first liver transplant, or the first lung transplant. Yet, which of us remembers the names of the surgeons who made those contributions? Which of those men, or groups of men and women, received the public attention and the accolades that were bestowed on Chris Barnard? The answer is clearly 'none'.

## Charisma and Celebrity

Let us consider the reasons for Chris's overnight celebrity when he carried out the first heart transplant in 1967. It was not only his major contribution to surgery that made him famous. If he had been a sedate, conservative, inarticulate man, he would have been rapidly forgotten and ignored by both media and public. However, Chris had that nebulous and indefinable quality known as charisma. It was more than good looks, it was more than personality (though he had both of these qualities); it was an appeal, a 'sparkle', that made others want to see him, listen to him, talk to him, and be with him.

I have met many good surgeons who have personality, but few with genuine charisma. In Chris's case, his charisma was made up of several facets that included a youthful and attractive physical appearance, an exciting energy, an excellent sense of humour, an intelligent and decisive mind, verbal articulacy, sexual appeal, an open (often naïve) honesty, and the unashamed expression of emotion—be it happiness, sadness, worry, relief, or grief. Chris Barnard, like the late John F. Kennedy and the young Muhammad Ali, undoubtedly had charisma. Although one or two of the pioneering heart transplant surgeons, such as Norman Shumway and Denton Cooley, had great personalities, none of them matched Chris's charisma.

Let us take a look again at his achievements and talents. Although he is best known to the public for performing the first heart transplant, his contributions to medicine were several. Suffice it to say that even without his work in heart transplantation, his reputation in the relatively small world of heart surgery would have been assured.

Although towards the end of his active career in Cape Town he was much less involved in the day-to-day care of patients than in his younger days, when his untiring attention to them was legendary, he still maintained a considerable interest in the research being conducted in his department's experimental laboratory. He encouraged some of the younger members of his department in their research activities (including me), which carried the field further. Their work was only possible because of the research facilities he had established, and so he deserves some credit for their contributions.

## Distractions and Divorces

Chris's last few years in Cape Town were not personally as productive as those that passed before. The worldly distractions that followed the first few heart transplants—travel, media commitments, social life, business endeavours, writing, and so on—steadily increased, causing him to spend more and more time away from the hospital and his surgical work. He was lured by the high life, perhaps not surprising for someone brought up when the good things in life were so scarce. In addition, he had worked long and very hard in his younger days and had received abundant recognition (if not financial reward) for his labours, and there is no doubt that his early ambition was no longer driving him relentlessly as it had for many previous years. This was a loss to his patients, a loss to his department, a loss to the hospital, and indeed, a loss to surgery as a whole.

It is a source of some regret to many of his friends and admirers that his interest in surgery began to wane at a relatively early stage when his social life and other interests began to expand inordinately. To understand how he allowed these distractions to affect his work, it is necessary to remember the relative deprivation of his childhood, the restrictions imposed upon him for many years by his geographic isolation and his dedication to his profession, and the immense temptations to enjoy the good life to which he was exposed after receiving worldwide recognition. He possibly could have contributed more to surgical science if he had not been distracted, but he had already contributed much.

The attractions of living in luxurious hotels as Chris often did on his travels, and which he admitted almost became an addiction, should not be minimised for someone of his relatively deprived childhood; even the usually critical Marius recognised this point.

Nevertheless, Chris regretted accepting so many invitations to lecture abroad. He travelled too extensively and too frequently, and the work of his own unit suffered accordingly, even though he was ably supported by his brother and several other very competent surgeons during much of that time. He should have handed over the day-to-day leadership of the heart surgery unit to Marius so that there would be more continuity in patient care, but Chris was not prepared to do this—a decision he later regretted.

To summarise his career and his contribution to medicine, let us conclude that for many years, he worked very hard and contributed far more than most doctors to the care of patients and the progress of medical science. As a doctor, his was a life well-spent, though possibly if Chris had stayed focused on it for longer it could have been even better. This opinion is echoed by others.

In 1989, I interviewed Donald Ross for a book I was editing on Chris. As Ross had known him since their medical student days, and followed the same career path as Chris, his opinion is worth repeating.

Up until the time of the transplant, I think he was one of the front-ranking open heart surgeons in the world, with a good knowledge and considerable experience. And he was making important contributions in congenital heart surgery ... He was in the front rank, like Walton Lillehei, Russell Brock, and several other surgeons—innovative, thinking, experimenting, and encouraging people ... His work made heart transplantation a clinical entity. Someone had to have the courage to do it, and he started the whole ball rolling. I believe his was a very important contribution in that respect.

But, afterwards, I think he was taken over by the media. He became a media man and clearly enjoyed himself. I don't blame him in any way. But that was the end of his surgery, as far as I know, and I think the end of a very attractive, magnetic era in Cape Town. He became a very attractive personality, but not a serious surgeon. As far as making further contributions to surgery, I believe he did not use the opportunities that the first transplant gave him. The authorities in Cape Town offered him excellent facilities, and he didn't utilise these as well as he might to produce good research. He made his decision, or it was made for him by the attractions of the media. I don't in any way criticise that. I think all of us have our special interests and desires—you might call them our 'pride'—and we go down the road that we find most suited to us.

Some of his activities, such as getting mixed up with anti-aging creams, have been negative, and have done harm. He has done himself harm in that respect. These activities have had the effect of reducing the value of his original work.

He has a brilliant personality. He has handled all sorts of adulation and anti-Barnard attacks very well indeed. He is a natural media man. He was born before television and the current fashion for public relations, but he was a natural in these areas.

I still think it is a little bit sad from surgery's point of view that he opted out. But otherwise, he is a man who is making his own destiny in society, and that's fine. I have no complaints about that.

Walt Lillehei, Chris's mentor in Minneapolis, always expressed a high regard for him, particularly for his innovation, 'prodigious' memory, 'intensity and seriousness', and courage. Yet he, like Ross, expressed some disappointment.

Judging him from the viewpoint of a former teacher and friend, and as an admirer of his qualities, I would say he accomplished a great deal in enhancing the technical and innovative aspects of surgery up until the transplant, and maybe for a year or two after. Since then he has not done much. But during the period before the first few transplants he did more than most surgeons ever accomplish in a lifetime ... He is very unconventional. For example, he created enemies with his comments on euthanasia. There are many good aspects of euthanasia but also some undesirable ones. It's like arguing about abortion; you're never going to convince everyone. Either you believe in it or you don't. But his high profile with regard to that cosmetic cream and, of course, the image of the playboy which he developed, I suppose detracted significantly from his medical image, particularly in the rather staid circles of the higher echelon of medical opinion-makers. I think the public enjoyed some aspects of his playboy image. I think he had a good time.

Looking over Chris's career, I would say that it's been a very successful one. He has lived well, has laughed a good deal, is loved much, and, most important, he has left the world a better place than it was when he arrived.

Sir Brian Barratt-Boyes perhaps went a step further by stating that he felt that in Chris's later life, he was no longer considered a member of the international fraternity of leading surgeons. Barratt-Boyes remembers that it was 'a pity that he spoiled it all with his later life, because he was virtually ostracised [from the surgical world]. The situation was a bit like that of Lillehei, who was ostracised at one stage, and then readmitted. But I don't think Chris was ever really readmitted to the clan.'

I would comment that I honestly do not think this bothered Chris very much. He had moved on from the world of surgery, and no longer needed—or desired—to be a member of 'the clan.'

Although it was his medical achievements and media appearances, and to a lesser extent his literary contributions, that brought him fame and renown, it was aspects of his private life and his forays into the world of business and advertising that made him a controversial figure, and to some extent tarnished his image as the brilliant surgeon.

He married three times, all ending in divorce. Many eminent and successful men have been married more than once; few people know, and few care. Perhaps the fact that the age gap steadily increased between Chris and his respective wives was a factor in drawing attention and comment, and even some criticism. 'Louwtjie married me because she loved me,' he wrote. 'My second wife married me because of my fame, and my third because of my fame and money. But I have no regrets.'

Although many thought that Chris's relationship with his second wife, Barbara, was the great love story of his life, one only has to read the memoirs of his daughter, Deirdre, to realise that this did not match the unconditional and undying love she had for her father throughout his life. The intense love of a daughter for her father is not uncommon; indeed, my own wife's love for her late father has been perhaps the greatest influence of her life.

Chris's attraction to beautiful young women and their attraction to him ensured that the paparrazi followed him avidly, and that his photograph appeared frequently in the world's periodicals and magazines. Stories and photographs published of him with beautiful women led to problems with his first marriage and its eventual break-up, partly through the publicity he received when in the company of other women, often famous women, usually beautiful women. On some occasions, he was a victim of his own innocence; on others, he probably was not. He frequently pointed out that if any normal healthy man, married or unmarried, were approached at a party and asked whether he would like to meet a beautiful film star, such as Gina Lollobrigida or Sophia Loren at that time, or some other beauty whom he had admired from afar, few would say 'no'. Most, if not all of us, would be delighted, even thrilled to meet the lady in question, and so was Chris. If we were then asked whether we would mind having our photograph taken with her, again, why would we refuse? Therefore, when that photograph appeared in a South African newspaper a few days later, was it fair for his wife to rage at him on his return? The answer is, of course, 'no', but possibly sometimes 'yes'.

Chris was fully aware how his courage to take that first surgical step had impacted his subsequent life.

> The operation, and its significance as the first of its kind, took me into another world. Not just professionally but personally and socially. I loved it. I'm a guy who loves people, I love the female sex and I like to enjoy life. You think I was under stress meeting with Gina Lollobrigida? Not on your life. I'm easy to get on with, to party with.

Chris's inability to rein in his sexual urges contributed to the failure of at least two of his marriages. Indeed, throughout life (even into old age), his activities had something of the Don Juan or Casanova image about them; the thrill of seduction was clearly important to him, at times a paramount, almost addictive, need. His second marriage failed at least in part because of his romantic indiscretions and deceptions. The failure of his third marriage was certainly the most unpleasant (from his perspective) of all.

He confided in me once that he had some doubts and misgivings when he married for the first and second times. On the first occasion, he was influenced partly by a sense of duty; he had been dating the same young lady (Louwtjie) for a couple of years, and felt morally committed to marriage. On the second occasion, he realised his lifestyle of incessant travelling and socialising was not to the liking of his nineteen-year-old fiancée (Barbara), and feared that the future would not be without incident. But whether these were genuine considerations that went through his mind before each marriage took place, or whether they had been seen only with the help of hindsight, probably even Chris Barnard was never sure.

## Abilities and Aptitudes

Chris Barnard was more than a doctor, more than a surgeon. He had many other talents, some of which have been underestimated, and many other facets to his personality, character, and life. He was a quite outstanding public speaker to both lay and medical audiences, and the range of topic on which he could speak was remarkable—far wider than the average surgeon. Over the years, he contributed a wealth of writings: medical and scientific papers, books on health for the layman, on the controversial subject of euthanasia, on the political situation in South Africa, newspaper articles, and even novels. To some extent, he used others to put his ideas and thoughts into words—Curtis Bill Pepper on his autobiography, Siegfried Stander to collaborate on his novels, Bob Molloy on the newspaper articles that appeared weekly in the *Cape Times,* and several surgical colleagues to write the scientific papers that emanated from his department. As a result of such collaboration, his talents as a writer are less easy to delineate than they might have been. Nevertheless, the subject matter and message of most of his writings came from him, not his collaborators. He wrote enough himself to demonstrate a genuine facility in this respect

A review of his several forays into the world of the printed page reveals the broad range of his interests. No fewer than half of his fourteen books were on matters of health and were aimed at the general public. There were four novels and, in addition to his two autobiographical texts, there was one book each in such fields as political commentary and ethics. Only one book was what might be called 'academic' and was aimed directly at specialists within the medical profession. This is perhaps surprising for one who made such major contributions to his field of expertise, and certainly reflects the degree to which other interests distracted him from surgery when he became a public figure. Another book aimed at the profession (the report of the heart transplant congress held in Cape Town in 1968) was instigated by Chris, but was actually edited by a colleague.

## Plusses and Minuses

At the end of anyone's life, we can look back and assess the positives (the contributions and successes) and the negatives (the lack of contributions and the failures) of that life. In other words, we can compare the plusses with the minuses. For Chris, the plusses included his contributions to medicine, the excellent care he gave to thousands of patients in need of heart surgery, his charitable work and philanthropy, the help his books gave to people suffering from heart disease or arthritis, and perhaps his positive contributions to the debate over apartheid.

The minuses are mainly related to his self-centredness (or selfishness) and included failing to provide his close family with the support they might have expected from him, such as his failure to visit either of his parents in their declining years; his infidelities; his lack of guidance and support for his oldest son, André; and his abandonment as a coach to his daughter, Deirdre, at a critical stage of her life. His decision not to remain at Barbara's bedside when she was dying because he could not resist a new overseas adventure is a minus that particularly surprises me as he was generally considered a very loyal friend. Chris's self-centredness was also seen in the extreme demands he made on his junior staff and in the priority he gave to the care of his own patients rather than those of his junior colleagues (although this is perhaps understandable and is not uncommon in medicine). His lack of judgment with regard to certain business ventures, in particular that relating to the marketing of Glycel, might also be considered a minus, though they did contribute very significantly to his financial well-being.

It is certainly not unknown for an ambitious man driven by a mission or major interest in life to spend less time with his family than perhaps he should. I well remember an acquaintance in Cambridge in the UK whose father had not only been a leading London surgeon but also a published authority on several writers of distinction in the world of literature. When I asked him how his father had found time for both his surgical career and his many literary contributions, with some bitternes in his voice he replied, 'by totally neglecting his children.'

In Chris's case, to society, the positives clearly outweighed the negatives. To individual members of his family and some of his professional associates, however, the negatives may have gained the upper hand. But overall, his life was one from which many, many sick people benefitted, either directly from his hands or indirectly from the lead he set for others. Some contemporaries found it difficult to distinguish Chris's good points from his bad. For example, the distinguished cardiac surgeon, John Kirklin, who pioneered open heart surgery in the mid-1950s at the Mayo Clinic, wrote, 'So Chris Barnard to me has always been as enigmatic as the human race itself. He is an accomplished, brilliant and lovable individual, who nevertheless seems often to be to a certain extent disappointing to himself and to those who value his friendship.'

## A Zest for Life: *Joie de Vivre*

We cannot summarise Chris Barnard very easily as he was a multifaceted character. He worked immensely hard, at least for the first fifty to sixty years of his life, but he played just as hard. He had been a surgeon, researcher, public speaker, author, novelist, journalist, restaurateur, farmer, rancher, husband, lover, father, traveller, and celebrity.

At the time of the first heart transplant, Bob Molloy wrote:

This was Barnard the winner, the one who laughed and loved the world. Barnard the softie. Barnard of the big heart and the warm smile. From that moment I became a Barnard-watcher and found that, behind the public face, there were many more Barnards. There was the cheeky kid who loved giving the finger to authority. The gentle doctor and soft touch for children. The scientist driven by a white-hot desire to achieve. The womaniser who needed good-looking females around him. The party-goer who loved the bright lights. The debater, after-dinner speaker, raconteur, media star—all powered by a razor-sharp mind that sliced through opposition and blazed ideas like a firework throwing off sparks. And in there somewhere the black despair, a kind of bottomless pit into which he descended on days when he lost hope of beating the arthritis which was seizing up his fingers and would one day bring an end to his career as a working surgeon.

I would remind you of the words of Bob Frater that I included in the introduction to this book. He wrote that Barnard 'was then, at once, rough-at-the-edges poor boy and charming sophisticate, democrat and tyrant, selfless healer and boorish egotist, lover and Don Juan, shrewd parvenu and naive acceptor of glitterati adulation—but, above all, surgical visionary and simply the most unforgettable character of the second generation of cardiac surgeons.'

These words draw attention to Chris's frailties (tyrant, egotist, and Don Juan) as much as to his strengths (democrat, healer, and visionary). There is no escaping Chris's faults, but to some extent, he was able to channel his self-centred and self-interested ambition to use his skills and compassion for the benefit of others.

To me, Frater's words most aptly sum up the Chris Barnard I knew: multi-talented, courageous, charismatic, and yet at times contradictory. He was an unforgettable blend of vision, intelligence, action, charm, warmth, and humour, tempered by human weaknesses. He exuded an intensity in, and an enthusiasm for, so many aspects of life—a true *joie de vivre*, a zest for life, despite suffering almost constant pain—until the last year or two of his life when his optimistic outlook was subdued. My experiences with him were numerous and varied, and remain indelibly imprinted in my mind, and I know this to be so for many of his former associates and friends.

Daughter Deirdre summed up my thoughts also.

When my father died that essence that made him the man he was died too. There are no letters, diaries or stories recounted that can even begin to capture the tiniest part of all those energies that surge together and make a human being quite unique and different from their fellows. That is what the sadness of death is really all about. That unique spark is gone and the fragile essence that makes up the person can never be recounted or recaptured no matter how hard we try. That is the pity of it.

She prefaced these comments by stating, 'There's something infinitely sad about this.' There is indeed. An indelible character has been lost to us.

When with Chris in Oklahoma, I learned of a Native American proverb that says, 'A man is not dead until the last person who remembers him dies.' If this is so, Chris Barnard will certainly be alive for many, many years.

I once asked him to write some words in my copy of his autobiography, *One Life.* He inscribed the phrase, 'One life is enough, if well lived.' Even with his very human faults and frailities, this is surely his own epitaph.

# Today:
# Progress in Alternative Forms of
# Heart Replacement

Heart transplantation was only the first step in surgeons' efforts to replace a failing heart. Subsequent approaches have centred largely on mechanical devices but, more recently, replacement by an animal heart is increasingly becoming likely.

## Mechanical Devices

The development and implantation of mechanical devices—ventricular assist devices and total artificial hearts—was the second step forward. Will they one day completely replace heart transplantation as the treatment of choice for patients with terminal heart failure? The answer is still uncertain but, in my opinion, this is unlikely. I believe a natural (biological) heart will always have an advantage over devices of man-made materials. One great advantage of a mechanical device, of course, is that there could be a limitless number of them. Unlike those waiting for a human donor heart, everybody who needs heart replacement or support could be treated.

The total artificial heart (TAH) and its close cousin, the ventricular assist device (VAD), have captured the public's imagination as being close to science fiction. In some ways, they represent the ultimate in the bioprosthetic man. Although their design and performance have improved markedly in recent years, they are still some way from becoming a routine replacement of a natural or biological heart. Chris Barnard also believed this. For this reason, my major research interest for the past thirty years has been cross-species transplantation (xenotransplantation).

Although both mechanical and biological hearts have advantages and disadvantages, he suggested that life would be much more limited if it depended on a mechanical device. With a well-functioning animal heart in his chest, a patient could go fishing as readily as any other person. With a mechanical heart, which was dependent on an outside source of energy (provided to the implanted device from an electric plug or batteries through a wire that entered the patient's body), doing something as simple as going fishing was much more difficult, if nigh impossible.

More than 10,000 patients have received some form of mechanical support of their hearts worldwide during the past decade. VADs that augment, rather than totally replace, the patient's heart are being implanted in increasing numbers and have achieved good reliability, many now functioning well for at least a year or two, and a few for considerably longer. Progress in the development of the TAH has been more variable, and a reliable mechanical device that can permanently replace the native heart without complications remains the goal of the future.

Dutchman, Willem Kolff, the creator and developer of the artificial kidney, was also the major pioneer in the field of mechanical hearts. However, it was the well-known surgeon, Michael DeBakey (Figure 15.iii), who, through his connections and influence in Washington, D.C., did much to ensure funding for this expensive area of bioengineering and surgical research. DeBakey influenced health care in the US through his friendship with Lyndon Johnson, who passed more health-related legislation, including Medicare, than any other US President.

DeBakey was the first surgeon to implant a VAD into a patient. (With this device, the heart is left in place, but the device augments its output of blood. The original VADs were large and cumbersome, but they have steadily become smaller, easier to insert in the patient, and increasingly efficient. When I met with Dr DeBakey in 1990, he told me:

> In 1966, I had proved with a clinical case for the first time that this concept was good. We had this girl who we couldn't wean off the heart-lung machine [after a 'routine' heart operation). After ten days of pumping [with an LVAD], we finally weaned her off and she recovered [i.e. her heart began beating strongly again and the LVAD could be removed]. [This was an operation Marius Barnard had witnessed while training in vascular surgery with DeBakey and Cooley in Houston.] She lived for six years and led a normal life in every way until she was killed tragically in an automobile accident.

The first implantation of a TAH was also in Houston in 1969, an event of great controversy that led to the permanent disruption of the hitherto productive collaboration between DeBakey and his junior colleague, the equally famous, Denton Cooley (Figure 14.i). This operation was planned as a 'bridge' to heart transplantation; the device was implanted with the aim of maintaining the patient's life until a human heart became available for transplantation, rather than as a permanent replacement of the native heart.

It was another thirteen years before attempts were made to permanently replace a patient's diseased and failing heart with an artificial device by Utah surgeon, William DeVries (Figure A1.i), with no plan to transplant a heart from a deceased human when one became available.

All of these initial operations in both Houston and Salt Lake City hit the headlines, and generated as much public interest as had Barnard's, Kantrowitz's, and Shumway's heart transplants a few years earlier. However, none of the key players had quite the boyish good looks or charisma as Chris Barnard, though some came close. Furthermore, none was as attracted to the celebrity circuit as Chris, and so did not become so well-known worldwide or remain in the limelight so long. Unlike Chris, their public fame was more transient and thereafter largely restricted to those within the medical profession.

As in every field of surgical endeavour, many have played major roles in the mechanical heart story, but here we shall concentrate attention on the two teams in Salt Lake City and Houston, in part because of their pioneering contributions and in part because of the personalities involved. The exciting pioneering efforts and the personalities of the surgeons involved have been fully described in my previous book, *Open Heart*.

## Willem Kolff

There are good reasons why Willem Kolff (Figure A1.ii) should be included in this chapter, even though he was never a heart surgeon, nor even a cardiologist. He was one of the most remarkable medical inventors of the twentieth century. He is most remembered for his development of the first truly functional dialysis machine, which remarkably he carried out in the Nazi-occupied Netherlands during World War Two. Observations he made at that time led him to develop a membrane oxygenator, a new type of oxygenator (that introduced oxygen into the blood and removed carbon dioxide), which would eventually be incorporated into standard heart-lung machines.

Kolff started work on the TAH in Cleveland in the USA in the spring of 1957. Ten years later, he moved his laboratory to the University of Utah in Salt Lake City. The basis of the TAH that Kolff and his colleagues designed and tested was a two-chambered structure that replaced the patient's ventricles (the pumping chambers of the heart) and that was sutured in place through connections with the two atria and the aorta and pulmonary artery (see Figure 4.i). Within each 'ventricle' was a polyurethane diaphragm, which was moved by air pressure pumped in and out from an external pneumatic pump through 'drivelines'. When air pushed the membrane upwards, the blood was ejected. When the membrane relaxed, the 'ventricles' filled with blood. The four artificial valves ensured that the blood only travelled in the correct direction. The drivelines could be connected to a portable power source at times to allow the patient some degree of mobility.

Well before the Kolff/Jarvik TAH was implanted into the first patient by DeVries, Denton Cooley took his controversial leap forward in 1969 by implanting a TAH that had largely been designed by his senior colleague, Michael DeBakey.

## Michael DeBakey: the 'Texas Tornado' or 'Black Mike'

DeBakey was a workaholic (hence the moniker, 'Texas Tornado') and a very difficult man to work with (hence 'Black Mike').

Like Kolff, DeBakey 'became interested in the artificial heart as an extension of the heart-lung machine.' He told me:

As we developed more experience with the heart-lung machine, my feeling was that there were high-risk patients who would only be able to be weaned from the machine if we could continue using it for, say, several hours. My reasoning was that, if you could support them for a longer period of time, perhaps the heart might recover. We began doing some laboratory work, and reviewed what had been done in the past, particularly the work by Kolff.

I commented to Dr DeBakey that there had been a big controversy when the first TAH was implanted in Houston in 1969. He agreed, and explained that, after several years of research, he did not feel the mechanical heart was ready to be tested in patients 'because we couldn't get survival in our animals for more than a few months. They all died.'

Yet his colleague, Denton Cooley, and one of DeBakey's research fellows felt otherwise. So, when DeBakey was out of town, the TAH was taken to Cooley, who was about to operate on a patient with a very sick heart. In Cooley's opinion, the heart would not recover from the operation, and so he removed it and implanted the TAH. Three days later, the device was replaced by a human donor heart, but this failed and the patient died.

DeBakey was naturally shocked and infuriated. He set up a committee to investigate the matter. The committee prepared a report in which they said it was a violation of ethics and was not standard procedure. Cooley had to resign from DeBakey's department. This controversy destroyed Cooley's relationship with DeBakey.

Returning to my interview with Dr DeBakey, I asked him about his subsequent work on the TAH.

'More and more, I became disillusioned about the total artificial heart and, in 1973, I stopped working on it. I became more interested in some kind of cardiac assistance—the left ventricular assist device [LVAD].'

## Denton Cooley: 'Dr Wonderful'

The surgically gifted and genial Denton Cooley (hence 'Dr Wonderful') was the other player in the first implantation of a TAH. He was one of the best known of the early cardiac surgeons, both within the medical profession and by the public. He epitomises the public's perception of the successful surgeon—or, at least, the media's perception—being tall and good looking, having a relaxed and charming manner, and a natural and exquisite gift for surgical dexterity. He became immensely wealthy through his surgical work and subsequent investments in his hometown of Houston, only to overextend himself financially during the period of the oil boom in the early 1980s, and see his business interests collapse when the boom dissolved. At one point, when he filed for bankruptcy, it was reported that his investment company owed $100 million. Remarkably, he recovered from this dramatic setback and my understanding is that he eventually paid off his debts.

Once open heart surgery had been introduced and established by such luminaries as Lillehei and Kirklin, Cooley rapidly became the busiest surgeon in this field, performing more surgical procedures than any other surgeon in the world. At one time, according to John Norman, a former colleague of Cooley, fully one-tenth of the open heart surgery in the US was being carried out by Cooley's group at the Texas Heart Institute in Houston.

On one occasion, when I met with Dr Cooley, I raised the topic of the controversial use of the first TAH. He responded:

It was evident to me that it was time to try the total artificial heart. We were having a number of frustrations in watching people die who could have been saved with a heart transplant ... Dr DeBakey was apparently not interested in going forward with its clinical application ... So I decided that the time had come to take a bold step. The opportunity arose to go ahead and do it, and suffer any repercussions that might follow. We did just that.

We had the ideal candidate who was dying and needed a cardiac transplant. We were just interested in seeing if you could sustain a human life with an artificial device. Sure enough, that proved to be the case. The patient did very well with the total artificial heart, but unfortunately he died following his transplant because of an infection. I have no regrets at all for having taken that step.

Although Cooley mentioned that the patient did well after insertion of the TAH, this is somewhat debatable. The device certainly maintained his life, but there were significant early complications. Norman Shumway was not so sure the TAH had been a success. He told me that 'this was the first time in medical history that a patient had a heart replacement done from one dead person to another. The patient was dead when they did it. By the time they got the heart transplant going, he was brain-dead.' Whether this is correct or not, I am uncertain, but the patient died less than two days after the heart transplant.

Of all the pioneers in heart surgery, Chris Barnard probably had his best relationship with Cooley, with the possible exceptions of his mentor, Walt Lillehei, and his medical school classmate, Donald Ross. Both Cooley and Barnard had excellent senses of humour and clearly enjoyed each other's company. His regard for Cooley as a surgeon is perhaps illustrated by his recommending his brother, Marius, should spend time training with Cooley.

While in Minneapolis, Chris had travelled to Houston to watch Cooley operate.

It was the most beautiful surgery I had ever seen in my life. No one in the world, I knew, could equal it. Dr Cooley's skill was matched by his grace and kindness toward me. He invited me into the theatre [operating room], showed me everything, and politely answered all questions. Dr DeBakey was more difficult to approach. When I finally obtained permission to watch him at work, he treated it as an intrusion and even shouted at me for being too close to the table. I thus learned little from him.

Marius came to the same conclusion. He was not impressed with DeBakey's surgery and he did not like him personally. 'If I'd thought Jannie Louw and Chris were difficult to work with,' he wrote, 'DeBakey was worse.'

## William DeVries

William DeVries was the surgeon who carried out the first real clinical trial using the TAH made by Kolff and and his junior colleague, Robert Jarvik.

Kolff and DeVries immediately hit it off because of their mutual Dutch heritage. They decided it was time to go ahead with the implantation of one of their mechanical hearts in a patient.

As a medical student in Utah, DeVries helped Kolff's group with their experiments. After a long surgical residency at Duke University, DeVries was appointed to the surgical staff in Utah. His practice there took some time to grow and, rather like Shumway, he found he had a lot of spare time on his hands. By this time, the animals [calves] with implanted TAHs were living for six or more months. He felt he had a mission to bring this technology into the clinic to benefit patients.

> I've had a lot of 'Come to Jesus' meetings about that, you know. I really was an evangelist. If you were to ask me what my part in this whole thing was, I was the one who really pushed it. The reason I pushed it was that I believed in it ... People were dying, and there was a way of doing it [helping them] ... There was a great need for it ... The more I got involved in it, the more of an evangelist I became.

## The First Patient: Barney Clark

It took Devries, Kolff, and Jarvik some further animal experimentation to be in a position to consider a clinical trial. Barney Clark, the first patient, was a dentist (like Philip Blaiberg, the second of Chris's patients). The implantation took place on 1 December 1982, fifteen years almost to the day after the operation on Louis Washkansky. The immediate media attention was comparable to that which Chris Barnard had received. Devries, who was a tall, good-looking thirty-eight-year-old, reflected on his situation at that time. He faced many of the same problems as had Chris.

> Suddenly, here I was like Christiaan Barnard. All of a sudden, I was debating Norm Shumway, Denton Cooley, DeBakey, and all of these guys. It was crazy. It was absolutely crazy. But I knew more about it than anybody else in the world at that time. That was an interesting time.
>
> We had the entire world breathing down our necks. These media guys were coming out of the woodwork and criticising. I was a little too sensitive about it those first few days, and I had to learn how to be thick-skinned. I realised that the best thing for me to do was not to read the newspapers, because I got hurt by what I read. It really hurt me what people were saying.
>
> There were an incredible number of mistakes made, but that's not unusual for a first try. Also, the media circus that was going on was

unbelievable. One-half of the students' cafeteria at University Hospital was cordoned off for television crews and reporters. If, in the middle of the night, I wanted to know how Barney Clark was doing, I called a reporter. The vice-president [vice-chancellor] of the university gave a news conference twice a day.

Shumway was really critical of it, and was really bad-mouthing me. I always asked myself the question, 'How can a guy who has changed the surgical world by his freedom and aggression be against this technology? Why do people like that fight against technology later in their life with the same strength that they fought for technology when they were younger?'

... [After a few weeks,] Barney Clark was just toughing it out ... At one stage he became discouraged with his progress. He realised he was in this thing and there was no way out, except to die. I continued in my mind thinking that this is an experiment, but the centre part of this whole thing is this patient. I wanted him to live ... Then we started getting into the issue of money. We hadn't charged the hospital, so how were we going to pay for this? Medical insurance can't pay for it. 'Barney, you're going to have to pay for it', which was crazy. The guy had to pay for an experiment on himself? Then he sold the rights [to his life story] for a million dollars to a newspaper, which meant that they had access to all of his [medical] charts. It got to be real bizarre.

About the same time, I started getting all kinds of legal things. The Attorney General's office started asking questions. 'How do you turn the patient's artificial heart off?' 'Who has the right to be assisted in suicide?' Am I a murderer? Things like that came up. The State of Utah was a very conservative state, and I realised the implications of this. Those were really hard issues. Am I prolonging death or prolonging misery, or am I accomplishing something? Those were the issues I dealt with daily.

Barney Clark died after 112 days. Kolff liked to quote what Chris Barnard said at the time. 'Barney Clark, the first patient with a total artificial heart, lived for one-hundred-twelve days. That's a lot longer than my first patient with a transplanted heart, who lived for only eighteen days.'

While trying to raise money to carry out a second artificial heart implantation, a hospital company, Humana, offered to fund the next hundred implants if DeVries moved to their hospital in Louisville in Kentucky. He decided to accept this offer and went on to carry out three more implants.

The first day after we did Bill Schroeder [the second patient], Wendell Cherry [the Humana CEO] said, 'Our name is now in every single newspaper in the world. This is the type of advertisement that you cannot buy. As far as I'm concerned, you've made your money for the next one hundred patients.' I realised what this was all about, but it was okay because it was for advancement.

Over a period of about two years, we consistently had one or two patients with an artificial heart the whole time. Mr Schroeder lived almost two years with the artificial heart [reminiscent of Dr Blaiberg]. And then we did Murray Haden, and he lived about a year and one-half. We did Jack Burton, who lived only ten days. He was too small, and it was difficult. It took me about two weeks of really pretty intense time to decide the best thing would be to turn the pump off, because it wasn't going to work. That's the first patient I turned off. It was prolonging his death. Then Mr Schroeder had a 'stroke' [a brain injury due to a clot of blood from the artificial heart]. That was the first time we had had a stroke. Then the pendulum for good, positive things was starting to turn back, and Humana started getting a little bit edgy about it; they didn't particularly like it.

By this time, one-hundred-one of these artificial hearts had been implanted all over the world, all as bridges to transplants, except for those I had done. The enthusiasm was exactly the same as it had been for heart transplants. The numbers rapidly went up, and then, as the strokes started occurring, the numbers went back down to about twenty to forty per year. Humana basically backed out. It was all money. When it costs more than it's worth, then you stop. That's basically what happened.

DeVries decided he had done enough and it was time to abandon his mission and return to routine heart surgery. His recollections of living in the public eye during this period, however, are of great relevance to those experienced by Chris Barnard.

## The Public Eye: the Price You Pay

It changed my life. I ended up flying all over the world—exactly the same scenario as Christiaan Barnard did. All of a sudden, here I am with President Reagan and King Hussain. You're on television. You realise that this is more than you did back in Utah. Your life is fast; it was just going, going, going. You get into that type of fast behaviour. You live in pretty heady air too. You go home, for example, and you've got Bryant Gumbel or Katie Couric wanting to come and talk with you. They want a piece of you. They want you to fly to Washington. You're doing this and this and this, and going back and forth. First of all, it takes time, and you have to be mentally sharp. I knew that all I needed to do was to crash out on something like this, and it would stop. So personally, you have to be attuned and ready to go. You can't come in unsharp. I realised that people would use me. I also realised I couldn't satisfy everybody. You get to a point where you can only go so far, and then it's time for you to stop.

I enjoyed it [being a celebrity], but got tired of it. It's initially highly attractive. It becomes unreal. You realise this. The next step is you ask, 'What do these people want from me? Are they wanting to use me? Does somebody want me for this or for that? I can live my life like this, but where's the end of it? Where's it going?' Philosophically, you're going to be that way until you're not useful to them anymore. Then you finally come to the realization of what you want out of life, what you need, and where you're going with it all. Those are the self-examinations you come to. I came to the realization that I couldn't please everybody. That was a very difficult thing to learn.

The other thing that was difficult was that, in the particular world and environment I was in, it was not appropriate to be a media doctor. You can lose the thing that is most important to you, and that is the respect of your colleagues. The media will say, 'You're famous,' but a lot of times it takes more out of you than it gives you back. These people will come out and suck the life out of you, and then they're gone back to New York, and you're back with the people here [in Utah or Kentucky]. I felt that my colleagues, the guys who were sending me my patients, were not happy with the fact that I was on television all the time. They made fun of people like that. That was before professional advertising came in. You can offend a lot of doctors, and they will cut you off.

The other thing is choices. I grew up in a very religious family. I never smoked a cigarette. I never drank alcohol. You have your first glass of champagne in a crystal glass, with all these exciting people. A normal person who's never been in that situation doesn't understand. All of a sudden you're meeting people who are exciting, whether they are men or women, and they're drawn to you and you're drawn to them. You have choices you never had before. Christiaan Barnard mentioned that to me. It eats you. It can totally consume you. In that type of environment, you can't survive. Going home at night, you are dead-ass tired, and you get up the next morning to keep your practice going. They're not paying for you to do this.

My mother didn't like it. My wife didn't like it either. I had six kids at the time ... My marriage had always been shaky. In Louisville, it lasted about two years, and dissolved. My mother wasn't happy with that as she was a good strong Mormon. She was very upset about that. I got married again about three years later, and it's been really good. But it has affected my children. It's taken awhile to get my relationships back with them, because I was never there.

When I was on the cover of Time magazine, I went out and bought a copy of the magazine for each of my kids. About six months later, I was in my daughter's room and she had ripped out the page and put on crayon marks; I had horns out of my head and a beard. She had made disparaging remarks on it. She would have been about thirteen or fourteen at the time. When I saw that, I realised, 'Hey, this is not without a price.'

These reminiscences could almost as readily be written by Chris, and there is no doubt that he also paid a price.

## The Other Alternative: The Transplantation of Animal Hearts

Today, there are several approaches being explored to provide alternative sources of organs for the purposes of transplantation. These include the development of organs from stem cells, which are very primitive cells with the ability to differentiate into many different types of cell, and by what has become known as 'regeneration' technology, where a suboptimal human or pig organ is stripped of its cells and seeded with healthy human cells, possibly from the intended recipient of the 'regenerated' organ. Neither of these techniques, however, has yet advanced to the point where it can be tested in human patients. Xenotransplantation (the transplantation of an animal heart) is much closer to clinical trials.

We have seen how the transplantation of an animal organ was attempted by James Hardy (who transplanted a chimpanzee heart), Donald Ross (pig heart), Denton Cooley (sheep heart), and by Chris and his colleagues (baboon and chimpanzee hearts), and finally by Len Bailey (baboon heart)—all rather unsuccessfully.

This field of research effectively began with the transplantation of chimpanzee kidneys into patients in the early 1960s by Keith Reemtsma, a surgeon then at Tulane University in Louisiana. Remarkably, one of his six patients, all of whom were in terminal kidney failure, returned to work as a schoolteacher before dying relatively suddenly nine months after the transplant (from what was believed to be an infection or an electrolyte disturbance, but not from rejection). This outcome was perhaps surprising when the immunosuppressive drugs available then were so limited and relatively weak. The other patients, unfortunately, died from rejection of the graft or infection within the first couple of months after transplantation.

Tom Starzl, who transplanted baboon kidneys, and several other surgeons in the 1960s, who transplanted monkey kidneys, reported similar results to those of Reemtsma, and so cross-species organ transplantation was largely abandoned as a clinically useful therapy.

More recently, for a number of good reasons, attention has been directed to the pig as a potential source of organs for humans. As Donald Ross found, a pig organ is rejected vary rapidly (within minutes, so-called hyperacute rejection) when transplanted into a human or nonhuman primate, but this problem has been overcome by genetic-engineering of the pig—the first time it has become possible to modify the donor rather than just treat the recipient of an organ transplant.

For those concerned about the use of pigs as sources of life-saving organs for transplantation, it could be pointed out that in the USA alone approximately 100 million pigs are used each year as a source of food. In China, 500 million pigs are killed each year to provide the natural anticoagulant drug, heparin. Worldwide, we have been implanting pig heart valves into patients with diseased valves for more than fifty years. These valves are treated with a chemical and therefore are rejected very slowly over years, but this is not possible if the organ has to remain truly alive and functioning.

Pigs with multiple (up to six) genetic manipulations are now available to us and auxiliary hearts (those that beat but do not support the blood circulation) from these pigs—together with the administration of new immunosuppressive drugs to the recipient—have functioned for more than two years in baboons. This is still not good enough to consider transplanting pig organs into humans, but it represents a great advance on the few minutes of graft survival that occurred thirty years ago. Indeed, progress has accelerated recently to the extent that researchers are beginning to plan the first clinical trials of testing pig organ transplants in patients for whom it is impossible to obtain an organ from a deceased human donor. Xenotransplantation, therefore, may be the future of heart transplantation, and, importantly, of the transplantation of all other organs.

When I first arrived in Cape Town in February 1980, I suggested to Professor Barnard that we begin some systematic research into the transplantation of organs between animals of different species, so that we could eventually carry out transplantation between animals (for example, pigs) and humans. He clearly thought my suggestion was premature. He said, 'We have enough trouble preventing rejection between man and man, let's not start thinking of transplanting animal hearts.' His scepticism regarding the likely success of such a research programme was in part due to his personal experience in xenotransplantation (involving the transplantation of baboon and chimpanzee hearts) that has been outlined elsewhere in this book. The failure of both of these animal hearts had clearly made a deep impression on him, and so my suggestion regarding a research project was shelved.

His negative attitude to the use of animal hearts in 1980 was perhaps surprising in view of opinions that he had expressed as early as 1968. In Peter Hawthorne's book, *The Transplanted Heart*, published in that year, Chris is quoted as saying that 'in twenty years or so, there would be 'spare-part farms' of specially bred animals to provide hearts, kidneys and livers for transplantation.' This vision of the future, expressed almost fifty years ago, has not yet become a reality, although it is becoming ever closer with the use of genetically engineered pigs.

If we had begun such a research programme in 1980, we might today be that little bit closer to solving the problems of xenotransplantation. However, many research endeavours have floundered because they were ahead of their time; the facilities, techniques, and background knowledge that might enable real progress to be made were just not available at the time, and the studies drew a blank. This field of research, however, remained in the back of my mind, and a year or two later, I initiated such a research programme in Cape Town.

New ethical questions will need to be answered. For example, in view of the greatly improving results obtained after the implantation of a VAD, is it ethical to transplant a pig heart? There are, however, some patients in whom, for anatomical or size reasons, a VAD cannot be implanted. In these patients, the choice for the patient may therefore be between a pig heart and a TAH, where the long-term results will not be so good. The transplantation of pig organs may well be the future of heart transplantation, and, I predict, a reality within the next few years.

# Chris Barnard: Biographical Outline, Degrees, Awards, and Honours

1922 8 November: born in Beaufort West, Cape Province, South Africa.

1940 Matriculated (first class) at Beaufort West High School.

1946 Qualified with the degrees Bachelor of Medicine and Bachelor of Surgery (MB, ChB) at the University of Cape Town.

1946–48 House appointments (internships) at Groote Schuur Hospital, Cape Town.

1948 Married Aletta (Louwtjie) Louw (two children: Deirdre and André).

1948–51 Family physician in Ceres, Cape Province.

1951–53 Senior resident medical officer, City Hospital, Cape Town, and registrar (resident), Department of Medicine (Prof. J. F. Brock), Groote Schuur Hospital, Cape Town.

1953 Took the degree of Master of Medicine (MMed) at the University of Cape Town.

1953 Awarded the degree of Doctor of Medicine (MD) by the University of Cape Town for a dissertation entitled 'The Treatment of Tuberculous Meningitis'.

1953 Registrar (resident) in the Department of Surgery (Prof. J. Erasmus), Groote Schuur Hospital, Cape Town.

1956 Received the Charles Adams Memorial Scholarship and a Dazian Foundation Bursary for two years' study in the USA.

1956–58 Training in cardiothoracic surgery in the Department of Surgery (Prof. O. H. Wangensteen, Dr C. W. Lillehei and Dr R. L. Varco), University of Minnesota, Minneapolis, Minnesota, USA.

1958 Awarded the degree of Master of Science in Surgery (MS) at the University of Minnesota for a thesis entitled 'The Aortic Valve: Problems in the Fabrication and Testing of a Prosthetic Valve'.

1958    Awarded the degree of Doctor of Philosophy (PhD) at the University of Minnesota for a dissertation entitled 'The Aetiology of Congenital Intestinal Atresia'.

1958    Awarded a United States public health grant for further research in the field of cardiac surgery.

1958    Returned to Groote Schuur Hospital, Cape Town, as a specialist in cardiothoracic surgery and full-time lecturer and Director of Surgical Research in the Department of Surgery at the University of Cape Town under Professor J. H. Louw.

1960    Received a bursary from the Oppenheimer Memorial Trust for overseas study.

1961    Appointed Head of the Department of Cardiothoracic Surgery at the teaching hospitals of the University of Cape Town.

1962    Promoted to Associate Professor, Department of Surgery, University of Cape Town.

1967    3 December: led the surgical team that performed the world's first human-to-human heart transplant

1967    Awarded the honorary degree of Doctor of Science (DSc honoris causa) of the University of Cape Town.

1969    Divorced.

1970    Married Barbara Zollner (two children: Frederick and Christiaan).

1972    Promoted to Professor of Surgical Science in the Department of Surgery, University of Cape Town.

1981    Began association (as a research advisor) with Clinque La Prairie in Clarens-Montreux in Switzerland.

1982    Divorced.

1983    Retired as Head of the Department of Cardiothoracic Surgery at the teaching hospitals of the University of Cape Town.

1984    Awarded the title of Professor Emeritus, University of Cape Town.

1985-87  Scientist-in-Residence, Oklahoma Transplantation Institute, Baptist Medical Center, Oklahoma City, Oklahoma, USA.

1988    Married Karin Setzkorn (two children: Amin and Lara).

2001    Divorced.

2001    2 September: died in Paphos, Cyprus.

# Awards

## *Honorary Fellowships*

American College of Cardiology
  American College of Surgeons (resigned 1986)
  New York Cardiological Society
  University of Cape Town

## *Honorary Degrees*

Doctorate of Medicine: Pahlavi University of Shiraz, Iran
  Doctorate of Science: Collegii Spei, Holland, Michigan, USA
  Doctorate of Science: Florida Southern College, Orlando, Florida, USA
  Doctorate of Science: Gama Filho University, Rio de Janeiro, Brazil
  Doctorate of Science: University of Cape Town, South Africa
  Doctorate: University of Uruguay

## *Honorary Memberships*

Brazilian College of Surgeons
  Cardiology Foundation and Society of Dominican Republic
  Dental College of Lima, Peru
  Lions International
  Montreal Clinical Society, Canada
  Order of the Knights Hospitalier of St. Thomas d'Acre
  Pan American Medical Association
  Research Center, Lagoa State Hospital of Rio de Janeiro, Brazil
  Societe de Medicine de Paris, France
  Venezuelan Society of Cardiology

## *Awards from Universities, Colleges, Academic Institutions*

Albert Einstein College of Medicine, New York, USA: Medal
  American College of Cardiology: Silver Medal
  American College of Cardiology: Diploma
  College of Surgeons of Ireland: Silver Medal
  Czechoslovakian University: Medal of Gregor Mendel Award
  Lombardi Medical Academy, Milan, Italy: Medal
  Pasteur Institute, France: Medal
  Rijks University, Leiden, The Netherlands: Presentation of two plaques

St. Boniface General Hospital Research Foundation, Winnipeg, Canada: International Award
Sydney University Medical Society, Australia: Medal
University of Caracas, Venezuela: Diploma Award
University of the Philippines Heart Institute and Transplant Foundation: Medal
University of Pretoria, South Africa: Gold Medal
University of Purkynianas Bkunensis: Diploma Award
Venezuelan National Academy of Medicine: Diploma of Honour

## Awards from Countries and States

Chile: Diploma and Gold Medal
China (Republic): Order of Brilliant Star with Violet Grand Cordon, Star Medal, Three Certificates and Violet Sash
Dominican Republic: Silver Cross
Ecuador: Order of Merit
France: Golden Cross of the Etoile Union Civique des Elites Francaises
Greece: The Decoration of the Commander of the Order of Phoenix
Italy: Cross of Grand Ufficiale in the Ordine: al Merito della Republica Italiana
Jordan: The Grand Cordon of the Order of Al-Kawkab Al-Urdini (First Class)
Lebanon: Cross of the National Cedar Decoration (presented by the President)
Paraguay: Honour Merito Salud Publica
Peru: Order of the Sun
Peru: Member of the Order 'Hipolito Unanuo' (presented by the President)
Philippines: Golden Heart Medal (presented by the President)
Rumania: Diploma de Onoare with Medal
South Africa: Hendrik Verwoerd Medal
South Africa: Order of the Southern Cross (Gold)
Spain: Blue Cross Award
Venezuela: Order of the Republic 'Andres Bello' (presented by the President)

## Freedom of the City

Beaufort West, South Africa
Cape Town, South Africa
Flint, Michigan, USA

Mayaguez, Puerto Rico
Republic of Bencento Lopez
San Juan, Puerto Rico
Santo Domingo, Dominican Republic
Sao Paulo, Brazil
Winterhaven, California, USA

## Honorary Citizenships

Birmingham, Alabama, USA
    Chatillon-les-Dombes, France
    Carpeta, Rome, Italy
    Island of Oinoussai, Greece
    Memphis Tennesee, USA
    New Orleans, Louisana, USA
    Riberao, Proto, Brazil
    State of Guanabara, Brazil
    Winnipeg, Manitoba, Canada

## Miscellaneous

Canada: Government of Quebec: Plaque
    Canada: Prime Minister of Canada: Certificate of Recognition by Pierre Trudeau
    Italy: Florence; Golden Spur of Florence
    Philippines: The Seal of the President
    USA: City of New York: Public Tribute by Mayor John V. Lindsay
    USA: Governor of New York: Document of Welcome by Nelson A. Rockefeller
    USA: Kennedy Foundation Award
    USA: President John F. Kennedy half-dollar presented by Robert Kennedy
    Vatican: Pope Paul VI: Medallions with inscribed book

## Associations and Societies

Academia Artistica Internazionale, Italy: Award of Honour
    Academia Della Scienze di Roma: Diploma Solenne and Certificate of Honour
    Bombay Medical Research Centre: Medal of First Tropical Conference on Surgery
    Brazil Ipase Hospital dos Servidores do Estado: Certificate Honouris Causa

Cape Provincial Council, South Africa: Medal
Certificado De Amparo, Bogota, Columbia: Certificate
Chris Barnard Fund, Cape Town: Gold Medal
Columbia Rotary International 'Socio Honourario': Diploma
Dag Hammarskjoeld Peace Prize
Dag Hammarskjoeld Internationa Prize: also the fifteenth Anniversary Prize
Eugan Moog Foundation of Germany and the USA: Cross of Merit and Certificate of Honour
Gold Medal inscribed with Hippocratic Oath, France
International Cardiological Symposium, Naples: Diploma with Gold Scalpel
International Federation of Arts, Letters and Sciences: Diploma of Honour
Knights of Humanity Award and Diploma of Honour, Italy
La Fundacion Cardio Infantil, Bogota, Colombia: Diploma
La Madonnina International Prize for Science
Lodovico Mina: Humanitarian Award
Lyon Administration Hospital, France: Medal
Medical Association of South Africa: Gold Medal
National Federation of Blood Donors: Medal and Scroll
New York Cardiological Society: Award of Honour
Premio Internazionale 'San Valentino D'Oro', Teni, Italy
Premio Via Veneto Literary Award for *One Life*, Italy
South African Academy of Arts and Sciences: Christo Veryers Award
South African Medical Journal: Blignault Medal for best article of 1975
Stritch Award: Plaque and Medal
Venezuela Fetrasalud Award
World Association of Military Surgeons: Award of Honour

# Books Written by Chris Barnard

The title, names of co-authors or co-editors, and publishers of Chris Barnard's books are listed below. In addition, certain of the following books, notably *One Life*, were translated and published in Eastern European countries.

## *Surgery of the Common Congenital Cardiac Malformations* (1968)

C. N. Barnard and V. Schrire
   Staples Press, London, UK
   Hober Medical Division, Harper and Row, New York, USA
   Springer-Verlag, Berlin, West Germany (in German; 1969)

## *One Life* (1970)

C. N. Barnard with Curtis Bill Pepper
   Howard Timmins, Cape Town, South Africa
   Harrap, London, UK
   MacMillian, New York, USA
   MacMillian, New York, USA (Book Club edition)
   Scherz, Bern, Switzerland (German)
   Presses de la Cite, Paris, France (French)
   R. Mohn, Gutersloh, West Germany, (German)
   Ullstein, Frankfurt-on-Main, West Germany (German)
   Plaza and Janes, Barcelona, Spain (Spanish)
   Bantam Books, New York, USA (paperback)
   Reader's Digest Association, Pleasantville, USA (Reader's Digest condensed books)

## *Heart Attack: All You Have to Know About It (You Don't Have to Die)* (1971)

C. N. Barnard
  W. H. Allen, London, UK
  Delacoste Press, New York, USA
  Mondadori, Milan, Italy (Italian)
  Boostan Mod, Tel-Aviv, Israel (Hebrew)
  Ullstein, Frankfurt-on-Main, West Germany (German)
  Ayma, Barcelona, Spain (Spanish)

## *The Unwanted* (1974)

C. N. Barnard with Siegfried Stander
  Tafelberg, Cape Town, South Africa
  Hutchinson, London, UK
  D. McKay, New York, USA (Book Club edition)
  Mondadori, Milan, Italy (Italian)
  Martinez Roca, Barcelona, Spain (Spanish)
  Arrow Books, London, UK (paperback)
  Scherz, Bern, Switzerland (German)
  Editions J'ai lu, Paris, France (French)

## *South Africa: Sharp Dissection* (1977)

C. N. Barnard
  Tafelberg, Cape Town, South Africa
  Books in Focus, New York, USA
  Hippocrene Books, New York, USA

## *In the Night Season* (1977)

C. N. Barnard with Siegfried Stander
  Tafelberg, Cape Town, South Africa
  Hutchinson, London, UK
  Popular Library, New York, USA (paperback)
  Scherz, Bern, Switzerland (German)
  Ediciones Martinez Roca, Barcelona, Spain (Spanish)
  Arrow Books, London, UK (paperback)

## The Best Medicine (1979)

C. N. Barnard (edited by Bob Molloy)
   Tafelberg, Cape Town, South Africa

## Good Life, Good Death (1980)

C. N. Barnard
   Howard Timmins, Cape Town, South Africa (English)
   John Malherbe, Cape Town, South Africa (Afrikaans)
   Owen, London, UK
   Prentice-Hall, Englewood Cliffs, New Jersey, USA
   Argos Bergara, Barcelona, Spain (Spanish)
   Hestia, Bayreuth, West Germany, (German)

## The Body Machine (1981)

C. N. Barnard (consultant editor) with John Illman (coordinating editor)
   Hamlyn, London, UK
   Crown, New York, USA

## The Junior Body Machine (1983)

C. N. Barnard (consultant editor) with Christopher Fagg (chief editor)
   Kestrel, London, UK
   Crown, New York, USA

## Christiaan Barnard's Programme for Living with Arthritis (1984)

C. N. Barnard with Peter Evans
   Michael Joseph, London, UK
   Simon and Schuster, New York, USA
   Bantam Books, Toronto, Canada and New York, USA (paperback)
   Stanke, Montreal, Canada (French)
   Grijalbo, Barcelona, Spain (Spanish)
   Also published under title *The Arthritis Handbook: How to Live With Arthritis*
   Panther, London, UK (paperback)
   Clio Press, Oxford, UK (large print edition)

## *The Living Body* (1984)

Karl Sabbagh and C. N. Barnard
  MacDonald, London, UK
  Plaza and Janes, Barcelona, Spain (Spanish)

## *The Faith* (1984)

C. N. Barnard with Siegfried Stander
  Hutchinson, London, UK

## *The Best of Barnard* (1984)

C. N. Barnard (edited by Bob Molloy)
  Molloy Publishers, Hout Bay, South Africa

## *Your Healthy Heart* (1985)

C. N. Barnard with Peter Evans
  MacDonald, London, UK
  McGraw-Hill, New York, USA
  Isis, Oxford, UK (Large print edition)
  Trecarre, Saint-Laurent, Quebec, Canada (French)
  Hotsaat Orbakh, Tel-Aviv, Israel (Hebrew)

## *The Second Life* (1993)

C. N. Barnard
  Vlaeburg, Cape Town

## *The Donor* (1996)

C. N. Barnard
  Penguin, London

## *50 Ways to a Healthy Heart* (2001)

C. N. Barnard
  Thorsons, London

# What Happened to the Other Players in the Heart Transplant Story?

Louwtjie Barnard died in 2006, aged eighty-four. She never remarried.

Marius Barnard died in Hermanus in South Africa on 14 November 2014, aged eighty-seven.

Denton Cooley died in Houston, Texas, on 18 November 2016, aged ninety-six.

Mr Edward Darvall, father of the first heart donor, Denise, died in Cape Town in 1970. He never regretted his decision to donate the organs from his daughter.

James Hardy died in Mississippi on 19 February 2003, aged eighty-four.

Adrian Kantrowitz continued in surgery and research, dying in Ann Arbor, Michigan, on 14 November 2008, aged ninety.

C. Walton (Walt) Lillehei died in Minneapolis on 5 July 1999, aged eighty.

Richard Lower retired from heart surgery in 1989 (before reaching the age of sixty), becoming a rancher in Montana for several years before returning to Richmond to carry out voluntary work as a general practitioner. He died in Montana on 17 May 2008, aged seventy-eight.

Donald Ross died in London, UK, on 23 July 2014, aged ninety-two.

After officially retiring, Norman Shumway continued to attend the department of cardic surgery at Stanford on an almost daily basis. He died in Palo Alto, California, on 10 February 2006, one day after his eighty-third birthday.

Nazih Zuhdi died in Oklahoma City on 7 February 2017, aged ninety-one.

Groote Schuur Hospital still carries out a small number of heart transplants each year, but the number is limited by financial constraints as South Africa has directed more of its resources to primary health care rather than tertiary health care.

# Selected Bibliography

The following books and articles have provided valuable sources of information on various aspects of this topic and I gratefully and readily acknowledge the information they have provided, some of which has been used in the preparation of this text.

Barnard C. N., and Schrire, V., *Surgery of the Common Congenital Cardiac Malformations* (London: Staples Press, 1968)

Barnard, C. N., and Pepper, C. B., *One Life* (London: Harrap, 1970)

Barnard, C. N., *The Second Life* (Cape Town: Vlaeberg, 1993)

Barnard, C. N., *The Best Medicine* (Cape Town: Tafelberg, 1979)

Barnard, C. N., *The Best of Barnard* (Hout Bay: Molloy Publishers, 1984)

Barnard, C. N., *The Donor* (London: Penguin, 1996)

Barnard, C. N., *South Africa: Sharp Dissection* (New York: Books in Focus, 1977)

Barnard, C. N., and Stander, S., *The Faith* (London: Hutchinson, 1984)

Barnard, C. N., and Stander, S., *The Unwanted* (New York: David McKay, 1975)

Barnard, C. N., and Stander, S., *In the Night Season* (Englewood Cliffs: Prentice-Hall, 1978)

Barnard, C. N., (with Evans, P.), *Christiaan Barnard's Program for Living with Arthritis* (New York: Simon & Schuster, 1983)

Barnard, C. N., *50 Ways to a Healthy Heart* (London: Thorsons, 2001)

Barnard, C. N., *Good Life, Good Death* (Englewood Cliffs: Prentice-Hall, 1980)

Barnard, C. N., *Heart Attack: You Don't Have to Die* (Cape Town: Tafelburg, and Hugh Keartland Publishers, 1971, and New York: Delacorte Press, 1972)

Barnard, C. N., *The Body Machine* (New York: Crown, 1981)

Barnard, C. N., *Junior Body Machine* (New York: Crown, 1983)

Barnard, C. N., and Sabbagh, K., *The Living Body* (London: MacDonald, 1984)

Barnard, D., *Fat, Fame and Life with Father* (Lansdowne, South Africa: Double Story Books, 2003)

Barnard, L., *Heartbreak* (Cape Town: Howard Timmins, 1971)

Barnard, M., *Defining Moments: An Autobiography* (Cape Town: Zebra Press, 2011)

Barr, B., *The Life of Nazih Zuhdi: Unchartered Voyage of a Heart* (Oklahoma City: Heritage Association, 2005)

Blaiberg, P., *Looking at My Heart* (London: Heinemann, 1968)

Brent, L., *A History of Transplantation Immunology* (London: Academic Press, 1997)

Calne, R., *The Ultimate Gift: The Story of Britain's Premiere Transplant Surgeon* (London: Headline Book Publishing, 1999)

Cooper, D. K. C., *Chris Barnard: By Those Who Know Him* (Vlaeberg, Cape Town: 1992)

Cooper, D. K. C., *Open Heart: The Radical Surgeons Who Revolutionized Medicine* (New York: Kaplan, 2010)

Digby, A., Phillips, H., Deacon, H., and Thomson, K., *At the Heart of Healing: Groote Schuur Hospital 1938–2008* (Auckland Park, South Africa: Jacana Media, 2008)

Hamilton, D., *A History of Organ Transplantation: Ancient Legends to Modern Practice* (Pittsburgh: University of Pittsburgh Press, 2012)

Hardy, J. D., *The World of Surgery 1945–1985, Memoirs of One Participant* (Philadelphia: University of Pennsylvania Press, 1986)

Hardy, J. D., *The Academic Surgeon: An Autobiography* (Mobile: Magnolia Mansions Press, 2002)

Hawthorne, P., *The Transplanted Heart* (Johannesburg: Hugh Keartland, 1968)

Logan, C., *Celebrity Surgeon: Christiaan Barnard, a Life* (Johannesburg, Cape Town: Jonathan Dole, 2003)

Louw, J. H., *In the Shadow of Table Mountain: A History of the University of Cape Town Medical School* (Cape Town: Struik, 1969)

Malan, M., *Heart Transplant* (Johannesburg: Voortrekkerpers, 1968)

McRae, D., *Every Second Counts: The Race to Transplant the First Human Heart* (New York: G. B. Simon & Schuster, 2006)

Moore, F. D., *A Miracle and a Privilege: Recounting a Half Century of Surgical Advance* (Washington, DC: Joseph Henry Press, 1995)

Murray, J. E., *Surgery of the Soul: Reflections of a Curious Career.* (Cape Cod, USA: Science History Publications, 2001)

Shapiro, H. (ed.), *Experience with Human Heart Transplantation: Proceedings of the Cape Town Symposium 13–16, July 1968* (Durban, South Africa: Butterworth & Co., 1969)

Starzl, T. E., *The Puzzle People. Memoirs of a Transplant Surgeon* (Pittsburgh: University of Pittsburgh Press, 1992)

Thorwald, J., *The Patients* (New York: Harcourt Brace Jovanovich, 1971)

Tilney, N. L., *Transplant; From Myth to Reality* (New Haven, Yale University Press, 2003)

*Wellcome Witnesses to Twentieth Century Medicine: Early Heart Transplant Surgery in the UK* (London: The Wellcome Trust, 1999)

# Index